Infective Endocarditis

INFECTIVE ENDOCARDITIS

LOUIS WEINSTEIN,

M.S., Ph.D., M.D.,
ScD. (Hon.), M.A.C.P.

**Professor of Medicine, Tufts University School
of Medicine (1958–1975) (Emeritus)
Visiting Professor of Medicine,
Harvard Medical School (1975–1982);
and
Senior Physician (Emeritus), Department of Medicine,
Brigham & Women's Hospital**

JOHN L. BRUSCH,

M.D., F.A.C.P.

**Instructor in Medicine, Harvard Medical School;
Attending Physician, Department of Medicine and
Infectious Disease Service, Cambridge Hospital;
Chief of Medicine and Director of Community Medicine,
Youville Hospital, Cambridge, Massachusetts**

New York   Oxford
OXFORD UNIVERSITY PRESS
1996

Oxford University Press

Oxford   New York
Athens   Auckland   Bangkok   Bombay
Calcutta   Cape Town   Dar es Salaam   Delhi
Florence   Hong Kong   Istanbul   Karachi
Kuala Lumpur   Madras   Madrid   Melbourne
Mexico City   Nairobi   Paris   Singapore
Taipei   Tokyo   Toronto

and associated companies in
Berlin   Ibadan

Published by Oxford University Press, Inc.
198 Madison Avenue, New York, New York 10016

Oxford is a registered trademark of Oxford University Press

Library of Congress Cataloging-in-Publication Data
Weinstein, Louis, 1909–
Infective endocarditis / Louis Weinstein, John L. Brusch.
p.   cm.   Includes bibliographical references and index.
ISBN 0–19–507395–9
1. Infective endocarditis.
I. Brusch, John L.   II. Title.
[DNLM: 1. Endocarditis, Bacterial.   WG 285 W424i 1996]
RC685.E5W45   1996   616.1'2—dc20
DNLM/DLC for Library of Congress   95–6079

1 3 5 7 9 8 6 4 2
Printed in the United States of America
on acid-free paper

This book is dedicated, with affection, to our wives, Ethel R. Weinstein and Patricia Brusch, whose continuous support and encouragement made it possible.

Preface

The disease now known as infective endocarditis was first described about 325 years ago. Pre- and postmortem studies defined some of its clinical and pathoanatomical features. Most important was the observation that the aortic valve was abnormal and that "caruncles" (vegetations) were present on its leaflets. Later reports confirmed these findings and presented additional information concerning the clinical and pathological features of the disease. Infective endocarditis was moderately frequent during this period and was associated with a high fatality rate because of the inability to identify its cause and the absence of effective therapy. It was not until the mid-nineteenth century that it became clear that some diseases were caused by microorganisms. When adequate microbiological-techniques became available, endocarditis finally became recognized as an infectious disease.

Among the physicians who were most prominent in defining and categorizing the features of the disease in the nineteenth and early twentieth centuries were Schottmuller, Osler, Libman, Blumer, and Keefer.

The poor prognosis of infective endocarditis disappeared with the development of effective antimicrobial agents in the early 1940s. First penicillin and later an increasing number of active antibiotics and other drugs altered the outcome of the disease by preventing complications and producing cure. More recently, echocardiography, arteriography, various scanning procedures, and sophisticated radiological methods have increased the frequency of exact diagnosis and permitted the detection of intracardiac complications. In some instances, medical therapy has not been very effective. The final approach to the cure of the endocardial infection in these cases has been surgery.

My first experience with infective endocarditis (L.W.) occurred in 1943 when I was an intern on the Medical Service at the Massachusetts Memorial Hospital (presently University Hospital) in Boston. Although penicillin was in very short supply at the time, Dr. Chester Keefer, Physician-in-Chief of the Medical Service of the hospital, was asked by the National Research Council to undertake a study of the effects of this agent in the management of endocarditis, a disease with which he had had broad experience. Ten beds on the Medical Service were vacated and, within a short time, were occupied by patients with infective endocarditis. Because of my previous training in microbiology, Dr. Keefer asked me to devote all my time to the study and care of these patients. The dose of penicillin used was 5,000 units every 3 hr a total of 10 doses administered intravenously. Twenty patients were included in the study; all died despite treatment with the antibiotic. To underscore the shortage of this agent at that time, Dr. Keefer brought to my attention the fact that we were about to run out of penicillin furnished by the National Research Council. He referred me to a paper from Oxford University indicating that, with some manipulation, penicillin could be recovered from urine. I collected the total daily urine output of 10 patients, treated it as suggested by the Oxford group, and was able to recover penicillin in small quantities. Fortunately, a new shipment of the antibiotic arrived before it became necessary to use that penicillin. I underscore this experience to emphasize the fact that this agent once scarce is now available enough to treat any number of patients with doses as large as 20 to 40 million units/day. Over the past 40 years, I have treated at least 10–15 patients with this infection every year. Because of this experience, infective endocarditis became the disease of greatest interest to me.

The Natural history of infective endocarditis has undergone remarkable changes over the past half century. Fifty or more years ago, the more common syndrome was subacute. The incidence of the acute form of the disease has been increasing in frequency. It is now equal to or even exceeds the subacute type. In addition, endocarditis was once most common in young women with rheumatic heart disease. At present, it occurs more often in elderly men with underlying atherosclerotic valvular disease. Very striking has been the increasing involvement of more than one valve. Recurrences of infective endocarditis are now relatively common.

Most striking has been a sharp decrease in the incidence of the so-called diagnostic signs of endocarditis. Among these are petechiae, subungual hemorrhages, Osler nodes, Janeway lesions, and Roth spots. These have markedly decreased in frequency in patients with subactue infections.

Although some of the factors involved in the acquisition of infective endocarditis were known many years ago, new ones have been recognized. These appear to play a very important role in the pathogenesis of the infection. For example, the present widespread use of illicit drugs, often administered intravenously, has been responsible for a marked increase in acute endocarditis, especially of the right side of the heart. Another problem, unknown years ago, is the acquired immunodeficiency syndrome (AIDS). This disorder may heighten the risk of acute endocardial infection, and it certainly leads to a high fatality rate despite appropriate therapy. Developments in cardiac surgery, especially the ability to implant prosthetic valves, have led to the cure of otherwise fatal cases of endocarditis but have also created new challenges in cardiac infections. There has been a sharp rise in the incidence of complications of endocarditis compared with the clinical experiences of the earlier years of this century. Some are due to the greater number of cases produced by highly invasive organisms such as *S. aureus* and *S. pyogenes*. Among these complications have been valular rupture, intraventricular abscesses, right-sided infection leading to pulmonary abscess, and repeated recurrences caused either by the organism initially involved or by different pathogens.

In this monograph I present, with Dr. Brusch, the history, pathophysiology, microbiology, diagnosis, treatment, and prevention of infective endocarditis. I do this from the perspectives of one who has treated the disease from the preantibiotic era to the age of AIDS, of the increasing resistance of bacteria to the available antibiotic agents, and of the growing problems of endocarditis of prosthetic valves and of intravenous drug abuse. We hope that this book continues the tradition of the physicians of the past who have contributed so much to our knowledge of infective endocarditis.

Boston   L. W.
February 1995

Contents

Infective Endocarditis

1

The Natural History of Infective Endocarditis Prior to the Availability of Antimicrobial Therapy

Early Observations

Lazare Riviere has been credited with providing the first precise clinical description of infective endocarditis in 1723.[1] The patient studied by Riviere complained of "palpitation of the heart." Examination disclosed a "small, irregular pulse with every variety of irregularity." Finally, dyspnea, edema of the legs, and hemoptysis developed and the patient died. The following findings were noted at autopsy: "In the left ventricle of the heart, round caruncles (? vegetations) were found like the substance in the lungs, the larger of which resembled a cluster of hazel nuts that filled up the opening of the aorta."

Morgagni[2] is usually credited with the first description of the disease, the clinical and pathological findings of which were highly suggestive of ulcerative endocarditis. In a treatise entitled *De Sedibus*, published in 1761, he wrote that the patient "fell into disease which seemed to be a dropsy of the thorax. His legs being swelled, his pulse being very low, and a virulent gonorrhea or ever afflicting, he died." At autopsy, the aortic valve was described as "swelled into short and unequal excrescences by the load of which being weighted down and brought so near together by this means, as to leave by a very narrow passage betwixt each other by which the blood might pass out. When I examined each valve in particular, I saw that the right had its borders much shorter than usual, or has become less transversy; and that the left was ruptured through the middle on the border quite lower to the parts; in it, from the very lips of the rupture, other excrescences were protuberant. I have seen these things, in other praeternatural appearances being look'd for in vain in the aorta and other vessels, I went on to examine the remaining parts." Morgagni also noted that the spleen was infarcted. The first report describing the pathoanatomical fea-

3

tures of endocarditis was published by Giovanni Maria Lancisi[3] in 1708 in a treatise entitled *De subitaneis mortibus.* He wrote that "the heart showed something hardening certainly rare to the human memory. Indeed at the surface there are uneven structures in the semilunar valves, and small fleshy nodules [sarcomata], which protruding in threads and fragments like condylomata, extended inside the aorta, nor was it possible to tear them off short of rupturing the valve, so that there was no doubt that these foreign bodies were wedged in the length and fibers and tissues of the valves and not by simple adhesion. Lastly, within the descending aorta there was discovered an irregular mass, to the nature of the polyp, filling up almost the entire cavity.

The first picture of the heart of a patient with endocarditis was published by Sandifort in 1777.[4] In an essay published in 1806, Corvisart[5] described "vegetations" found at autopsy in a 39-year-old man. He noted that "there were many kinds of rather irregular, rather long vegetations and resembled such certain venereal excrescences from the mitral valves." Corvisart[5] believed that these were syphilitic in origin. Laennec[6] noted this and stated that "I have besides encountered some of these excrescences in subjects who, according to all probability, had a venereal disease."

In a book describing disease of the heart published in 1824, Bertin and Bouillaud[7] wrote that "induration and vegetations of the valves of the heart and stenosis of its different orifices" were present in patients who died with endocarditis. The terms *endocardium* and *endocarditis* were introduced by Bouillaud[8] in 1841 in his *Traité Clinique des Maladies due Coeur,* in which all the well-known clinical and pathoanatomical features of endocarditis were described.

Pathophysiological and Microscopic Studies

The relation between blood-borne infection and endocarditis was first pointed out by Virchow[9] in 1847. He described one of the earliest cases of the disease complicated by an embolism. The association of systemic emboli with infection of the cardiac valves was confirmed by Kirkes[10] in 1852. A microscopic study by Virchow[11] 4 years later disclosed "numerous granules, smaller than the nuclei of leukocytes, within many of the valvular thrombi." These were insoluble in potassium hydroxide, acetic acid, or nitric acid. He named them *virions* and suggested a "possible close association with endocarditis." Almost simultaneously, von Rokitansky[12] "observed small, round, oblong, cylindric, and sausage-shaped bodies" within the vegetations on a valve of a patient with endocardial infection. In 1870, Winge[13] described such formations in the valvular lesions of 27 patients. Heiberg both confirmed these observations and added a case of his own.[14] In 1875, Klebs[15] suggested that all cases of endocarditis were due to infection.

There was considerable debate concerning the pathogenesis of infective endocarditis. A basic question was whether or not normal cardiac valves contained blood vessels. In 1852, Luschka[16] suggested that the cardiac valves were susceptible to infections in the course of bacteremia. This theory was based on the assumption that normal valves possessed an extensive vascular network arising from the coronary circulation. On the basis of his experiments in rabbits, Rosenow[17] concluded that endocarditis following intravenous injection of streptococci was due to an embolic process and that the bacteria invaded the valves via a network of fine capillaries present within the valves. Other investigators[18,19] reported that blood vessels were present in the cardiac valves of pigs.

However, several years before the publication of Luschka's paper,[17] Virchow[11] and Klebs[15] documented that human valvular leaflets were avascular. The result and long-lived controversy was due, in part, to the lack of appreciation of the fact that the cardiac valves of many animals, including pigs, cows, sheep, and horses, were normally vascularized. Early investigators were also misled by their failure to recognize that the growth of blood vessels into the valvular leaflets was related to the organizational stage of healing following a variety of inflammatory disorders such as rheumatic valvulitis. It was not until 1909 that Coombs[20] described the histological features that distinguished the valvular response to rheumatic fever from that present in infective endocarditis. This controversy was finally settled during the first half of the twentieth century when Gross[21] demonstrated that in humans the cardiac valves are normally not vascularized and that if blood vessels are present, they are the result of an inflammatory process in the valvular leaflets. In 1945, Harper[22] presented the results of his studies, as well as an extensive review of those by other investigators. He pointed out that "normal human heart valves, like those of rabbits, are largely nonvascular and contain no lymphatic vessels. In diseased valves, blood vessels are found as part of the inflammatory response. Primary embolism cannot be considered a factor in the genesis of endocarditis in the man or rabbit." Several new experimental procedures to induce endocarditis in animals were developed over the following years. Most common were (1) the intravenous injection of organisms, with or without the addition of inert material; (2) traumatic injury to three cardiac valves, followed by the injection of organisms into the bloodstream; and (3) multiple exposures to an organism leading to the development of immunity. In 1912, Rosenow[17] produced endocarditis in rabbits by the intravenous injection of streptococci recovered from a patient with chronic endocarditis. In 1886, Ribbert (cited by Rosenow) produced infection in the cardiac valves of animals by injecting an emulsion of staphylococci and "particles" of potatoes. Based on the results of these experiments, he suggested that the development of endocarditis is, in some cases, due to the direct implantation of bacteria on the leaflets of the valves.

In 1886, Wyssokowitch[23] and Orth,[24] using the technique developed by Rosenbach,[25] traumatized leaflets of the aortic valve of animals and then injected saline suspensions of staphylococci or streptococci recovered from patients with endocarditis. They correlated the development of new cardiac murmurs and embolic complications with the findings at necropsy and concluded that this was a valid model for human disease.

Studies of the role of immunization in the pathogenesis of endocarditis were carried out by Wadsworth[26] in 1914. Horses that he had used to produce pneumococcal antibody developed endocarditis during the course of immunization. He injected the animals initially with killed organisms and then with live pneumococci. Although a high titer of antibody developed, pneumococcal bacteremia occurred. Despite this, some of the animals were afebrile. Acute fatal endocarditis developed in seven of the eight horses 6 to 21 months after they were immunized. Examination of the valves at autopsy disclosed "evidence of complete healing and restitution of the tissues, but with thickening and some contraction causing roughening or sclerotic conditions of the endocardium." Most important was the presence of subacute, chronic, and healed lesions in the involved valvular leaflets, a picture identical to that seen in human disease. On the basis of this finding, Wardsworth concluded that "there are no fundamental differences in the anatomical changes—or lesions—which are practically identical in men and in the horse."

Endocarditis began to be reported with increasing frequency in the latter part of the nineteenth century. In a discussion of the relationship of intermittent fever to endocarditis, Von Leyden[27] described the development of subacute endocarditis involving a previously damaged valve that was infected by streptococci.

Eichorst[28] published the first clinical classification of endocarditis in 1883. He defined the presentations as acute (*septic*), subacute (*endocarditis verrucosa*), and (*chronic retrohans*).

Osler's Contributions

The next important event in our understanding of endocarditis was the three Goulstonian Lectures delivered by Sir William Osler in 1885. According to his biographer, Harvey Cushing,[29] Osler discussed endocarditis by presenting "the first comprehensive account in English of the disease, and did much to bring the subject to the attention of the clinician." Osler was 35 years old and just 13 years out of medical school when he was asked to be the Goulstonian Lecturer. The series was then 250 years old[30] and was intended to be presented by one of the four youngest members of the Royal College of Physicians of London. The data on which Osler based his historic observations came from two major sources: a series of cases gathered from publications of other authors and 23 cases from his own clinical experience in Montreal.

Osler presented the first description of the clinical manifestations of what he called *acute* or *malignant* endocarditis. He made the following comments:[31] "With a view of obtaining data upon which to base statements regarding the etiological relations of malignant endocarditis, I have gone over the records of 209 cases . . . 37 of these occurred in connection with pyaemia, traumatic or puerperal septicemia with metastatic abscesses. Doubtless, this number could have been very greatly increased had I examined files of special gynaecological and surgical journals, but my investigation did not lie so much in these directions. In 45 cases, there was no record of any previous disease with which the cardiac trouble could, with a greater or less degree of probability, be associated." The infection was first detected at postmortem examination in the majority of patients and was usually secondary to a primary infection at some other site in the body. Osler emphasized the frequency (75%) with which endocarditis affected previously damaged cardiac valves; described the clinical and pathological findings of the disease; commented that "micrococci are constant elements in the vegetations"; and recorded the now classic features of infective endocarditis, including embolic phenomena, mycotic aneurysms, valvular perforations, and rupture of papillary muscles, septum, or valves.

Osler stated that "The general symptoms are those of a febrile affection of variable intensity, which may be ushered in, like any acute fever, with rigors, pain in the back, vomiting, headache, etc." "Cardiac symptoms may be marked from the outset: pain, palpitation, sense of distress, and murmur; in many instances, there has been old valvular disease, but in a considerable number of cases the heart symptoms remain in the background, hidden by the general condition and giving no indication; or they may be so slight that they are not even detected on special examination. The embolic processes give a special prominence to local symptoms, which may divert attention from the general malady. Thus, delirium, coma, or paralysis may arise from implication of the brain or its membranes; pain in the side and local peritonitis from involvement of the spleen; bloody urine and pain in the back from affection of the kidneys; loss of vision from retinal hemorrhage; and suppression in various organs or gangrene from the distribution of emboli.

"First let me direct your attention . . . to those cases in which the endocarditis is merely a part of a septic or pyaemic state, the result of an external wound, a puerperal process, or an acute necrosis. Somewhat over 18 percent of the cases I have analysed were of this nature, the majority of them occurring in connection with puerperal fever—11 per cent of the others in association with various wounds and injuries or acute necrosis of bone."

In referring to ulcerative endocarditis following trauma or surgical procedures, Osler pointed out that "Many of the cases occur after very slight injuries, as paring a hangnail or a corn, a sloughing pile, or the passage of a sound through a stricture. In acute necrosis of bone or acute osteomyelitis, a secondary endocarditis may develop and, in some instances, the clinical features may strongly resemble malignant endocarditis."

The clinical syndromes of endocarditis were classified by Osler into two main groups—*cardiac* and *cerebral*.[31]

The cardiac group. "Under this heading may be arranged as suggested by Dr. Bramwell, those cases in which patients, the subjects of chronic valve disease, are attacked with febrile symptoms and evidences of a recent endocarditis engrafted upon the old process. I have already remarked on the great frequency with which ulcerative changes are found in connection with sclerotic endocarditis. Many of such cases present features of the pyaemic, typhoid or cerebral types, and may be of the most acute character; but in others the process appears much less intense, and the cause more chronic. In a considerable series of cases, the history is somewhat as follows: the patient has, say, aortic valve disease, and is under treatment for failing compensation, when he begins to have slight irregular fever, an evening exacerbation of two or three degrees, some increase in cardiac pain, and a sense of restlessness and distress. Embolic phenomena may develop; a sudden hemiplegia; pain in [the] region of [the] spleen, and signs of enlargement of the organ; or there is pain in the back, with bloody urine. In other instances, peripheral embolish may take place, with gangrene of [the] foot or hand. There may be hebetude (obtuseness) or low delirium. Instances such as these are extremely common; and while in some the process may be very intense, in others it is essentially chronic, and may last for weeks and months, so that the term malignant seems not at all applicable to them; still in a large series of cases, all gradations can be seen between the most severe and the milder forms. I have known the febrile symptoms to subside for weeks, to recur again with increased severity, and there are cases which render it probable that the process may subside entirely. The ulcerative destruction in these cases may be most extensive, and it is to be carefully distinguished from the atheromatous changes. In very many instances, there is no history of rheumatic fever or other constitutional disorder but the endocarditis appears to attack the sclerotic valves as a primary process, and a very considerable number of the most typical cases are of this kind."

The Cerebral Group. "Certain clinical features may be specially referred to in a few words. The fever, as will have been gathered from the previous statements, is of a very variable character. Irregularity is the prominent feature; periods of low may alternate with periods of high temperature, or a remittent may become an intermittent. A remittent type is most frequently met with, but the remissions do not occur with any regularity. Occasionally, there may be a continuous high fever, the thermometer not registering below 103° for a week at a time. The pyaemic and anguish (painful) types have been sufficiently noted. The occurrence of a rash has been described by many observers, and, in some instances, has led to errors of diagnosis. The most common form is the hemorrhaging, in the form of small petechiae, distributed over the trunk, particularly the abdomen, less often on the face and extremities. They may be most abundant over the whole body, and at times are large and present small white centres. When severe, nervous symptoms are also present. The resemblance of the cases of cerebrospinal meningitis or typhus may be very close. In one instance, the case was thought to be hemorrhagic variola. An erythematous rash has also been observed. The mental symptoms may be of very varied character. By far the most frequent conditions are low delirium and a dull semi-conscious, apathetic state. There may be, at the outset, active delirium, or even maniacal outbursts. When there is extensive meningitis there is usually a condition of deep coma. Sweating is a very frequent symptom, and is worthy of special notice, from the peculiarly drenching character, which is second only to ague, and usually far beyond the average mark of phthisis or pyaemia. The diarrhoea is not necessarily dependent on any recognizable lesion, and may not be very marked, even when the infarcts on the mucosa are more abundant. As noted in several of the cases, it may be profuse, and still further add to the resemblance which some of the cases bear to typhoid fever. Jaundice may be present, but appears to be a rare symptom. The heart symptoms may early attract affection, from the complaints of pain and palpitation; but, as a rule, they are latent, and unless looked for are likely to be overlooked. In those cases with chronic valve disease, there is usually no difficulty, but where the attention sets in with marked constitutional symptoms, the local trouble is very apt not to attract attention. Even on examination, there may be no murmur present, with extensive vegetations, or it may be variable. There are many instances on record, by careful observers, in which the examination of the heart was negative.

"The course of the disease presents many variations. . . . Very acute cases may run their course within the week, while in others the duration may be even two or three months. Except in certain cases in which the patients are the subjects of chronic valvulitis, the course is rarely prolonged beyond four or five weeks. Some of the pyaemic group, particularly those with intermittent pyrexia, appear very prolonged, even two or three months."

Osler made the point that there are "no various essential differences in the various forms of acute endocarditis. Between the small capillary excrescences and the huge fungating vegetation with destructive changes, all gradations can be traced, and the last may be the direct outcome of the first; the two extremes, indeed, may be present in the same valve. They represent different degrees of intensity of one and the same process."

Osler also noted that "The micrococci are constant elements in the vegetation. . . . Some times, the smaller vegetations seem made up exclusively of them. . . . The microorganisms found in connection with the malignant endocarditis are not all of the same kind." Osler was impressed by the fact that micrococci are not peculiar to the vegetations of the ulcerative form of endocarditis, but exist in small bead-like outgrowths of the rheumatic and other varieties of the disease. . . . "So far as my observation goes, the micrococci do not exist in the blood during the course of the malady."

It is clear from these descriptions that, while the title of Osler's paper was "Malignant Endocarditis" (or *ulcerative,* a term used to describe some of the cases), in fact, he described both the acute and subacute forms of the disease. It is difficult to distinguish these as they are described, but reference to cases that survive for "even two to three months" indicates that both types of the disease were included and classified as "malignant." It was not until 1909 that Osler[32] defined the syndrome of subacute infective endocarditis (see below).

Osler's outstanding talent as a clinical observer and his exceptional knowledge of morbid anatomy were insufficient to allow him to fully comprehend this disease. His awareness of his shortcomings became evident when he presented his "Outline for Our Ignorance" in his final Goulstonian

Lecture. Pathological and microbiological advances over the next two decades would provide the tools for arriving at the modern understanding of infective endocarditis.

In 1899, Heubner[33] described five patients with fever that persisted for 3 to 9 months. At necropsy, all were found to have endocarditis and splenic infarction. In the same year, Lenhartz[34] identified cases of endocarditis caused by staphylococci, streptococci, pneumococci, and gonococci. He noted that patients with acute streptococcal endocarditis were extremely ill; had a high, irregular temperature with frequent chills; and experienced an acute, stormy course. The ordinary streptococcus was not isolated from these patients. Instead, a delicate, fine steptococcus, characterized by its slow growth, the formation of a greenish zone around individual colonies, and a lack of virulence for animals, proved to be the cause of infection in these patients. In 1899, Harbitz[35] also emphasized the clinical and pathological differences between acute and chronic endocarditis.

In 1903, Schottmuller[36] noted that the ordinary streptococcus produced hemolysis when grown on blood agar, while the small streptococcus produced a greenish pigment. He named the latter organism *Streptococcus mitior seuviridans* and emphasized its importance in the etiology of chronic and subacute endocarditis. Later, he proposed that the type of valvular disease caused by this organism was a specific clinical entity that he named *endocarditis lenta*.

Horder[37] emphasized the importance of cultures of the blood in the diagnosis and treatment of bacteremia. After analyzing more than 100 cultures, he noted that the results were positive in 85% of cases of "undoubted septicemia" and pointed out that the diagnosis of septicemia was often impossible to make on clinical grounds alone. He also stressed the fact that blood culture may yield organisms from patients who are not very ill and suggested three methods for examining blood for the presence of organisms: (1) blood smears (bacteria must be present in large numbers in the circulation to be detected by this method), which may be very useful when organisms difficult to grow are responsible for disease; (2) inoculation of suitable animals with blood; and (3) cultures of blood obtained by venipuncture.

By 1910, the bacteriological and clinical information accumulated over a number of years had clearly delineated the major clinical syndromes of endocarditis associated with infections of the cardiac valves. One form was marked by an acute, stormy, and rapidly fatal clinical course and was caused primarily by the pneumococci, *Streptococcus pyogenes* or *Staphylococcus aureus* or the gonococcus labeled *ulcerative* or *acute bacterial endocarditis*. It usually developed from bacteremia that originated in a focus of infection in another area of the body. Another type, *chronic infective endocarditis*, was associated with a protracted clinical course and was caused, in most instances, by organisms with a low capacity to produce disease.

The subacute and chronic forms of bacterial endocarditis were described in great detail by Osler in 1909.[32] He noted that

The anatomical condition in these cases is quite unlike that of the ordinary ulcerative endocarditis. In three specimens I have had an opportunity of studying, there was no actual ulceration, but large proliferative vegetations, firm and hard, greyish yellow in colour, projected from the endocardium of the valves like large condylomata, encrusting the chordae tendineae, and extending to the endocardium of the auricle. The condition is quite unlike the globose vegetations of the pneumococcal and gonorrhoeal endocarditis or the superficial ulcerative erosions of the acute septic cases.

"With carefully made blood-cultures, one should now be able to determine the presence of septicaemia. This was easily done in three of my more recent cases. . . . The blood-cultures and the presence of the painful erythematous nodules and the occurrence of embolism furnish the most important aids [to diagnosis]." Osler pointed out that the disease was of "chronic character, not marked especially by chills, but by a protracted fever, often not very high but from four to twelve month's [sic] duration."[32]

This paper contains the first comment concerning the nature of the murmur associated with this disease. Osler remarked that "one of the most striking circumstances is the *very slight change in the character of the heart murmur* in spite of the most extensive vegetations and alterations in the valves. In several cases, the absence of any change in the character of the heart murmur and the remarkably quiet vegetative state of the organ urged strongly against evidence of endocarditis."

Osler also noted embolic occlusion involving the brain, retinal arteries, spleen, and kidneys. The first description of the lesions that later became known as *Osler's nodes* is presented in this communication. "One of the most interesting features of the disease and one to which very little attention has been paid is the occurrence of ephemeral spots of a painful nodular erythema, chiefly in the skin of the hands and feet, the *nodosites cutanees ephemeres* of the French. My attention was first called to these in the patient of Dr. Mullen of Hamilition whose description is admirable. . . . The spots come out at intervals as small swollen areas, some the size of a pea, others a centimetre and a half in diameter, raised, red, with a whitish spot in the center. I have known them to pass away in a few hours, but more commonly they last for a few days or even longer. The commonest situation is near the tip of the finger which may be swollen." It is important to emphasize that, as early as 1909,[32] Osler knew that "from beginning to end no heart murmur has been present." It is interesting that this has been considered one of the *recent* changes in the clinical picture of subacute infective endocarditis. The following were described by Osler as the characteristic features of this type of endocardital infarction: "The presence of an old valvular lesion, embolic phenomena, splenomegaly, sudden onset of hematuria, the presence of a dermal lesion such as purpura and particularly the painful erythematous nodules, progressive cardiac signs including gradual enlargement of the heart, changes in the character of mitral murmur and the appearance of a loud rasping, tricuspid murmur of the development, under observation, of an aortic diastolic bruit."

Osler's observations were confirmed by many European clinicians. For example, the French literature contains references to subacute bacterial endocarditis as *Jacoud's disease* or *la maladie d'Osler-Jacoud*.[38]

Further Observations

One year after Osler's description, the classic paper describing the clinical features of subacute infective endocarditis, as it was observed in the United States, was published by Libman and Celler.[39] They reported the results of their studies of 43 cases of the disease and added descriptions of findings not mentioned by Osler. They described this type of endocarditis as follows: "The duration of our cases varied from four months to a year or a year and a half. The longer cases may be grouped as the chronic type. Although the cases differed from one another in certain respects, the picture, as a whole, is a characteristic one resembling that described by other writers on the disease. In nearly all the cases, the disease began insidiously; it was often difficult to determine, with any degree of accuracy, the date of onset. Fever was present in all cases, at times quite low, at times (usually later in the disease) high, and with or without chills. In the cases in which splenic infarction dominated the clinical picture, the temperatures were usually high and markedly intermittent. Malaise and gastric or intestinal disturbances were frequently present; sweats occurred in nearly all the cases, usually during the latter part of the disease. In all of the cases, there was progressive weakness and emaciation. The spleen was nearly always enlarged and palpable. Pain was quite constant. In some cases, it was localized in the bones, joints or muscles; in others, they seemed to be neural in origin. Mild joint pains were not infrequently met with. At times, the pains were due to the development of embolic aneurysms which are so apt to develop in this type of disease. The painful, erythematous, cutaneous nodules, the diagnostic value of which has been particularly emphasized by Osler, seem to be pathognomonic. A symptom to which no attention has been paid is the tenderness of the lower sternum that was present in nearly all our cases. It is present at times even before the anemia is sufficiently developed to account for it.

"The progressive anemia of the disease and the color of the face (waxy, dirty waxy or whitish) are noteworthy features. The leucocytes were not particularly increased to any degree except when the disease was advanced and various secondary lesions occurred. Petechiae occurred in nearly all cases at some time or other. At times they were abundant, and were scattered over a large part of the body. At times, they were few in number but few crops appeared. Hematuria, microscopic or macroscopic, occurred quite commonly. None of the cases that we succeeded in following recovered."

Many detailed studies of the microbiological, pathological, and clinical features that defined the nature of the disease were carried out over the next 30 years. Two of the best reviews of the subject are the monographs published by Libman and Friedberg.[40,41]

Four peripheral stigmata, when present, have been considered suggestive or, in some instances, diagnostic of subacute or chronic infective endocarditis. These are the Osler node, the Roth spot, the Janeway lesion, and splinter hemorrhages. The initial description of the Osler node has been presented. The first description of a specific retinal lesion in patients with valvular infections was published in 1872 by Roth.[42] He described "cotton wool" exudates consisting of aggregates of cytoid bodies and thought they were due to "varicose hypertrophy" of the retina. This lesion, the Roth spot, was erroneously described as a boat-shaped hemorrhage by Doherty and Trubek,[43] who suggested that it was produced by recurrent crops of petechiae. In a paper entitled "Certain Clinical Observations upon Heart Disease" that appeared in 1899, Janeway[44] was the first to describe lesions on the palms and soles in patients with endocarditis. "Several times I have noted small hemorrhages with slightly nodular character in the palms of the hands and soles of the feet, and possibly the arms and the legs and but a scanty crop in malignant endocarditis—." In one case, he noted "a very profuse, reddish eruption on the palms of the hands and the soles of the feet which was slightly nodular." This is now known as the *Janeway lesion*. However, more recent descriptions have defined it as a pink, painless, nontender, irregular macular rash usually present on the hypothenar eminences of the hands and soles. However, in some cases, it may be present as a diffuse rash over other areas of the body. *Splinter hemorrhages* were first mentioned in 1926 by Blumer.[45] He wrote that "In a series of forty-eight cases, I have observed two in which a very interesting hemorrhagic lesion occurred under the nails. The name 'splinter hemorrhage' is suggested for these lesions because it exactly describes them. The patient complained of a sore finger, just as is usually the case in connection with the development of an Osler node, and examination, instead of showing the common Oslerian lesion, shows a linear hemorrhage beneath the nail, usually about 4 or 5 millimeters in length and several millimeters removed from the growing edge of the nail. These lesions so exactly simulate the appearance of a splinter that were it not for the fact that the patient is usually in bed and that the lesion is several millimeters from the growing nail edge, one would suspect that a splinter had been accidentally introduced."

By the early 1940s, the clinical description and understanding of the pathogenesis of endocarditis seemed complete. However, the patients' outlook remained dismal. Less than 1%[46] recovered spontaneously from the subacute disease. By 1940, sulfapyridine and sulfathiozole were available and were employed for treatment. However, the rate of cure was only 4–6%.[47]

The effect on a patient with endocarditis was related in the diary of a fourth-year Harvard medical student who developed the disease.[48] He described what it was like to live with rheumatic heart disease, stressing the discomfort of the palpitations, the symptoms of aortic insufficiency, and the profound physical discomfort associated with each ventricular systole. In January 1931, he experienced an early forboding that he was suffering from endocarditis because he recognized one of the early signs of the disease, namely, clubbing of the figners. He consulted several specialists, who told him that he had one of the manifestations of the disease. At 11:45 P.M. on May 29, he knew, without doubt, that he had endocarditis and would die. He wrote: "No sooner had I removed the left arm of my coat, than there was on the ventral aspect of my left wrist, a sight which I shall never forget until I die. It greeted my eyes about 15–20 bright red, slightly raised hemorrhagic spots about one mm in diameter which did not fade on pressure which stood defiant, as if they were challenged from the very gods of Olympus. I had never seen such a sight since, and I hope I shall never see such a sight again. I took one glance at the pretty, little collection of spots and turned to my sister-in-law, who was standing nearby, and calmly said 'I shall be dead in 6 months.' There was no mistaking what the sign was, it only had to be read." He then proceeded to describe the relief he experienced when a definite diagnosis was established by recovery of *Strep. viridans* from cultures of his blood. Initially, he dealt with the strain with a great deal of intellectualization in a valiant attempt to be objective about his illness. However, he was willing to try any treatment. He wrote that "By this time I was quite reconciled to my fate, but never the less seeking new treatment. I am entirely sincere when I say I sought new treatment, not in a serious endeavor to cure the disease or prolong my life, but simply to satisfy the urge that something be done." Treatment with intravenous Pregl's solution, an iodine-containing compound as well as a polyvalent antistreptococcal medication, was ineffective.

Surgical Therapy

The first surgical approach to the heart was reported by Rehn[49] in 1897. He saw a patient with a stab wound of the heart. Approaching the organ through the lateral chest, he closed the laceration; the patient survived. In 1900, Bruton[50] first called attention to and speculated about the potential for cardiac surgery as an approach to the cure of mitral stenosis, a common form of heart disease for which medical therapy was then not available. He expressed frustration regarding the inability of physicians to alleviate the distress of patients with this disorder and suggested a surgical technique for relieving the stenosis. He stated that "mitral stenosis is not only one of the most distressing forms of cardiac disease, but in a severe form it resists all treatment by medicine. On looking at the contracted mitral orifice in a severe case of this disease, one is impressed by the hopelessness of ever finding a remedy which will enable the auricle to drive the blood in a sufficient stream through the small mitral orifice, and the wish unconsciously arises that one could divide the constriction as easily during life as one can after death."

It was not until 1923, 23 years after Bruton's paper appeared, that the first surgical treatment of mitral stenosis was reported by Cutler and Levine.[51] The patient was a 12-year-old girl who had "growing pains" but, as far as could be ascertained, had not had an episode of acute rheumatic fever or chorea. A valvulotome, an instrument somewhat similar to a slightly curved tonsil knife, was used to cut the stenosed valve. The surgeons reported that "the knife was inserted into the left ventricle about one inch from the apex and then pushed about 2.5 inches until it encountered what seemed to us to be the mitral valve." An incision was made in the aortic leaflet of the valve. Although the postoperative course was stormy, the patient recovered and had no hemodynamic problems.

The first successful surgical treatment of a patent ductus arteriosus was accomplished by Gross and Hubbard[52] about 3 years before penicillin became available for clinical use. A similar case was treated successfully by Touroff and Vessel[53] at about the same time.

References

1. Riviere, L: *Opera omnia*. Venice, Viezzin, 1723, p 526.
2. Morgagni JB: *The Seats and Causes of Diseases*, Vol I, tr Benjamin Alexander. London, Millar and Candell, 1769, Book II, Letter XXIV, Article 18, p 730.
3. Lancisi GM: *De subitaneis mortibus*. Venice, Poleti, 1708, p 225.
4. Sandifort E: *Observations Anatomico-Pathologicae*. Leyden, v.d. Eyk and Vygh, 1777–81.
5. Corvisart JN: *Essai sur les maladies et les lesions organiques du coeur*. Paris, Migneret, 1806, p 220.
6. Laennec RTH: *De l'auscultation mediate*, Vol II. Paris, Brosson and Chaude, 1819, p 334.
7. Bertin RJ, Bouillaud J: *Traité des maladies du coeur*. Paris, Bailliere, 1824, p 169.
8. Bouillaud J: *Traité clinique des maladies du coeur*, Vol II. Paris, Bailliere, 1841, p 1.
9. Virchow F: Ueber die acute Entzundug der Arterien. *Arch Pathol Anat Physiol Klin Med* 1847;I:272.
10. Kirkes W: On some of the principal effects resulting from the detachment of fibronous deposits from the interior of the heart and their mixture with the circulating blood. *Med-Chir Tr*, London, 1852.
11. Virchow R: *Gesammelte Abhandlugen zur wissenschaftlichen Medicin*. Frankfurt, Meidinger, 1856, pp 709–710.
12. Von Rokitansky C: *Lehrbuch der pathologischen anatomie*, Vol 31. Berlin, 1855, p 387.
13. Winge EFH: Mycosis endocardii. *Hygiae Med Farmaceut Monad* 1870;XXXII:172.
14. Heiberg H: Ein Fall von Endocarditis ulcerosa puerperalis mit Pilzbildungen im Herzen (*Mycosis endocardii*). *Virchows Arch F Pathol Anat Physiol Klin Med* 1872;LV:407.
15. Klebs E: Weitere Beitrage zur Entstehungsgeschicte der Endocarditis. *Arch Exp Pathol Pharmakol* 1878;IX:52.
16. Luschka H: Das endocardium imd die endocarditis. *Arch Pathol Anat Physiol* 1852;4:171.
17. Rosenow EC: Experimental infectious endocarditis. *J Infect Dis* 1912;11:210.
18. Bayne-Jones S: The blood vessels of the heart valves. *Am J Anat* 1917;21:449.
19. Kerr WJ, Mettier SR: The circulation of the heart valves: Notes on the embolic basis for endocarditis. *Am Heart J* 1925;1:96.
20. Coombs C: The histology of rheumatic endocarditis. *Lancet* 1909;11:1377.
21. Gross L: Significance of blood vessels in human heart valves. *Am Heart J* 1937;13:275.
22. Harper WF: The structure of the heart valves with special reference to their blood supply and the genesis of endocarditis. *J Pathol Bacteriol* 1945;57:229.
23. Wyssokowitsch W: Beatrage zur lehre von der endocarditis. *Arch Pathol Anat* 1886;103:21.
24. Orth J: Ueber die aetiologie der esperimentellen Mycotischem endocarditis. *Arch Pathol Anat* 1886;103:23.

25. Rosenbach O: Ueber artificielle herzklappenfehler. *Arch Exp Pathol* 1878;9:1.
26. Wadsworth AB: A study of the endocardial lesions developing pneumococcal infection in horses. *J Med Res* 1914;39:279.
27. Von Leyden E: Ueber intermitterendes fieber und endocarditis. *Z Klin Med* 1882;IV:323.
28. Eichorst H: *Handbuch der speciellen pathologie und therapie,* Vol 1. Vienna and Leipzig, 1883, p 97.
29. Cushing H: *The life of Sir William Osler,* Vol I. Oxford, Oxford University Press, 1925.
30. Pruitt R: William Osler and his Goulstonian Lectures on malignant endocarditis. *Mayo Clin Proc* 1982;57:8.
31. Osler W. *The Goulstonian lectures on malignant endocarditis. Br Med J* 1885;1:467.
32. Osler W: Chronic infective endocarditis. *Q J Med* 1909;2:219.
33. Heubner O: Ueber langdauernde Fieberzustande unklaren Ursprungs. *Deutsch Arch Klin Med* 1899;LXIV:33.
34. Lenhartz H: *Die septischen Erkrankungen.* Vienna, Holder, 1903.
35. Harbitz F: Studien uber endocarditis. *Deutsch Med Wchnschr* 1899;XXV:121.
36. Schottmuller H: Die Artunterscheidung der fur den Menschen pathogenen Streptokokken durch Blutagar. *Munchen Med Wchnechr* 1903;L:849.
37. Horder RJ: Infective endocarditis with an analysis of 150 cases with special reference to the chronic form of the disease. *Q J Med* 1909;2:289.
38. Jacoud S: *Leçons de clinique medicale faîtes a l'Hôpital de la Pitié (1885–1886).* Paris, Delahaye and Lecrosnier, 1887, p 1.
39. Libman E, Celler HL: The etiology of subacute infective endocarditis. *Am J Med Sci* 1910;140:516.
40. Libman E, Friedberg CK: *Subacute Bacterial Endocarditis.* Oxford, Oxford University Press, 1941.
41. Libman E, Friedberg CK: *Subacute Bacterial Endocarditis.* Oxford, Oxford University Press, 2nd ed 1948.
42. Roth M: Ueber Netzhautaffectionen by Wundfiebern. *Deutsch Chir* 1872;1:471.
43. Doherty WB, Trubek M: Significant hemorrhagic retinal lesions in bacterial endocarditis (Roth spots). *JAMA* 1931;97:308.
44. Janeway EG: Certain clinical observations upon heart disease. *Med News* 1899;LXXV:257.
45. Blumer G: The digital manifestations of subacute bacterial endocarditis. *Am Heart J* 1926;1:256.
46. Lichtman S: Treatment of subacute bacterial endocarditis: Current results. *Ann Intern Med* 1943;19:787.
47. Long PH, Bliss EA: *The Clinical and Experimental Use of Sulfanilimide, Sulfapyridine and Allied Compounds.* New York, Macmillan, 1939.
48. Weiss S: Self-observations and psychologic reactions of medical student A.S.R. to the onset and symptoms of subacute bacterial endocarditis. *J Mount Sinai Hosp* 1941–42;816:79–94.
49. Rehn L: Ueber penetrirende harzwunden im herzneht. *Arch Klin Chir* 1897;55:315:327.
50. Bruton L: Preliminary note on the possibility of treating mitral stenosis by surgical methods. *Lancet* 1900;1:352.
51. Cutler EC, Levine SA: Cardiotomy and valvulotomy for mitral stenosis. Experimental observations and clinical notes concerning an operated case with recovery. *Boston Med Surg J* 1923;188:1023.
52. Gross RE, Hubbard JP: Surgical ligation of patent ductus arteriosus. *JAMA* 1939;112:729.
53. Touroff ASW, Vessell H: Subacute *Streptococcus viridans* endocarditis complicating patent ductus arteriosus. *JAMA* 1940;115:1270.

2

The Historical Development of Antimicrobial and Surgical Therapy of Infective Endocarditis

The concept and the attempt to use substances derived from one organism to kill another (antibiosis) are almost as old as the science of microbiology. In fact, the use of antimicrobial therapy is considerably older. The Chinese were aware 2,500 years ago of the therapeutic properties of mold and soybeans applied to carbuncles, boils, and other infections and used this as standard treatment for these disorders. For centuries, the medical literature had described the beneficial effects of soil and various plants, many of which were sources of antibiotic-producing molds.

The first studies suggesting that microorganisms produced antimicrobial substances were reported by Pasteur and Joubert in 1877.[1] They noted that *Bacillus anthracis* grew rapidly when inoculated into sterile urine but failed to multiply and died when one of the common bacteria in the air was introduced in the urine at the same time.

Treatment with antibiotics represents the practical, controlled, and direct application of organisms that occur naturally and continuously in soil, sewage, water, and other habitats. During the late nineteenth and early twentieth centuries, several antimicrobial agents were identified in some cultures of certain organisms. Substances elaborated by *Chromobacter prodigiosum* (*Serratia marcescens*) and *Pseudomonas aeruginosa* were found to inhibit the growth of some organisms, but were too toxic for clinical use and were discarded.

The development in 1936 of the first sulfonamide, sulfanilamide, ushered in the modern era of effective antimicrobial therapy. However, despite impressive results in the management of some infections, the sulfonamides were of little importance in the treatment of infective endocarditis.

The Medical Therapy of Endocarditis

The discovery of penicillin led to the first successful treatment of infective endocarditis. It remains the drug of choice in most instances of the disease.

In 1928, while studying staphylococcal variants in the laboratory of St. Mary's Hospital in London, Fleming[2–4] noted that a mold that had contaminated one of his cultures lysed bacteria that had grown in the vicinity of the fungus. The fluid in which the mold grew was bactericidal in vitro for many common pathogenic organisms. Because the fungus belonged to the genus *Penicillium,* Fleming named the antibacterial substance *penicillin.* He applied filtrates of the growth to infected wounds. The clinical results were not encouraging because the potency of this crude material was low and it was unstable. Very little was made of Fleming's discovery for nearly a decade. A few microbiologists used the active broth as a selective agent in differential culture media, mainly to isolate *Haemophilus influenzae* from mixtures of gram-positive microorganisms that might be present in cultures of secretions from the respiratory tract.

Penicillin was developed as a systemic therapeutic agent by the brilliant concerted activities of a group of investigators, headed by H.W. Florey, working in the Sir William Bunn School of Pathology at Oxford University. Starting in 1939, work on the biosynthesis and extraction of penicillin from broth cultures of *Penicillium notatum* was pursued. Within a few months, many of the chemical and physical properties of the antibiotic, its antibacterial spectrum, its potency, and its low order of toxicity for animals were established. In May 1940, the crude material then available produced dramatic therapeutic effects when administered parenterally to mice with experimental streptococcal infections. The in vitro activity of penicillin, its very high therapeutic index, and its activity even in the presence of blood, pus, or tissue autolysates were factors that focused the attention of the Oxford group on the potential value of the antibiotic as a systemic chemotherapeutic agent, especially in treating soldiers during World War II. Despite many obstacles to the production of penicillin in the laboratory, enough was accumulated by 1941 to treat several patients desperately ill with staphylococcal or streptococcal infections refractory to all other therapies. At this point, crude amorphous penicillin was only about 10% pure. Almost 100 liters of broth in which the mold was grown was required to obtain enough antibiotic to treat one patient for 24 hr. Herrell (1945) pointed out that bedpans were used by the Oxford group to grow cultures of *P. notatum.* Case 1 in the 1941 report from Oxford described a policeman who was suffering from a severe, mixed staphylococcal and streptococcal infection. He was treated with penicillin, some of which had been recovered from the urine of patients who had received the drug. It is said that an Oxford professor referred to penicillin as a remarkable substance grown in bedpans and purified by passage through the Oxford police force.

Extension of the clinical program required larger quantities of penicillin than could be produced in the laboratory. Commercial manufacture of the antibiotic on a large scale was impossible in Great Britain because of the exigencies of war. As the direct result of a visit by the Oxford team in 1941, a broad research program was initiated in the United States in which governmental, university, and industrial laboratories cooperated. In 1942, 122 million units of penicillin was made available. The first clinical trials were conducted at Yale University and the Mayo Clinic. By the spring of 1943, 200 patients had been treated with the antibiotic. The results were so impressive that the Surgeon General of the U.S. Army authorized a trial of the antibiotic in a military hospital. Penicillin was soon adopted throughout the medical services of the U.S. armed forces.

In 1943, the deep fermentation process for the biosynthesis of penicillin developed at the Northern Regional Research Laboratories of the Department of Agriculture, in Peoria, Illinois, marked a crucial advance in the large-scale production of the antibiotic. From total production of a few hundred million units per month in the early years, the quantity manufactured increased to 800 billion units per month by January 1949.

To use the limited supplies to the maximum, the National Research Council gave control of penicillin to the Committee on Penicillin Therapy under the direction of Chester S. Keefer, M.D. In 1943, the committee reported its experience with the treatment of 500 patients with a variety of infections.[4] Of the 17 patients with infective endocarditis treated by Keefer, 16 died, 2 had transient improvement, and 1 was cured. The total dose of penicillin ranged from 240,000 to 1,760,000 units administered over 9 to 26 days.

In this period, it was common practice to add heparin to therapeutic regimens in order to decrease the size of the valvular vegetations. It was thought that this might permit better penetration of antimicrobial agents. In 1944, Loewe[5] reported the results of a study in which patients with subacute infective endocarditis were treated with penicillin plus heparin. Five of seven patients were infected by *Streptococcus viridans*. The dose of penicillin ranged from 40,000 to 100,000 Florey units/day. The organisms were sensitive to 0.007 to 0.01 Florey unit/ml. The duration of treatment ranged from 2 to 4 weeks; when a relapse occurred, patients were treated for 4 weeks. It gradually became clear that heparin was not a necessary component of the therapy. In 1951, Cates[6] reviewed 492 cases of infective endocarditis and described a number of adverse prognostic factors that are still true. Among these were (1) the presence of congestive cardiac failure, (2) advanced age, (3) delay in the institution of treatment, and (4) rheumatic injury to the aortic valve.

In the early 1950s, chloramphenicol and the tetracyclines were used to treat subacute bacterial endocarditis. Although significant symptomatic improvement was produced while the drugs were being administered, the majority of patients relapsed rapidly after therapy was discontinued.[7] Experience with these drugs provided support for the concept that bactericidal antibiotics were required to cure infective endocarditis.

Recognition that therapy of enterococcal endocarditis with penicillin alone is often ineffective led to clinical trials with penicillin plus streptomycin; the latter was discovered by Schatz, Bugie, and Waksman[8] in 1944 in a program designed to discover new antibiotics. The combination of these antibiotics produced a high rate of success against a very resistant organism.[9,10] In the same period, it was noted that the relapse rate after 2 weeks of therapy of endocarditis with penicillin plus streptomycin caused by *S. viridans* was much lower than in patients treated with penicillin alone for 4 weeks.[11] The results of these studies contributed greatly to the concept of antimicrobial synergism.

Most classes of antimicrobial agents have been used to treat infective endocarditis. Many of the basic principles of therapy of this disease were established in the early 1950s.

The Surgical Treatment of Infective Endocarditis

The first report of the importance of surgery in the therapy of endocarditis that failed to respond to intensive antimicrobial therapy was published by Wallace, Young, and Osterhourt in 1965.[12] The patient was a 45-year-old man who had had chills and fever for 1 month, during which *Klebsiella* was recovered from his blood. He developed a loud diastolic murmur, splinter hemorrhages, and petechiae. Despite appropriate treatment with colistin and kanamycin for 3 weeks, his fever persisted and aortic regurgitation became more marked. Because cardiac failure became increasingly severe and refractory to medical management, the patient underwent surgery for removal of the infected valve and the placement of a Starr-Edwards prosthesis. Large, soft vegetations were present on the perforated left and right coronary cusps from which *Klebsiella* was cultured. The patient recovered without sequelae and remained free of disease over the following 15 months. Of special importance was an observation by Wallace et al. that the presence of active infection was not a contraindication to surgical replacement of an infected valve. They concluded that "when uncontrolled heart disease develops during the course of antibiotic therapy, surgical correction of the hemodynamic defect may become urgent." The results of a combined program of intense antimicrobial therapy, and resection of the infected valve produced encouraging results in the correction of the hemodynamic abnormality. These authors did add the qualifying statement that, "in selected cases, active endocarditis need not be considered a reason for valvular replacement." The case for surgical intervention was echoed 2 years later by other physicians.[13–15] Windsor and Shanahan[16] pointed out that "It has become apparent that, in a certain number of cases, valve destruction is rapid and medical therapy cannot control the resultant cardiac disease."

As surgery for the management of hemodynamic problems became common, it became clear that although surgery is successful therapy in patients with or without valvular infection, it may also be responsible for the introduction of organisms and the initiation of infection involving the prosthesis or the tissues to which it is attached.[12] The surgeon wields a double-edged scalpel that, on the one hand, cures disease and, on the other, is responsible for inducing infection.[15]

Almost all surgical maneuvers—including mitral and aortic valvulotomy, the Blalock procedure, operations that do not involve cardiopulmonary bypass, the insertion of prosthetic valves, replacement of homograft valves, application of patches to repair ventricular septal defects, placement of pacemakers, and procedures involving open-heart surgery—have been complicated by infection. The incidence of infective endocarditis induced by these manipulations has varied from 0.1% to 2.7%, with an average of about 1%. Infection may appear immediately after surgery or may be delayed for periods ranging from several months to 5 to 6 years. A high fatality rate, despite appropriate antimicrobial therapy, emphasizes the dangers of this type of disease.

The mechanisms involved in the pathogenesis of postoperative infective endocarditis are multiple and operate alone or in combination. Windsor and Shanahan[16] have pointed out that "Beginning with the possibility of the introduction of organisms during diagnostic cardiac catheterization, each additional step in the course of surgical treatment adds an increment of risk of bacterial infection. Among the factors that may be involved are the use of contaminated blood, deposition of organisms from the environment into the heart, the presence of an intracardiac foreign body, the introduction of infectious agents during suturing, prolonged placement of venous catheters and the exposure to antimicrobial agents."

The development of cardiopulmonary bypass has made it possible for surgery to solve two major problems associated with infective endocarditis. One is the cure of infection of natural valvular leaflets, prostheses, or infected sutures situated in the myocardium. The other is the control of intractable cardiac failure, a common sequel of the destruction of cardiac valves that may occur in the course of acute infective endocarditis. A large number of studies have underscored the success of surgical intervention in these situations. These studies have now cured infection and controlled cardiac failure in enough patients to make it clear that surgery may be the final and critical maneuver in an increasing number of patients with infective endocarditis.

References

1. Pasteur L, Joubert J: Charbonne et septicemie. *C hebd Seanc Acad Sci* (Paris) 1877;85:101.
2. Weinstein L: Antimicrobial agents (continued) penicillins and cephalasporins, in Goodman, Gilman (eds): *The Pharmacology and Basis of Therapeutics*, ed 5. New York, Macmillan, 1975, chap 57.
3. Durack D: Review of early experiences in the treatment of bacterial endocarditis 1910–1955, in Bismo AC (ed): *Treatment of Infective Endocarditis*. New York, Grune and Stratton, 1981, p 1.
4. Keefer CS, Blake FG, Marshall EK, et al: Penicillin in the treatment of infectious endocarditis: A report of 500 cases. *JAMA* 1943;122:1217.

5. Loewe L, Rosenblatt P, Green HJ, et al: Combined penicillin and heparin therapy of subacute bacterial endocarditis: Report of seven consecutive successfully treated patients. *JAMA* 1944;124:14.
6. Cates JR, Christie RV: Subacute bacterial endocarditis. *Q J Med* 1951;20:93.
7. Kane LW, Finn JJ: The treatment of subacute bacterial endocarditis with aureomycin and chloromycetin. *N Engl J Med* 1953;244:623.
8. Schatz A, Bugie E, Waksman SA: Streptomycin, a substance exhibiting antibiotic activity against gram-positive and gram-negative bacteria. *Proc Soc Exp Book Med* 1944;55:449.
9. Moellering RC, Weinberg A: Studies on antibiotic synergism against enterococci. II. Effect of various antibiotics on the uptake of 4C-labelled streptomycin 64 enterococci. *J Clin Invest* 1971;50:2580.
10. Geraci J, Martin W: Antibiotic therapy of bacterial endocarditis. IV. Successful short term (2 weeks) combined penicillin dihydrostreptomycin therapy in subacute bacterial endocarditis caused by penicillin sensitive streptococci. *Circulation* 1953;8:494.
11. Wallace AG, Young WG Jr, Osterhout J: Treatment of acute bacterial endocarditis by valve excision and replacement. *Circulation* 1965;31:450.
12. Bahnson HTM, Spencer FC, Bennett IJ: Staphylococcal infections of the heart and great vessels due to silk sutures. *Ann Surg* 1957;146:399.
13. Brannif BA, Shumway NE, Harrison DC: Valve replacement in active bacterial endocarditis. *N Engl J Med* 1967;271:1964.
14. Scott SM, Fish RG, Crutcher JC: Early surgical intervention for aortic insufficiency due to bacterial endocarditis. *Ann Thorac Surg* 1967;3:158.
15. Weinstein L: The double-edged scalpel. Editoral. *N Engl J Med* 1968;279:775.
16. Windsor HM, Shanahan MX: Emergency valve replacement in bacterial endocarditis. *Thorax* 1967;22:25.

3

Epidemiology

Incidence and Age Distribution

The precise incidence of infective endocarditis is difficult to determine. Only autopsy reliably differentiates bacteremia associated with endocardial infection from that arising from other sources. When strict definitions were applied to 123 patients with documented infective endocarditis studied at a university hospital, less than 50% of the diagnoses were classified as definite or probable.[1] The progressive decline in the frequency of autopsies has increased the problem of accurate diagnosis. Newer investigative techniques have not been an effective substitute for the postmortem examination. The incidence of endocarditis in any hospital depends on the clinical profiles of its patients.[2,3]

Facilities that care for large numbers of intravenous drug abusers, as well as for patients who require replacement of congenitally abnormal valves or who suffer from rheumatic cardiac disease, experience a disproportionately large number of cases of infective endocarditis. A study of patients in community hospitals or medical centers with infective endocarditis has indicated that age is an important risk factor. Patients older than 65 years are nine times more likely to develop infective endocarditis than younger patients. S. aureus causes infective endocarditis more often in patients admitted to community hospitals; the reverse is true for disease caused by enterococci.[1]

The recent tendency to discard the long-standing classification of infective endocarditis as *acute* or *subacute* in favor of characterizing it in relation to the causative organism has led to epidemiological confusion.[4] From a therapeutic standpoint, this makes it difficult to compare recent experiences with older ones and minimizes significant differences in the pathogenesis, clinical course, and outcome of infective endocarditis. These factors not only depend on the involved organism but are often the result of a variety of time-related immune phenomena. The results of a number of studies have identified an increase, no change, or a decrease in the incidence of infective endocarditis over the last several decades.

The total number of cases of infective endocarditis in the United States in 1936 was reported by Hedly[5] to be approximately 4,000 to 5,000, or 4.2 per 100,000 person-years. This is similar to the annual average number of cases in Great Britian during 1929 to 1942 and in 1964.[6] There is little evidence to indicate that the introduction of antimicrobial agents has led to a significant decrease in the incidence of endocardial infection.[6-8] However, the incidence did decrease during the 1950s and 1960s.[9] The factors thought to be responsible were (1) the widespread use of antimicrobial agents that cured many extracardiac infections before they produced bacteremia and infection of the cardiac valves or endocardium; (2) the widespread use of prophylaxis in patients with rheumatic and congenital cardiac disease; and (3) the tendency to admit patients with endocardial infection to referral hospitals. In addition, fewer patients were admitted to large municipal hospitals, according to studies conducted by Afrenow[10] and Finland and Barnes.[11]

A low incidence of endocardial infection, 1.3 cases per 100,000 admissions, was noted in Australia between 1962 and 1971;[12] this has not been verified. Surveys conducted by Uwaydah and Weinberg,[13] Lerner and Weinstein,[14] and Wilson[8] found no change in the incidence of infective endocarditis following the introduction of effective antimicrobial agents. Autopsy studies carried out in the United Kingdom yielded similar results.[15,16] In 1977, Durack and Petersdorf[17] performed an extensive review of the incidence of infective endocarditis in the periods before and after the introduction of antibiotics. They concluded that it had remained essentially unchanged over the preceding 30 years. More recent investigations have confirmed this finding.

In 1984, Newsom[18] reported that the incidence of bacterial valvulitis had changed very little since the 1930s. It averaged 3.8 cases per 100,000 person-years between 1950 and 1981. However, there had been an increase in the incidence of staphylococcal endocarditis over this period. Griffin and colleagues[19] reported that there had been 78 cases of valvular infection in Olmstead County, Minnesota, between 1950 and 1981. Based on stricter definitions, 50 cases were considered definite, 27 probable, and 14 possible examples of endocarditis. The mean incidence was 3.8 per 100,000 person-years, despite the almost doubling of the population over the same period. The incidence of the disease in this area was 4.3 (1950–1959), 3.3 (1960–1969), and 3.9 (1970–1981) per 100,000 person-years. Currently, infective endocarditis accounts for 0.16 to 5.4 cases per 100,000 admissions to hospitals.[20,21]

Overwhelming evidence indicates that there has been no change in the incidence of infective endocarditis. Perhaps during the early days of antimicrobial therapy, before the increase in bacterial resistance to these drugs, the appearance of suprainfection, and the rise in thoracic surgery, there may have been a true, short-lived decrease in the frequency of this disease.

The ratio of acute to subacute endocarditis was 1.1 : 6 in the preantibiotic era; it is now about 1 : 3.[13,14,22,23] This change is related to an increase in the frequency of cardiac surgery, the high incidence of the intravenous drug abuse, and the increasing number of cases of atherosclerotic valvular disease and prolapsed mitral valve syndrome. As these predisposing factors continue to increase in importance, cases of acute disease will expand in number. Lack of appreciation of the difference between subacute and acute endocarditis has led to diagnostic errors.

Studies of the age distribution of infective endocarditis have indicated that the disease has undergone considerable change from the 1940s to the present.[14,24,25–33] Before antimicrobial agents were available, the disease involved primarily young adults. The mean age of patients with subacute disease increased from 30.6 years prior to 1923 to 32 years in the 1930s and 1940s, 46 years in the 1950s, and 50 to 56 years in the 1960s. Currently, the average age of patients is 57 years. Prior to 1923, fewer than 2% of patients with infective endocarditis were older than 60 years. Early in the antibiotic era, only 12% of the cases involved elderly individuals. Currently, 55% of these patients are 60 or more years of age.[3,23,34–36] Individuals with infective endocarditis caused by group D streptococci range in age from 61 to 67 years.[37] A major exception to this "graying" phenomenon is the syndrome that involves intravenous drug abusers (mean age, 27 years).[26]

There is undeniable evidence that the incidence of infective endocarditis has increased in the elderly. Patients with this disease studied by Thayer[33] in 1926 were, on average, less than 34 years of age; a large number were younger than 30 years. Of 123 cases studied by von Reyn and his colleagues in 1981,[1] 55% were 60 years or older. In 1984, Cantrell and Yoshikawa[38] commented that "infective endocarditis has become a disease affecting primarily elderly persons." A report by Newsom in 1984[18] indicated that the mean age of patients with valvular infection was 51.6 years; 135 of 544 were 65 years of age or older.

Lerner and Weinstein[14] pointed out in 1966 that the increasing age of onset of endocarditis posed a serious problem in older patients because their clinical presentation might not be suggestive of the presence of this disease. Even when appropriate therapy is administered, the prognosis is generally poorer than it is in the young. In 1976, Gladstone and Rocco[39] noted that elderly patients were more susceptible to infective endocarditis and other potentially lethal infections, the clinical manifestations of which were so subtle that a specific diagnosis was difficult early in the course of the disease. They suggested that this increased susceptibility was probably related to a decrease in the activity of the immune system and to dysfunction of various organs.

Kaye[40] has pointed out that "there has been a significant trend toward an increase in age of patients with endocarditis, and it seems likely that the age of these patients will continue to increase as the population ages." Durack and Petersdorf[17] have suggested several reasons that might explain this phenomenon. Among these are the following: (1) atherosclerotic cardiovascular disease provides a large number of sites that may be infected in the course of a bacteremia; (2) there has been a marked increase in the frequency of cardiac surgery and the placement of intravascular lines in severely ill elderly patients; (3) two-thirds of individuals with nosocomially acquired staphylococcal bacteremia have been elderly, as opposed to 30% of those with community-acquired infections over the same period;[41] (4) the incidence of rheumatic fever has decreased and is now more common in the older population;[42] (5) patients with congenital cardiac disease now live to old age and are likely to require placement of a prosthesis, which may become infected.

Endocarditis in children is rare.[43,44] The incidence of the disease is approximately 0.55 per 100,000 admissions to large pediatric hospitals.

A study of the sexual distribution of infective endocarditis by Lerner and Weinstein[14] indicated that the disease occurs twice as often in men as in women. This increases to a ratio 9:1 in patients 50 to 60 years old and to 6.5:1 in those 61 to 70 years old. A statistically singnificant increase in the incidence of endocarditis caused by *S. viridans* had been documented in older men.[45] The ratio of male to female patients generally is not related to the nature of the organism responsible for the disease. However, women younger than 35 are disproportionately represented when endocarditis is caused by enterococci.[23,46]

Predisposing Cardiac Lesions

The type of cardiac pathology underlying endocardial infections depends on the characteristics of the patient with respect to age, history of drug abuse, and prior cardiac surgery, as well as the nature of the organism responsible for the infection. Bacteria with a low level of pathogenicity, such as *S. viridans*, require a previously damaged valve to produce endocardial infection. Classically, *S. aureus* invades normal or damaged valves. Enterococci may behave similarly to *S. aureus*.

Durack and Petersdorf[17] reviewed the literature describing the changes in the types of cardiac disease involved in the development of infective endocarditis before and after the introduction of antimicrobial therapy (Table 3.1). They concluded that there has been no change in the importance of congenital heart disease with respect to the pathogenesis of infective endocarditis. Bicuspid aortic valves account for 20% of cases of endocarditis in patients older than 60 years. Other congenital cardiac abnormalities, including ventricular septal defects, patent ductus arteriosus, and tetralogy of Fallot, play important roles in the development of infective endocarditis.

The prevalence of rheumatic cardiac disease has decreased strikingly over the last 40 years and is now a minor risk factor. Effective antimicrobial prophylaxis of rheumatic fever has sharply decreased the risk of infective endocarditis and other microbial infections. A report of one study[23] has pointed out that the risk of endocardial infection in patients with rheumatic fever is about 6%[47] (Table 3.2). The mitral valve alone is involved (85% of cases). In this situation, women predominate.

Mitral valve prolapse occurs in about 30% of patients with endocarditis

Table 3.1. Changing Prevalence of Various Conditions Predisposing to Infective Endocarditis

	Preantibiotic Era (1944)	Early Antibiotic Era (1944–1965)	Recent Antibiotic Era (1965)
Congenital heart disease	+ +	+ +	+ +
Rheumatic heart disease	+ + + +	+ + +	+ +
Degenerative heart disease	+	+	+ +
Compromised host	+	+	+ +
Cardiac surgery	0	+	+ +
Drug addiction	0	+	+ +
Intravascular catheters, dialysis, hyperalimentation, pacemakers, etc.	0	+	+ +

Source: Adapted from Ref. 17.

Table 3.2. Lesions Predisposing to Endocarditis

	Number of Patients	Percent of Patients
Mitral valve prolapse	18	29
Prolapse with redundancy	15	24
Prolapse without redundancy	1	2
Prolapse with partial flail leaflet with redundancy	2	3
None	17	27
Drug abuse	7	11
No drug abuse	10	16
Degenerative calcific valvular lesions	13	21
Aortic sclerosis	9	14
Mitral annular calcification	4	6
Congenital heart disease	8	13
Rheumatic heart disease	4	6
Hypertrophic cardiomyopathy	3	5
Total	63	100

Source: Adapted from Ref. 47.

involving the natural valves.[47] Most of these infected valves (about 97%) are redundant. This abnormality has now replaced rheumatic valvular disease as the primary precursor of infective endocarditis in young patients.

Degenerative valvular disease is present in about 20% of patients with endocardial infection. This is probably the most common valvular lesion among the elderly. Several published studies have indicated that 33–50% of individuals older than 60 years have degenerative aortic valvular disease. Most present with no past history of cardiac disease.[36,48,49]

About 5% of cases of asymmetric septal hypertrophy eventually develop infective endocarditis.[50] This usually occurs among patients with the greatest level of obstruction (highest peak systolic pressures). Most cases involve the mitral valve, some the aortic valve, and, rarely, both valves. About one third of patients develop a new murmur. *S. viridans* causes approximately 75% of these infections. About 29–50% of patients have no underlying cardiac disorder. Many are intravenous drug users.[2,51]

Fifty-four percent of patients with degenerative valvular disease have other significant medical illnesses.[38] This accounts for the increased fatality rate among these patients. Excluding intravenous drug abusers, 40% of individuals free of underlying cardiac disease, except for prolapse of the mitral valve, have associated medical illnesses including renal failure, diabetes mellitus, and chronic pulmonary disease. Von Reyn et al.[1] noted that predisposing events differ with age, the nature of the infecting organism, and whether the patient acquired the infection in the community or in a hospital. About 15% of patients with infective endocarditis acquire the disease in the process of dental manipulation.[52] Many cases with long periods of incubation may be due to *S. viridans* bacteremia, the source of which is poor oral hygiene, rather than to dental procedures. There is a strong association between enterococcal endocarditis and surgical manipulation of the genitourinary tract.[53] The site at which *S. aureus* enters the circulation can be identified in about 50% of patients.[22] The portal of entry of the invading organism may be determined in about 20% of individuals with subacute infective endocarditis.[54]

Although it has been suggested that the immunocompromised state is associated with an increased risk of infective endocarditis,[55] Durack and Petersdorf[17] have concluded that this is only partially true. Infective endocarditis in patients with leukemia is rare, despite a high incidence of bacteremia. In this situation, the low frequency of endocardial infection may be due to thrombocytopenia, which may interfere with the function of platelets in the development of a noninfected thrombus, an essential step in the pathogenesis of endocarditis.

Congenital cardiac disease accounts for 80% of the conditions leading to the development of infective endocarditis in children[56] (see Chapter 11). Ventricular septal defect is the most important congenital abnormality (36%). Aortic stenosis (19%) is the second most common predisposing factor, followed closely by the tetralogy of Fallot (16%). Patent ductus arteriosus and pulmonary stenosis account for less than 10% of cases. Rheumatic heart disease is the underlying cause in only 8%. Various types of cardiac surgery, especially those involving placement of a prosthesis, have become much more important factors. Intravenous drug abuse has become very important in the pathogenesis of endocardial infection.

About 40% of cases of infective endocarditis involve the mitral valve alone; 5–36% are restricted to the aortic valve. Less often, both valves are involved. The tricuspid and pulmonary valves are rarely infected. The incidence of endocarditis of the aortic valve increased from 5% in 1938 to 39% presently.[27] Of these patients, 61% were males and 31% were females.

Nosocomial Infections

Finland and Barnes[11] were among the first to call attention to an increase in the incidence of infective endocarditis caused by *S. aureus,* gram-negative bacilli (excluding shigella and salmonella), enterococci, and *S. epidermidis.* This appears to have resulted from the widespread use of antimicrobial agents and was predominantly nosocomial in origin. A study by von Reyn et al.[1] of patients with valvular infection disclosed that 72 cases developed in a community setting and 16 followed outpatient dental manipulation. The disease was acquired by 14 hospitalized individuals. An episode of infective endocarditis was considered nosocomial in origin when it appeared 48 hr. or more after hospitalization or when it followed a hospital-based procedure carried out 4 weeks prior to the development of symptoms. Fourteen individuals (13%) were 62 years or older. Friedland and his colleagues[57] compared the clinical and other features of 14 patients with infective endocarditis that developed in a hospital with the features of 90 individuals who acquired the disease outside. Individuals with nosocomial infections were older, more often women, had a higher incidence of cardiac valvular disorders, and experienced episodes of bacteremia associated with a variety of invasive procedures. These characteristics were present in 93 individuals with nosocomial infections but in only 50% of those who developed infective endocarditis in the community. The fatality rate of disease acquired in the hospital was 43% compared to 11% in the community.

The organisms responsible for this type of disease reflect the site of origin. The skin is most often the source of staphylococci, the urinary tract of enterococci. Friedland et al. emphasized that "Nosocomial endocarditis occurs in the definable subpopulation of hospitalized patients and is potentially preventable." Weinstein and Rubin[46] and Kaye[23] noted that nosocomially acquired bacterial valvulitis involved women more often than men. The opposite was true of community-acquired disease. The former group exhibited a higher incidence of underlying valvular abnormalities and an increased fatality rate. The results of a study by Cantrell and Yoshikawa[38] emphasized that when gram-negative organisms were responsible for infective endocarditis in the elderly, the bacteria were frequently acquired in a hospital or in a chronic institutional setting. There was also a high rate of association with diseases of the gastrointestinal and urinary tracts of the elderly.

In an analysis of 103 patients with bacteremia caused by *S. aureus,* Finkelstein and colleagues[58] identified several fundamental differences between nosocomial and community-acquired infections. Staphylococcal disease that originated in the community was usually not associated with a primary extracardiac focus of infection, and was more likely to lead to infective endocarditis and metastatic infections. In contrast, a portal of entry was often identified in patients with staphylococcal bacteremia that developed in a nosocomial setting; endocarditis was less common. Regardless of the epidemiological background of staphylococcal bacteremia, the fatality rate was high, especially in nosocomial infections, because of the high frequency of underlying disorders that, by themselves, were associated with an increased risk of death.

Van den Broek and colleagues[59] have reported a hospital outbreak of endocarditis caused by *S. epidermidis* that involved prosthetic valves. The source of the organism was a cardiac surgeon who was identified as a healthy carrier. During the investigation, a second group of patients was discovered to have been contaminated by staphylococci in the course of open cardiac surgery performed by a different surgeon, who was found to carry the same organism. Neither of these doctors developed infection.

Microbiology

In addition to the striking changes in the epidemiology of infective endocarditis over the last 40 years, it is clear that over the same period, remarkable qualitative and quantitative changes have occurred in the profile of the infecting organisms. The introduction of many potent antibiotics over the years has played a major role in altering the microbial etiology of infective endocarditis.[11] It is clear that these drugs, when administered early, have been highly effective in eradicating extracardiac infections produced by a number of organisms, including *S. pneumoniae, Neisseria gonorrhoeae,* and *S. pyogenes,* common causes of acute infective endocarditis. However, the role of these organisms in the pathogenesis of infective endocarditis has decreased markedly.

There is no doubt that the administration of antimicrobial agents exerts a profound effect on the indigenous microbial flora that may lead to overgrowth and eventual invasion by *S. aureus, S. epidermidis,* gram-negative bacteria, yeasts, and fungi. Many of these are innately resistant to the usual antibiotics. Resistance is more likely to occur when two or more antibiotics are administered simultaneously.[60] Both the widespread use of intravenous drugs and cardiac surgery have increased the frequency of infective endocarditis caused by uncommon organisms.

Cardiac surgery may produce paradoxial effects.[61] It is often used as a last resort in patients in whom treatment with antimicrobial agents fails to eradicate an infection. The surgical procedure itself may be followed by a suprainfection caused by opportunistic organisms including *Pseudomonas,* species of *Serratia,* yeast, or fungi.

Many investigators have pointed out that there has been a relative, but not an absolute, increase in the involvement of certain streptococci in the pathogenisis of infective endocarditis since antibiotics became available. An increase in the frequency of valvular disease caused by *S. aureus* occurred simultaneously. In 1970, Finland and Barnes[11] reported an appreciable decrease in the incidence of infective endocarditis caused by *S. viridans* and streptococci. Accompanying this was an increase in the number of patients with infections caused by enterococci, a group rarely involved in the preantibiotic era. More recent studies have confirmed these observations. Of 544 instances of infective endocarditis studied by Bayliss et al.,[54] 63% were produced by streptococci, 19% by staphylococci, and 14% by "bowel organisms." Sixty-three percent of 340 instances of endocardial infections described by Newsom[18] in 1984 were caused by streptococci; 46 were group D and 27 were enterococci. In the same year, Cantrell and Yoshikawa[38] pointed out that, in their experience, *S. bovis* was the organism most commonly involved in patients older than 55 years. This organism is important because it often indicates underlying gastrointestinal pathology, including carcinoma. Because these lesions are often asymptomatic, a search for colonic neoplasm is indicated when *S. bovis* is identified.

Kaye[40] suggested that because of our aging population, the incidence of infective endocarditis caused by streptococci or enterococci might be expected to increase. Cherubin and Neu[7] proposed that the older age at which patients are presently developing infective endocarditis is a major reason for changes in the microbial etiology of the disease. They noted that *S. viridans* infects younger patients more often then older ones. Age appears to increase the susceptibility to invasion by enterococci and *S. aureus*. The frequency with which these organisms produce valvular disease has not changed significantly over the past 30 years. However, it is known that the incidence of infective endocarditis caused by *S. aureus, S. epidermidis,* gram-negative bacteria, yeasts, and fungi has grown dramatically since the introduction of antimicrobial agents.

Durack and Petersdorf[17] questioned the results presented above. They analyzed the microbiological information in 1,328 cases of infective endocarditis reported over three periods: prior to 1944, 1944–1965, and after 1965. The data indicated that there had been a decrease in the frequency of infection by *S. viridans* and an increase due to enterococci and *S. aureus*. They stated that "the apparent decrease in *S. viridans* bacterial endocariditis and an apparent increase in enterococci are partly artifacts." However, other recently recorded experiences have not agreed with these observations. There is presently no doubt that *S. epidermidis* has increased in frequency because of its significant involvement in the infection of prosthetic valves. It is presently thought to be the organism most often involved in this infection.

The increasing use of illegal intravenous drug abuse has led to an expanding number of cardiac infections produced by gram-negative bacteria, yeasts, and common fungi greater than that appreciated by Durack and Petersdorf.[17] Experience over the last 10 years has indicated that unusual organisms are now increasingly responsible for endocarditis. This trend will probably continue as larger numbers of bacteria become resistant to presently available antibiotics. Another very important factor altering the microbiology of infective endocarditis is the increasing age of the population and the accompanying atherosclerosis, with its degenerative effect on valve leaflets and their supporting structures. These are now the common lesions that predispose to the development of endocardial infection.

S. viridans has been the most common organism causing infective endocarditis among children. *S. aureus* is becoming the most important pathogen, especially following cardiac surgery.

References

1. Von Reyn C, Levy B, Arbeit R: Infective endocarditis: An analysis based on strict case definitions. *Ann Intern Med* 1981;94 (Part I):505.
2. King J, Nguyen L, Conrad S: Results of a prospective statewide reporting system for infective endocarditis. *Am J Med Sci* 1982;31:517.
3. Kim E, Ching D, Plen F: Bacterial endocarditis at a small community hospital. *Am J Med Sci* 1990;299:487.
4. Kaye D: Infective endocarditis, in JB Wyngarden, LH Smith Jr (eds): *Cecil Textbook of Medicine*, ed 11. Philadelphia, WB Saunders, 1982, p 1457.
5. Hedley OF: Rheumatic heart disease in Philadelphia hospitals. III. Fatal rheumatic heart disease and subacute bacterial endocarditis. *Pub Health Rep* 1940;55:1707.
6. Gates JE, Christie RV: Subacute bacterial endocarditis. A review of 442 patients treated in 14 centers appointed by the Penicillin Trials Committee of the Medical Research Council. *Q J Med* 1951;20:93.
7. Cherubin CE, Neu HC: Infective endocarditis at the Presbyterian Hospital in New York City from 1938–1967. *Am J Med* 1971;51:83.
8. Wilson LM: Etiology of bacterial endocarditis: Before and since introduction of antibiotics. *Ann Intern Med* 1963;58:946.
9. Kaye D, McCormack RC, Hook EW: Bacterial endocaditis: The changing pattern since the introduction of penicillin therapy. *Antimicrob Agents Chemother* 1961;3:37.
10. Afrenow ML: Review of 202 cases of bacterial endocarditis. III. *Med J* 1955;108:67.
11. Finland M, Barnes MW: Changing etiology of bacterial endocarditis in the antibacterial era: Experiences at Boston City Hospital 1933–1955. *Ann Intern Med* 1970;72:341.
12. Bailey IK, Richards JG: Infective endocarditis in a Sydney teaching hospital 1962–1971. *Aust NZ Med J* 1975;5:413.
13. Uwaydah NM, Weinberg AN: Bacterial endocarditis: A changing pattern. *N Engl J Med* 1965;273:1231.
14. Lerner PI, Weinstein L: Infective endocarditis in the antibiotic era. *N Engl J Med* 1966;274:199.
15. Hayward GW: Infective endocarditis: A changing disease. *Br Med J* 1973;2:706.
16. Hughes P, Gauld WR: Bacterial endocarditis: A changing disease. *Q J Med* 1966;35:511.
17. Durack DT, Petersdorf RG: Changes in epidemiology of endocarditis. Infective endocarditis. *Am Heart Assoc Monogr* 1977;52:3.
18. Newsom SWB: The treatment of endocarditis by vancomycin. *J Antimicrob Chemother* 1984;14:79.
19. Griffin M, Wilson W, Edwards W: Infective endocarditis, Olmstead County, Minnesota, 1950 through 1981. *JAMA* 1985;254:1199.
20. Watanakunakorn C: Changing epidemiology and newer aspects of infective endocarditis. *Adv Intern Med* 1977;22:21.
21. Oakley C: Infective endocarditis. *Br J Hosp Med* 1980;22:232.
22. Freedman LR: *Infective Endocarditis and Other Intravascular Infections*. New York, Plenum, 1982.
23. Kaye D: Definitions and demographic characteristics, in Kaye D (ed): *Infective Endocarditis*. Baltimore, University Park Press, 1976, p 1.
24. Garvey GJ, Neu HC: Infective endocarditis—an evolving disease. *Medicine (Baltimore)* 1978;57:105.

25. Kelson SR, White PD: Notes on 250 cases of subacute bacterial (streptococcal) endocarditis studied and treated between 1927 and 1939. *Ann Intern Med* 1940;22:40.
26. Stimmel B, Donoso E, Dack S: Comparison of infective endocarditis in drug addicts and non-drug users. *Am J Cardiol* 1973;32:924.
27. Nager F: Changing clinical spectrum of infective endocarditis in *Infective endocarditis*. D Horstkotte, E Bodnar (eds). ICR Publishers, London, 1991, p 25.
28. Hamburger M: Acute and subacute bacterial endocarditis. *Arch Intern Med* 1963;112:1.
29. Wedgwood J: Early diagnosis of subacute bacterial endocarditis. *Lancet* 1955;2:1058.
30. Kerr A Jr: *Subacute Bacterial Endocarditis*. In Pullen RL (ed.). No. 274, in Am Lecture Series, Monograph of Bannerstone Division of Am Lectures in Internal Medicine. Springfield, IL, Charles C Thomas, 1955.
31. Linde M, Hinrichsen H, Schubert J, et al: Infective endocarditis at a hospital of the University of Kiel. *Klin Wochenschr* 1990;68:921.
32. Mandell G, Kaye D, Levenson M, et al: Enterococcal endocarditis. An analysis of 38 patients observed at the New York Hospital Cornell Medical Center. *Arch Intern Med* 1970;125:258.
33. Thayer WS: Studies on bacterial (infective) endocarditis. *Johns Hopkins Hosp Rep* 1926;22:1.
34. Robbins N, De Maria A, Miller MH: Infective endocarditis in the elderly. *South Med J* 1980;73:1335.
35. Rabinovich S, Evans J, Smith I, et al: A long term view of endocarditis. *Ann Intern Med* 1965;63:185.
36. Venezio F, Westenfelder G, Cook F: Infective endocarditis in a community hospital. *Arch Intern Med* 1982;142:789.
37. Morgan WL, Bland EF: Bacterial endocarditis in antibiotic era. *Circulation* 1959;19:753.
38. Cantrell M, Yoshikawa TT: Infective endocarditis in the aging patient. *Gerontology* 1984;30:316.
39. Gladstone JL, Rocco R: Host factors and infectious disease in the elderly. *Med Clin North Am* 1976;60:1225.
40. Kaye D: Changing pattern of infective endocarditis. *Am J Med* 1985;78:157.
41. Terpenning M, Buggy B, Kauffman C: Infective endocarditis: Clinical features in young and elderly patients. *Am J Med* 1987;83:626.
42. Land M, Bisno A: Acute rheumatic fever: A vanishing disease in suburbia. *JAMA* 1983;249:89.
43. Coutlee F, Carceller A, Deschamps L: The evolving pattern of pediatric endocarditis from 1960 to 1985. *Can J Cardiol* 1990;6:169.
44. Samet SM, Weinstein L: Host factors as determinants of the syndrome of subacute bacterial endocarditis. *Proc N Engl Cardiovasc Soc* 1958;17:16.
45. Sussman J, Baron E, Tenebaum M: Viridans streptococcal endocarditis: Clinical, microbiological and echocardiographic correlations. *J Infect Dis* 1986;154:597.
46. Weinstein L, Rubin RH: Infective endocarditis 1973. *Progr Cardiovasc Dis* 1973;16:239.
47. McKinley D, Ratts T, Bisno A: Underlying cardiac lesions in adults with infective endocarditis. *Am J Med* 1987;82:601.
48. Weinstein L: Infective endocarditis, in Braunwald E (ed): *Heart Disease, a Textbook of Cardiovascular Medicine*, ed 3. Philadelphia, WB Saunders, 1988, p 1098.
49. Mansur A, Grinberg M, Bellotti G: Infective endocarditis in the 1980s: Experience at a heart hospital. *Clin Cardiol* 1990;13:623.
50. Chagnac A, Loebel H, Rudnicki C: Endocarditis in idiopathic hypertrophic subaortic stenosis: Report of three cases and review of the literature. *Chest* 1982;81:346.
51. Weinstein L: "Modern" infective endocarditis. *JAMA* 1975;233:260.
52. Guntheroth W: How important are dental procedures as a cause of infective endocarditis? *Am J Cardiol* 1989;54:797.
53. Maki D, Agger W: Enterococcal bacteremia: Clinical features, the risk of endocarditis and management. *Medicine* 1988;67:248.
54. Bayliss R, Clarke C, Oakley CMM: The microbiology and pathogenesis of infective endocarditis. *Br Heart J* 1983;50:513.

55. Johnson A, Rosenthal A, Nadas A: A forty year review of bacterial endocarditis in infancy and childhood. *Circulation* 1978;51:581.

56. King H, Harkness J: Infective endocarditis in the 1980's. Part I: Aetiology and diagnosis. *Med J Aust* 1986;144:536.

57. Friedland G, von Reyn CF, Levy B: Nosocomial endocarditis. *Infect Control* 1984;15:193.

58. Finkelstein R, Sobel JD, Nagler A, et al: *Staphylococcus aureus* bacteremia and endocarditis: Comparison of nosocomial and community-acquired infection. *J Med* 1984;15:193.

59. Van den Broek PJ, Lempe AS, Berbe S: Epidemic of prosthetic valve endocarditis caused by *Staphylococcus epidermidis. Br Med J (Clin Res)* 1985;291:949.

60. Weinstein L, Goldfied M, Chang TW: Infections occurring during chemotherapy. A study of their frequency, type and predisposing factors. *N Engl J Med* 1954;251:247.

61. Weinstein L: The double-edged scalpel. Editorial. *N Engl J Med* 1968;279:775.

4

Microbiology of Infective Endocarditis
and Clinical Correlates:
Gram-Positive Organisms

Infective endocarditis has been classified as acute on the basis of the invasive capacity of the organism responsible for the disease.[1,2] *S. aureus, Neisseria meningitidis, N. gonorrhoeae, S. pyogenes, Haemophilus influenzae,* and *S. pneumoniae* are generally involved in the development of acute infective endocarditis. *S. viridans* and *S. epidermidis* are usually the causative agents of subacute disease. It is important that the presentations of the disease be differentiated because their clinical courses are strikingly different. However, it must be emphasized that, on occasion, infection by *S. aureus* may produce subacute disease, while invasion by *S. viridans,* an organism with a low invasive capacity, leads to the development of acute infection. Lerner and Weinstein[1] have pointed out that the distinction between the two types may be altered by antimicrobial therapy. The administration of an anti-infective drug may cause the acute disease to become chronic and the subacute infection to be life-threatening.

Information concerning the etiology of infective endocarditis is usually passed from the microbiology laboratory to the physician. This includes the morphological and staining characteristics of the organism recovered from a positive blood culture. The data obtained are often sufficient to allow initiation of potentially effective antimicrobial therapy. More definitive identification may require an additional 24 to 72 hr. of incubation at 37°C. When acute, severe disease is present, clinicians are often forced to initiate therapy based on the microscopic characteristics of the organism recovered from the bloodstream. Delay in the initiation of appropriate treatment while awaiting definitive identification and sensitivity to antimicrobial agents of the organisms recovered from the circulation often leads to a high incidence of morbidity and mortality. Although any organism may produce infective endocarditis, those listed in Tables 4.1 and 4.2, appear to be responsible most often for the development of the disease.

Table 4.1. Microbiology of Endocarditis

GRAM-POSITIVE COCCI

S. viridans	Responsible for 50% of all cases of endocarditis and 70% of subacute disease. Three instances of progressive, invasive disease. Predisposing factors: trauma, dental manipulations (extractions, flossing, gingivectomy, periapical abscess, use of Water-Pik). May produce disease in edentulous patients. Usually produces subacute disease; rarely, acute.
Enterococcus	Member of group D streptococci. May produce a, B, or y hemolysis. Species: *S. liquefaciens, S. zymogenes, S. faecalis, S. faecium, S. durans.* Source of organism: GU and GI tracts and oral cavity. Causes 3–17% of cases of endocarditis. Course of the disease may be acute or subacute.
S. bovis	Member of group D but not enterococcus. Responsible for about 50% of cases caused by group D streptococci. Fails to grow in medium containing 6.5% saline. Sensitive to penicillin G. Survival rate higher than with enterococcus. Strong association with endocarditis accompanying cancer of the colon, Crohn's disease, ulcerative colitis.
Peptostreptococcus	Anaerobe; causes 3.85% of cases. Requires culture under anaerobic conditions (thioglycollate broth). Produces mostly subacute disease, occasionally acute.
S. pyogenes (group A, beta-hemolytic)	Currently an uncommon cause of endocarditis, probably because of high rate of successful treatment of pharyngitis, cellulitis, and other extracardiac foci of infection. Although organism usually produces beta hemolysis, some strains may be alpha-hemolytic on surface of blood agar. Clinical course of valvular infection is acute. May produce intracardiac complications, e.g., rupture of valve leaflets.
S. pneumoniae	Frequency of endocarditis decreasing because of highly successful therapy of pneumonia and other extracardiac infections caused by this organism. Current incidence about 5–6%. Disease is usually acute. High frequency of destructive intracardiac complications. Increased risk of valvular infection in patients with multilobar pulmonary involvement and bacteremia.
Other species of streptococci	*S. mutans,* group G, group C—uncommon acute disease with destruction of valves. Organism may be tolerant to penicillin G. *S. constellatus*—only one case reported. Group B involves mitral valve most commonly; next is aortic valve. Groups D, G, K, and L.
Nutritionally deficient ("satelliting") streptococci	Uncommon. Requires pyridoxine for growth. Thioglycolate broth plus pyridoxine is good medium. Colonies group around colonies of *S. aureus* (satelliting). Grow in ordinary broth but cannot be subcultured from this or from agar.

Table 4.1. (*Cont.*)

S. aureus	Most common organism producing acute endocarditis. Predisposing factors: cardiac surgery, intravenous drug use, infections of the skin, osteomyelitis, peripheral sepsis, rheumatic carditis (rare). No underlying disease in 50–60% of cases. No murmurs in presence of endocarditis in about one-third of patients. High frequency of intracardiac complications: rupture of valvular leaflets, septal abscesses, aneurysm of sinus of Valsalva, myocardial abscesses. Disseminated extracardiac infections common. Proved staphylococcal bacteremia in absence of evidence of endocarditis associated with risk of valvular infection in 30–65% of cases. Most strains are resistant to penicillin G. Treatment with a penicillinase-resistant penicillin or an active cephalosporin is required. Some strains are methicillin resistant (tolerant) and fail to be killed by penicillins and cephalosporins. Replacement of infected valve with a prosthesis is often required. Average fatality rate about 50%.
S. epidermidis (albus)	Incidence has increased over the past 25 years. Occasionally involves normal valves; most patients have underlying valvular disease. Common in intravenous drug addicts. Thought to be most common organism infecting prosthetic valves. Produces subacute and chronic endocarditis. High incidence of recurrence after appropriate antimicrobial therapy. May require replacement of involved valve. Organism variably sensitive to antibiotics. Fatality rate high.

GRAM-POSITIVE BACILLI

Erysipelothrix insidiosa	Acquired from fish, birds, cats. May involve normal heart. Disease is acute. Fatality rate about 50%.
Lactobacillus	Dental procedures are a predisposing factor. Underlying cardiac disease may exist.
Listeria monocytogenes	Rare. Involves natural and prosthetic valves. High incidence of systemic embolization.
Corynebacteria	Aerobic diphtheroids and anaerobic *Propionibacterium acnes*. Uncommon cause of endocarditis.
Corynebacterium diphtheriae	Rare cause of endocarditis. Only eight reported cases (1944–1980). Not all strains produce toxin. Increased susceptibility with congenital heart disease.
Bacillus cereus	Only two reported cases. Has involved only prosthetic valves.
B. subtilis	Only one reported case. Drug addict; right heart involved.
Rothia dentocariosa	Only two reported cases of endocarditis. Produces subacute disease.

GRAM-NEGATIVE COCCI

N. gonorrhoeae	Caused 10–14% of cases of endocarditis in preantibiotic era; now uncommon. Not always related to genital

(Continued)

37

Table 4.1. Microbiology of Endocarditis (*Cont.*)

	infection. Aortic and mitral valves involved most often. High incidence of infection of right heart. Arthritis in 50% of cases. No underlying heart disease in most patients. One patient with prolapsed mitral valve described. Frequent intra- and extracardiac complications requiring surgery. Recent increase in number of penicillin-resistant strains.
N. meningitidis	Rare. Always secondary to bacteremia, with or without meningitis. Acute endocarditis.
Other gram-negative cocci	*Neisseria flava, N. catarrhalis, N. pharyngis, N. mucosa, Megasphaera elsdenii* (anaerobe).

GRAM-NEGATIVE BACILLI

Escherichia coli	Responsible for about 3–10% of endocarditis. For a recent detailed review, see Ref. 59. Murmur not always present. Mitral valve most often involved.
Enterobacter	Uncommon. Manipulation of GU tract is a predisposing factor in 50% of cases.
Klebsiella pneumoniae	Very rare. Preceding infection of GU tract.
Proteus	Rare. Both indole-positive and indole-negative strains involved. Infection of GU tract is a predisposing factor.
Pseudomonas aeruginosa	Most common in drug addicts. In nonaddicted patients, occurs most often during therapy of another infection (superinfection). Emboli produce necrosis of walls of bloods vessels. Tricuspid valve commonly involved. Infection of more than one valve not uncommon.
Other species of *Pseudomonas* and *Salmonella*	*Ps. multophilia, Ps. cepacia.* Uncommon cause of endocarditis. Most patients over 50 years old. Underlying cardiac disease in most instances. Course often acute. GI tract source of organism in <50% of patients. Fatality rate high even when treated.
Haemophilus	Responsible for about 0.5% of cases of endocarditis. Three species involved: *H. influenzae, H. parainfluenzae,* and *H. aphrophilus.* High frequency of embolization with *H. parainfluenzae.*
Brucella	Rare. Species involved: *Br. abortus, Br. suis, Br. melitensis.* Underlying heart disease in most cases. Mitral valve most often involved. Occasionally acute. Bulky vegetations.
Pasteurella	Rare. Usual source is animal bite or scratch. Cats and dogs carry organism. Three species: *P. multocida* (most common), *P. pneumotropica, P. hemolytica.*
Acinetobacter	May involve normal heart. Acute or subacute disease. Cardiac failure and embolization in >50% of cases. Fatality rate 50–75%.
Serratia	Causes 75% of cases in drug addicts. Infection of prosthetic valves common. Subacute course most

Table 4.1. *(Cont.)*

	common. Large emboli in most instances. Fatality rate about 70%.
Campylobacter (Vibrio)	One species: *C. fetus.* May involve normal heart. Dental manipulation a predisposing factor. Aortic valve usually affected.
Streptobacillus moniliformis	Rare. Endocarditis occurs during course of rat bite fever.
Cardiobacterium hominis	Uncommon. Organism present in pharynx of 70% of normal people. Usually involves abnormal valves. Course subacute. Emboli in 50% of cases.
Actinobacillus actinomycetemcomitans	Most common in middle-aged and older men. Normal valves involved in two-thirds of cases. Course subacute. Organism grows slowly.
Flavobacterium	Only one case reported. Ulceration of aortic valve.
Edwardsiella tarda	Single case report.
Citrobacter diversus	Single case.

YEASTS AND FUNGI

Yeasts	Species of *Candida involved: C. albicans, C. parapsilosis, C. guilliermondii, C. krusei, C. stellatoidea,* and *C. tropicalis* (most common cause in drug addicts). One-third of cases follow cardiac surgery; 20% related to superinfection. Course subacute. Emboli in 50% of patients—occlude large arteries. Blood cultures negative in 75% of cases.
Histoplasma capsulatum	Uncommon. Most cases in eastern United States occur in Ohio and Mississippi River Valley. Involves natural and prosthetic valves. Embolus to large artery may be first sign. Cultures of blood usually negative.
Aspergillus	Various species involved. All cases occur in debilitated or immunocompromised patients or those treated with antibiotics. Prosthetic valves most commonly involved. Infection of mural endocardium common. Blood cultures rarely positive.
Other yeasts and fungi	*Penicillium, Phialophora, Hormodendrum, Paecilomyces, Curvilacea, Saccharomyces, Mucor, T. glabrata, Trichosporon cutaneum, Cryptococcus, Rhodotorula.*

OTHER ORGANISMS

Mycobacterium chelonei	Porcine bioprostheses involved. Organisms cultured from the valve prior to insertion.
M. gordonae	An atypical mycobacterium—one instance of infection of a prosthetic valve.
M. tuberculosis	Usually involves only natural valves as a complication of disseminated tuberculosis. Infection of homograft valves reported.
Coxiella burnetii (Q fever)	All cases of endocarditis have occurred in the course of Q fever. Very few reported from the United States;

(Continued)

39

Table 4.1. Microbiology of Endocarditis (*Cont.*)

	all others in Australia and New Zealand. Duration of Q fever before development of endocarditis: 1 to 20 years. Diagnosis made by detection of rising titer of phase 1 complement-fixing antibody.
Actinomyces israelii (bovis)	Infection by this organism very rare. Both natural and prosthetic valves involved.
Nocardia israelii	Very rare. Both natural and prosthetic valves involved.
Bacteroides	Several species involved. Only 11 reported cases. Usually subacute but may be acute. Infects both prosthetic and natural valves.
Fusobacterium	Only 10 reported cases. May be fulminant.
Chlamydia psittaci	Infection not proved by isolation of the organism. Contact with birds important. Diagnosis made by staining endocardial biopsy specimen with fluorescein-labeled specific antibody.
Cell wall–deficient organisms	Possible but not proved cause of endocarditis. Thought to be responsible for fever persisting despite appropriate therapy. Most common in drug addicts and in patients undergoing cardiac surgery.
Polymicrobial infection	Incidence ranges from 1 in 250 to 1 in 10. More than two organisms in some cases. Most mixtures of gram-positive cocci, or the latter with gram-negative rods or yeast.
Virus	Indirect evidence. One case of serologically proved coxsackievirus B endocarditis.
Legionella sp.	Usually involves prosthetic valves, both mechanical and bioprosthetic.

Gram-Positive Cocci

The viridans streptococcus encompasses all streptococcal species except groups A, B, and D. These organisms exhibit a wide variety of cultural and biochemical characteristics. In the past, they were classified as nonhemolytic or alpha-hemolytic, hence the term *green strep*. However, it is now clear that some strains may produce beta-hemolysis.[3] Present in their cell wall are peptidoglycans, teichoic acids, and lipipoteichoic acid. Unlike the pyogenic streptococci, there is no relation between the Lancefield serogroups and the biochemical reactions of these organisms. An isolate of one species may belong to several serogroups or to none. There is considerable confusion in the classification of these bacteria.[4] A detailed discussion of the serological and biochemical characteristics of these streptoccocci is beyond the scope of this text. Our purpose is to present the features that are relevant to clinical disease.

Many species of viridans streptoccocci have been identified as the etiological agents of infective endocarditis. These were responsible for

Table 4.2. Frequency of Etiological Organisms in 211 Episodes of Active Infective Endocarditis of Natural Valves

Organism	Frequency		(%)
Streptococci	106	(50)	
Viridans streptococci			56
S. bovis			24
Enterococci			15
Beta-hemolytic streptococci (groups A, B, C, G)			9
Pneumococci			2
Staphylococci	74	(35)	
S. aureus			64
Coagulase-negative staphylococci			10
Fastidious gram-negative coccobacilli*	10	(5)	
Gram-negative bacilli†	6	(3)	
Multiple bacteria‡	4	(2)	
Fungi§	3	(1)	
Negative cultures	8	(4)	

Actinobacillus actiomycetemcomitans, three cases; *Cardiobacterium hominis*, two; *Hemophilus influenzae*, *H. parainfluenzae*, *H. aphrophilus*, *Kingella kingae*, *Neisseria flavescens*, one each.

†*Escherichia coli*, *Proteus mirabilis*, *Pseudomonas aeruginosa*, *Achromobacter* species, *Campylobacter intestinalis*, *Bacteroides fragilis*, one each.

‡*S. aureus* and group F streptococococcus, one; *Mima polymorpha* and *Pseudomonas cepacia*, one; *P. aeruginosa* and *Peptostreptococcus micros*, one; *Streptococcus bovis*, *S. faecalis*, and *S. faecium*, one each.

§*Candida albicans*, *C. tropicalis*, *Torulopsis glabrata*, one each.

Source: Adapted from DiNubile MJ, Calderwood SB, Steinhaus DM, et al: Cardiac conduction abnormalities complicating native valve active infective endocarditis. *Am J Cardiol* 1986;58:1215.

more than 90% of subacute disease and 70% of all instances of valvular infection in the preantibiotic era.[2,5-9] Other serotypes of streptococci have replaced those described above as the major cause of infective endocarditis. There has been increasing recognition of the role of microaerophilic and anaerobic streptococci in the pathogenesis of endocardial infection. These organisms produce a subacute syndrome similar to that caused by the classical green strep.[2,10-12] Enterococci have recently become more important as causative agents of endocarditis (see below). In the 1950s and early 1960s, the involvement of *S. viridans* decreased to 50% of all cases and to 70–80% of subacute disease.[12-14] Currently, these organisms are responsible for less than 50% of valvular infections.[2,5,15-18]

Among the more common members of this group of organisms are *S. salivarius*, *S. sanguis* I, *S. sangiuis* II, *S. mitis*, *S. intermedius-MG-anginosus*, *S. milleri*, and *S. mutans*. Although most of these bacteria are sensitive to the penicillins, a species highly resistant to this class of antibiotics, *S. constellatus*, has been recovered from a patient with endocardial infection.[19]

Infective endocarditis caused by viridans streptococci is classically subacute. Occasionally, however, these organisms are highly invasive.[20] They are usually present in the microflora of the normal mouth, upper respiratory tract, and upper intestinal tract.[21] *S. mitior, S. sanguis, S. milleri, S. salivarius,* and *S. mutans* constitute 30–60% of the normal oral microflora. *S. mutans* and *S. sanguis* I are present most often on the surface of the teeth; *S. mitis* and *S. sanguis* II on dental surfaces and the oropharynx; and *S. salivarius* on the tongue, pharynx, and hard palate.

The production of extracellular dextran by viridans streptococci is associated with increased adherence of bacteria to dental enamel and valvular endothelium.[22] The microbial species that adhere most readily to dental enamel are responsible for the highest incidence of endocarditis.[23–25] *S. sanguis* I and II are involved in 16.4% and 72% respectively, of all instances of streptococcol endocarditis. *S. mutans* has been recovered from 8–10% of patients with endocardial disease and from 14.2% of all patients with streptococcal valvular disease. Synthesis of dextran is not the only mechanism involved in invasion of the valves by streptococci. Isolates of *S. mitor* fail to produce dextran and are involved in 13.2% of cases of infective endocarditis. About 7.3% of infection are caused by organisms that produce dextran.[26]

The antimicrobial prophylaxis of rheumatic fever has led to a change in the sensitivity patterns of the oral streptococci.[27] About 5% of strains of *S. viridans* recovered from blood cultures are relatively resistant to penicillin. Roberts and colleagues[25] have pointed out that the minimal inhibitory concentration (MIC) of penicillin is 0.1–0.2 μg/ml in 8% for *S. viridans* and more than 0.2 μg/ml in 9%. However, the prophylactic use of this antibiotic does not lead to an increased incidence of endocardial infection.[28] Oral prophylaxis appears to produce a higher incidence of resistant streptococci than does monthly administration of benzathine penicillin.[28] Twelve percent of *S. mitior,* 9% of *S. sanguis,* and 5% of other streptococcal species have an MIC above 0.1 mg/ml.[29] About 15% of *S. mutans* strains are tolerant to penicillin. The MIC is low but the (MBC) is higher by a factor of 10.[30,31]

Among the factors that predispose patients to invasion of the bloodstream and infection of the cardiac endothelium by viridans streptococci are (1) accidental or surgical dental trauma (particularly extractions); (2) periodontal disease; (3) periapical dental abscesses associated with devitalized teeth; and (4) occasionally, the use of Water-Pik. Despite the important role of dental disease in the pathogenesis of infective endocarditis, valvular infection caused by these organisms also occurs in edentulous patients.[32–36] This has raised some concern regarding the advisability of whole-mouth dental extractions in an attempt to prevent subacute endocardial infection.[37,38] However, periapical abscesses or significant periodontitis in patients receiving therapy for endocarditis should be treated with an appropriate dental procedure before antimicrobial therapy is completed.

The *S. intermedius* group (*S. milleri, S. anginosus,* and *S. MG*) differ from other strains of *S. viridans* in several respects. They are often microaerophilic and may produce small colonies on agar. These organisms were initially designated *minute hemolytic streptococci*.[39] Unlike other speices, isolates of *S. intermedius* tend to invade tissues and produce abscesses.[39] The factors that contribute to this process are unknown but may be related to the presence of a polysaccharide capsule.[40] Some strains of *S. intermedius* are less likely to attach to cardiac valves than are other serotypes of *S. viridans* and may produce myocardial abscesses.[41] This group of streptococci can lead to brain abscesses (75% of cases) and may be recovered from hepatic abscesses or empyema.

Nutritionally Variant Streptococci

Nutritionally variant streptococci (NVS) were first discovered in 1961.[42] These organisms have become increasingly important in the pathogenesis of infective endocarditis.[42–45] Although readily identified in Gram-stained smears of positive broth cultures, these organisms fail to grow when subcultured on solid media. They require the presence of cystine or pyridoxine for multiplication. The medium must contain thiol compounds, cysteine, or the active form of vitamin B_6 (pyridoxal or pyridoxamine) but not pyridoxine.[46] It appears that NVS are unable to take up pyridoxine from the media. Another method of demonstrating the presence of these organisms is *satellitism*, the ability of NVS to grow in an area adjacent to colonies of *S. aureus*. In all other respects, NVS are quite similar to *S. mitior*. *S. defectibus*, the major species recovered from NVS-associated endocarditis, binds specifically to the extracellular matrix of fibroblasts and endothelial cells. *S. mutans*, *S. mitis*, *S. sanguis*, and *S. faecalis* bind to the extracellular matrix. Other species of *S. viridans* are unable to do this.

NVS account for about 5% of streptococcal endocarditis.[47,48] These organisms require more than 0.1 μg/ml of penicillin for inhibition. This accounts, in part, for the higher fatality rate of infective endocarditis caused by these organisms compared with disease caused by *S. viridans* (17% vs. 5%). The incidence of relapse produced by NVS is also higher (8% vs. 1%). These organisms usually produce subacute disease on previously damaged valves. The incidence of embolization is high. Failure to eradicate the organism is a problem in 41% of patients despite the fact that in vitro the pathogen is sensitive to the administered antibiotic. Treatment with penicillin and an aminoglycoside produces a more favorable effect. The fatality rate is high even when the infected valve is excised. It has been suggested that the long generation time for NVS (2–3 hr compared to 50 min for *S. viridans*) underlies the relative ineffectiveness of antimicrobial therapy. Treatment of endocarditis caused by other slowly growing organisms (*Corynebacterium JK* and *Haemophilus aphrophilus*) may require longer periods of therapy. NVS are a common cause of culture-negative endocarditis. A major clue to their presence is the fact that although they multiply, they cannot be subcultured on agar without the addition of thiol compounds.

Group D Streptococci

Group D streptococci are presently responsible for fewer cases of infective endocarditis than are viridans strains. *S. faecalis* var. *zymogenes, S. faecalis* var. *liquefaciens, S. faecium,* and the nonenterococcal species, *S. bovis,* and *S. equinus.* Of these, *S. faecalis* is the most common. It has been estimated that group D streptococci cause 10–20% of cases of infective endocarditis.[5,10,11,49–51] These organisms were responsible for 2% of all instances of endocardial infection at the Massachusetts General Hospital between 1944 and 1958; 6% occurred between 1958 and 1964 and 8% between 1964 and 1973.[52] It is possible that the increasing incidence of endocardial infection caused by the enterococci reflects a decrease in the frequency of disease produced by viridans streptococci.

Although they may produce acute endocarditis, enterococci usually cause subacute disease.[53–55] Nonspecific symptoms may be present for as long as 6 months before the presence of endocardial infection is established. Forty percent of patients are free of underlying cardiac disease. Only a minority exhibit the typical peripheral manifestations of infective endocarditis. Endocardial infection is most common in young adult women and older men (the male:female ratio is 2:1). The primary portal of entry of the organism is the genitourinary tract.[56] Any gynecological or obstetrical procedure (e.g., insertion of an IUD) increases the risk of infection. Enterococci may cause prostatitis, as well as bacteremia and infection of the urinary tract. Other portals of entry of these organisms are the biliary tract and the oropharynx. Forty percent of enterococcal bacteremias have no identifiable source. The marked increase of enterococcal disease in the last decade was primarily nosocomial in origin.[57,58] This was related to many factors, among which were older and sicker patients and the widespread use of third-generation cephalosporins.[59] Up to 43% of enterococcal bacteremias are polymicrobial.[60] Enterococci account for about 5% of positive blood cultures. Intravenous drug use is an increasing risk factor for the development of infective endocarditis. Eight percent of addict-related valvular infections are caused by this group of organisms.[61] Unlike disease produced by *S. aureus,* enterococcal infection does not involve the tricuspid valves and does not lead to the development of septic pulmonary emboli.[56]

Physicians often find it difficult to distinguish uncomplicated enterococcal bacteremia from enterococcal endocarditis. Among the features that differentiate the latter from the former are (1) acquisition of the organism in the community; (2) no recognizable portal of entry; (3) the absence of polymicrobial bacteremia; and (4) preexisting valvular disease.

Because the antimicrobial therapy of enterococcal endocarditis differs markedly from that of other streptococcal infections, precise microbiological diagnosis is critical.[62,63] Not all group D organisms are enterococci. Some of the microbiological techniques used to identify group D strains may fail to distinguish these organisms from nonenterococcal species such as *S. bovis.* Enterococci may produce alpha, beta, or gamma hemolysis on blood agar. Many cases of infective endocarditis caused by these organisms are characterized by an acute fulminant course that may be associated with severe intra- and extracardiac complications. Appropriate antimicrobial therapy of disease produced by enterococci mandates the administration of a cell wall–active antibiotic, such as penicillin or vancomycin, with an aminoglycoside. The survival rate in enterococcal disease is lower than that caused by either alpha-hemolytic streptococci or *S. bovis*. The incidence of relapse is higher than that associated with disease caused by other streptococcal species.[53]

Streptococcus bovis

Precise microbiological studies indicate that an appreciable number of group D streptococci are *S. bovis*, not enterococci. This suggests that the apparent increase in the incidence of enterococcal endocarditis may be lower than has been reported. Of 29 cases of infective endocarditis in which group D streptococci were recovered, 15 were caused by *S. bovis*.[64] A study of 11 patients with group D enterococcal endocarditis at Mt. Sinai Hospital in New York in 1972 and early 1973 disclosed that eight infections were due to *S. bovis* and only three to enterococci.[65] Several reports describing the role of penicillin-susceptible streptococci in the pathogenesis of endocardial infection have indicated that nonenterococcal group D strains or *S. bovis* were identified most often. These accounted for 15 episodes of endocardial disease reported by Garvey and Neu,[66] 18 of 99 instances studied by Karchmer et al.,[67] and 21 of 91 cases that came to the attention of Wilson and his colleagues.[68]

Early studies failed to distinguish enterococci from *S. bovis*. More recent ones indicated that the feature differentiating these species is the failure of *S. bovis* to grow in *S. faecalis* broth (sodium azide, S.F. broth).[55] Because of variations in its manufacture some strains of *S. bovis* are able to multiply in this media. Several biochemical and physiological studies are carried out to permit accurate identification of these bacteria.[69–71] Both *S. bovis* and enterococci possess a group D antigen, multiply in 40% bile, and hydrolyze esculin. Five percent of *S. viridans* share these traits. Unlike enterococci, *S. bovis* fails to grow in media containing 5% sodium chloride and hydrolyzes starch but not arginine. Enterococci metabolize the latter but not the former. The ability to ferment lactose distinguishes *S. bovis* from *S. equinus*, a nonenterococcal group D organism that rarely causes human infection. *S. bovis* is susceptible to the semisynthetic penicillins (methicillin, oxacillin, cloxacillin), clindamycin, and lincomycin. Enterococci are resistant to all of these agents. Susceptibility to methicillin and clindamycin distinguishes *S. bovis* from enterococci. The ability of the enterococcus to hydrolyze L-pyrrolitonyl-beta/-naphthylamide (PYR reaction) is a reliable, rapid test that identifies this organism.[72] Because *S. pyogenes* also hydrolyzes this compound, it is necessary to perform a bacitracin susceptibility test simultaneously. *S. pyogenes*, but not the enterococcus, is sensitive to bacitracin.

S. faecalis adheres to valvular endothelium more avidly than any other gram-positive or gram-negative organism[73] and stimulates the production of fibronectin by the endothelial cell.[74] This leads to the development of more luxuriant, rapidly growing vegetations that protect the bacteria from the activity of antibiotics. Some investigators have suggested that endocarditis produced by *S. bovis* may be treated in the same manner as disease produced by penicillin-susceptible viridans streptococci. Moellering and his associates[64] noted that 12 of 13 patients with valvular infection caused by *S. bovis* who were treated appropriately (primarily with penicillin) survived. Only 8 of 15 individuals with endocardial disease caused by enterococci were cured when appropriate antimicrobial therapy was administered.

In a retrospective study of bacteremic *S. bovis,* Murray and Roberts[75] discovered gastrointestinal lesions or a history of recent manipulation of the intestinal tract in 22 of 36 patients; 9 of the 22 had a colonic neoplasm. Wilson and his colleagues[68] identified abnormalities in the large intestine of 13 of 21 persons with infective endocarditis caused by *S. bovis.* Fourteen individuals with definite or probable endocardial infection studied by Klein and colleagues[76] were found to have colonic neoplasms (adenocarcinoma); two had esophageal cancer. Aggressive evaluation of the gastrointestinal tract, especially the colon, in patients with bacteremia or endocarditis caused by *S. bovis* is mandatory.[76–82] Valvular infections caused by this organism may also originate from a primary focus in the genitourinary tract.

Although *S. bovis* is usually very susceptible to penicillin G, strains resistant to this agent have been isolated from individuals with infective endocarditis.[83,84] The MIC for this organism was 100-fold lower than the MBC. The significance of this is not clear. Some strains of *S. bovis* are resistant to the aminoglycosides.

Anaerobic Streptococci

Anaerobic streptococci (peptostreptococci) are occasionally involved in the pathogenesis of infective endocarditis. Three of 100 cases studied by Lerner and Weinstein,[1] and as many as 8.2% of patients reported by others, have had peptostreptococcal infection.[15–18] Peptostreptococci may produce alpha, beta, or gamma hemolysis. Although cardiac disease caused by this organism is usually subacute, the clinical course may, in some cases, be rapidly progressive. Massive doses of penicillin G (60–80 million units/day) administered intravenously may be required to cure some patients because of high-grade resistance of the organism.[85] Routine anaerobic cultures are not useful for the isolation of peptostreptococci. Although some strains may multiply aerobically in thioglycolate broth, culture under strict anaerobic conditions is more likely to yield growth of the organism.

Streptococcus pyogenes (Group A Beta-Hemolytic)

In sharp contrast to the experiences in the preantibiotic era, group A beta-hemolytic streptococci (GABHS)[86–90] are now a very uncommon cause of infective endocarditis. The decreased incidence of this disease may be related to the successful treatment of extracardiac infections such as pneumonia, erysipelas, cellulitis, and pharyngitis that predisposed patients to valvular invasion by this organism.[85–89] GABHS bacteremia now occurs primarily in individuals with chronic debilitating diseases such as cancer, renal failure, and alcoholism, as well as those undergoing treatment with corticosteroids. Diabetes mellitus has been present in one-third of patients with infective endocarditis caused by GABHS. Intravenous drug abuse has been recognized as a risk factor. GABHS are not members of the normal microflora. Endocarditis produced by *S. pyogenes* is, with rare exceptions, acute. In many ways it resembles the infection caused by *S. aureus*. Rupture of valvular leaflets, myocardial abscesses, and localized infections at sites of embolization are common. Although *S. pyogenes* is considered the prototype of the beta-hemolytic streptococcus, not all strains of this organism produce this type of hemolysis. In some instances, alpha rather than beta hemolysis is present. When grown on a pour plate, these strains induce the beta hemolysis. The isolation of an alpha-hemolytic streptococcus from the blood of a patient with acute infective endocarditis not only suggests the presence of a viridans streptococcal or enterococcal infection but also raises the possibility that an alpha-hemolytic strain of *S. pyogenes* is involved.[90] This mandates subculture in deep agar and serological grouping of the organism. It must be kept in mind that many species of streptococci other than group A may produce beta hemolysis.

The bacitracin test has been used to speciate beta-hemolytic streptococci. The presence or absence of an appropriate zone of inhibition of microbial growth around a paper disc that contains 0.02 to 0.04 unit of bacitracin is diagnostic. All beta-hemolytic streptococci, the growth of which is inhibited by bacitracin, are members of group A. This test indentifies 94.6–99% of Lancefield group A streptococci. However, a number of other groups (B, C, and G) may also be sensitive to this concentration of bacitracin.[91–95] Thus, precise identification of beta-hemolytic streptococci is best determined by the Lancefield method.

Other Streptococci

Although much less often involved in the pathogenesis of infective endocarditis than the organisms described above, other streptococcal species occasionally produce this disease. One of these is the group B streptococcus *S. agalactiae*.[96–100] This organism infects the mitral valves most often and the aortic valve less frequently. Antecedent cardiac disease is present in more than 50% of patients. Infection of prosthetic valves by group B streptococci has been reported.[101] *S. agalactiae* produced rapidly progressive endocarditis almost exclusively in pregnant women in the preantibiotic era. Currently, the clinical course of this disease may be either acute or subacute. Group B streptococci produce valvular disease primarily in patients with a median age of 50 years. Group B streptococcal endocarditis in young patients has recently been reported.[99] Patients with diabetes mellitus or alcoholism, as well as pregnant women, are at high risk of developing endocardial infection caused by group B streptococci. Major systemic emboli have been noted in 40% of patients. Evidence of arterial thrombi alerts the clinician to the possibility of endocarditis caused by *S. agalactiae*. This organism may be responsible for a fulminant infection that requires valvular replacement. Precise microbiological identification of group B streptococci is mandatory because, with the exception of the enterococcus, this organism is less susceptible to penicillin G than are any of the other streptococci. The overall fatality rate of this disease is 43.5%.

Group C streptococci (*S. equi*, *S. zooepidemicus*, and *S. dysagalactiae*) have often caused infection in animals. However these organisms have also been recovered from the skin, nose, throat, and vagina of healthy persons[102] and have been implicated in puerperal sepsis, wound infections, cellulitis, tonsillitis, glomerulonephritis, pulmonary disease, infections of the urinary tract, and bacteremia. Group C streptococci rarely cause infective endocarditis.[103,104] They may be less susceptible to penicillin G than are many other types of streptococci. A strain tolerant to penicillin (MBC 128-fold higher than the MIC) has been the cause of at least one instance of infective endocarditis.[105] Disease caused by group C streptococci is acute and most often involves normal aortic and mitral valves.

Group C streptococcal bacteremia and infective endocarditis are rare. In a 10-year survey of 150,000 cultures of blood collected at the Mayo Clinic, Mohr et al.[106] identified a bacteremia in only eight patients. One individual had infective endocarditis. A review of the characteristics of patients with group C streptococcal endocarditis[102] indicated that 5 of 17 had frequent contacts with animals. Among them were two farmers, a cattle truck driver, a butcher, and the owner of a factory that processed animal hides. Probable initiating events in those patients were septic abortion, infection of the skin and soft tissues, gastroenteritis, and addiction to heroin. Group C streptococci were not recovered from any of the areas where these patients worked. One patient had infective endocarditis that involved a prosthetic valve. Nine individuals were free of underlying valvular disease. Forty-eight percent of the patients died. This exceeded the fatality rate of enterococcal endocarditis. Eighty percent of individuals treated with 10–20 million units of penicillin survived; three required valvular replacement. Some patients were treated concurrently with an aminoglycoside for 4 to 6 weeks.

The predisposing factors responsible for infection caused by *S. mutans* have been urethral dilatation, surgical procedures involving the gallbladder or vocal cords, and dental manipulation.[107] This organism may be confused with enterococci.[26,108–111] It grows on S.F. agar and enterococcal broth and multiplies in the presence of 40% bile. It hydrolyzes esculin and is susceptible to penicillin. The treatment and prognosis of endocarditis caused by this organism are similar to those of disease produced by other strains of viridans streptococci. *S. mutans* can be differentiated from the latter by its inability to grow in 6.5% sodium chloride broth. It is sensitive to lincomycin and, unlike *S. bovis,* does not contain a group D antigen but hydrolyzes starch.

Group F streptococci are an uncommon cause of endocarditis. Two percent of beta-hemolytic streptococci were recovered from blood cultures at the Mayo Clinic between 1970 and 1980.[112] These organisms are members of the normal microflora of the oropharynx, gastrointestinal tract, and perineum. Most bacteremias with group F organisms are associated with underlying pathology of the gastrointestinal tract. Polymicrobial bacteremia is common, probably due to the fact that the intestinal tract is the primary portal of entry of group F streptococci. Thirty-nine percent of individuals with bacteremia have had infections caused by a different organism.[112] Suppurative disease is a hallmark of invasion by group F organisms and leads to the development of lesions in the chest, abdomen, and skin. Group F streptococci is capable of causing fulminant infective endocarditis.[113]

Group G streptococci have been recovered from the human pharynx, sinuses, abscesses, vagina, skin, and feces. Infective endocarditis is occasionally caused by these organisms.[114–118] Most, but not all, patients have underlying cardiac disease. This bacterium is highly sensitive to penicillin G. A positive hippurate test may lead to confusion with group B streptococci. In this situation, serological studies are required to differentiate the two organisms. The clinical course of valvular infection caused by group G streptococci may be more aggressive than that produced by uncomplicated group G bacteremia. Endocarditis occurs typically in elderly patients with multiple risk factors including diabetes mellitus, underlying valvular disease, alcoholism, and squamous cell carcinoma of the tonsils. Individuals with uncomplicated group G bacteremia are young (median age, 37.8 years) and have fewer risk factors.

A fatal case of endocarditis caused by group G streptococcus has been reported by Bouza et al.[114] This experience, together with the observation that 7 of 11 individuals with infective endocarditis caused by group G streptococcus died, has led to the conclusion that this is a more aggressive infection. However, careful analysis of the data indicates that five of those who died were not treated with optimal doses of antibiotic.[115–118]

Group L streptococci have caused infective endocarditis.[119] Infection of cardiac valves caused by group I streptococci, as well as by nongroupable strains, has been reported by Dismukes et al.[120]

Aerococcus viridans causes infective endocarditis. This organism differs from other streptococci because it is weekly catalase positive and produces tetrads rather than chains in broth.[121] It also tolerates exposure to 40% bile or salt. Unlike the enterococci, this organism does not contain group D streptococcal antigen and is susceptible to many antibiotics. The clinical course of the disease caused by this organism is similar to that produced by *S. viridans.*

Stomatococcus mucilaginosus is a member of the normal oral flora. It has caused endocarditis, usually in association with catheterization of the heart or prior cardiac surgery.[122] The lack of catalase activity differentiates this organism from coagulase-negative staphylococci and micrococci.[121]

Gemella haemolysans, a member of the family Streptococcacea, produces infective endocarditis. This organism resembles diphtheroids because it is pleomorphic and exhibits a variable reaction to the Gram stain. It is sensitive to penicillin G.[123]

Staphylococcus aureus

Staphylococci are responsible for about 20% of all instances of infective endocarditis; 50% are acute.[5,14,124–127] Although *S. aureus* is the leading cause of acute disease, it may produce a subacute infection as well. The incidence of endocardial infection caused by this organism has increased in frequency over the past 30 years. Finland and Barnes[128] noted that prior to 1941, *S. aureus* was only occasionally responsible for infective endocarditis. It has been suggested that the widespread use of penicillin has played a role in increasing the incidence of staphylococcal bacteremia and endocarditis and has also been responsible for the increase in the resistance of the organism to penicillin. The frequency of infection caused by staphylococci increased from 6% in 1932–1943 to 16% in 1944–1966.[129] The incidence of acute valvulitis produced by this organism appears to have reached a plateau and has declined only slightly. It has been suggested that "these cases of bacterial endocarditis are part of what is to be called a Staph pandemic which was presumably reflected in large hospitals and all the highly developed countries."[127] An increase in the incidence of this disease has been associated with the intravenous use of narcotics and other illicit drugs, as well as with cardiac surgery.

S. aureus possesses several properties that permit it to produce acute infective endocarditis. Teichoic acid, a phosphate-containing polymer, is a major component of the bacterial cell wall and facilitates binding of the organism to the nasal mucosa.[130] This process is augmented by estrogen use, viral infection, and the use of intravenous drugs. Employing the nares as "a base of operations," the organism sets up a "beachhead" on the skin. At any given time, about 20–30% of patients carry *S. aureus* on the skin. Invasion of the bloodstream by this organism is related to its ability to break through the barriers of the mucous membranes and skin.[131]

A tear in the skin produced by trauma or placement of an intravascular catheter may be the point of entry of organisms into the microcirculation. Prostatic infection or pneumonia caused by *S. aureus* permits an organism to enter the small venules, primarily via the lymphatics, when the normal defenses are impaired.[132–134] When it reaches the microcirculation, *S. aureus* produces infection of the endothelium (endotheliosis). Fibronectin, a glycoprotein produced by the endothelial cells, anchors *S. aureus* to the lining of the venules and initiates its aggregation. Clumps of bacteria are then ingested by the endothelial cells by a mechanism similar to pinocytosis.

Bacteremia develops when the concentration of organisms released into the circulation exceeds the capacity of the phagocytes to ingest them.

Several components of *S. aureus* are involved in the ingestion and killing of the organism by monocytes and polymorphonuclear leukocytes.[135] Protein A, present in the outer peptidoglycan layer, binds to the Fc terminal of IgG and produces immune complexes that destroy complement. It may also attach to the Fc portion of specific antistaphylococcal antibodies already attached to the organism and prevent the linkage of this complex to the Fc receptor on the surface of the phagocyte. This protein may bind and inactivate nonspecific antibodies.

Catalase produced by *S. aureus* destroys the hydrogen peroxide generated by the organism within phagocytic cells. Unless destroyed, it becomes rapidly bactericidal. This organism produces alpha, beta and gamma toxins.[136] The clinical importance of these toxins has not been defined. However, it is clear that they injure the membranes of many types of cells, including platelets and red and white blood cells. Another toxin, leukocidin, produces significant granulocytopenia by severely injuring the membranes of white blood cells.[136]

Fifty percent of strains of *S. aureus* have a poorly defined capsule. When this structure is present, antibodies specific for it are required for effective phagocytosis.[137] Most pathogenic strains of the organism elaborate a clumping factor that produces aggregation and binding of the organism to the membrane of endothelial cells. This facilitates uptake by these cells.[138]

The resistance of *S. aureus* to a variety of antimicrobial agents is an essential part of its pathogenicity. About 80% of strains of this organism recovered from patients produce penicillinase. The resistance of the organism to various penicillins and cephalosporins may be due to altered binding proteins (methicillin resistant *S. aureus*—MRSA).[139] *S. aureus* may be tolerant.[140] Tolerance defines an organism that requires a much higher concentration of an antibiotic to destroy it rather than merely suppress its growth. Thus, while the MIC and MBC of a penicillin or a cephalosporin for a nontolerant organism are either the same or similar, in tolerant strains they may differ by as much as 128 times higher than the MIC. Some strains of *S. aureus* are tolerant to penicillinase-resistant penicillins, cephalosporins, and vancomycin. Most important is the determination of the MBC of the antibiotic initially selected on the basis of its MIC. Combined antimicrobial therapy may be required to eradicate staphylococci in patients with tolerant strains of the organism.[141]

Endocarditis caused by *S. aureus* is often secondary to a bacteremia originating in an extracardiac focus. Among these bacteremias are infections of the skin or subcutaneous tissues, abscesses in various organs, osteomyelitis, and puerperal sepsis, as well as infection due to the use of contaminated intravascular catheters. Although the pathogenic mechanism is unknown, acute staphylococcal valvular disease may develop early in the course of acute rheumatic carditis.

Infective endocarditis caused by *S. aureus* may present diagnostic problems because it often develops in patients with no preexisting valvular disease or with murmurs that are not detectable early in the course of disease in about one-third of patients. The clinical distinction between uncomplicated staphylococcal bacteremia and endocarditis may be difficult. It has been suggested that when *S. aureus* is recovered from the blood of a patient with an extracardiac infection, the incidence of endocarditis is relatively high.[142] Conversely, it has been suggested, but not proved, that when a removable focus of staphylococcal infection is the source of bacteremia, the incidence of valvular infection is low.[143]

It has been reported that infection of human valvular endothelium leads to the production of tissue factors of the extrinsic clotting system.[144] This explains the development of endocarditis involving normal heart valves. From 30% to 40% of individuals with this disease have normal valves. *S. aureus* may initiate the production of procoagulating factors by endothelial cells that provide platelet-fibrin in which a nidus of bacteria may multiply in an environment protected from host defenses. *S. aureus* produces vegetations by interfering with the activity of thrombomodulin and the normal fibrinolysins.[138]

Forty percent of intravascular catheters are infected. Although *S. aureus* was once thought to be the primary infecting agent, later studies indicated that *S. epidermidis* is most often involved.[145] The initial event in infection of these lines is bacterial invasion of the dermal tunnel through which the catheter is passed. From 24 to 48 hr later, a sheath of fibrin forms in and around the lumen. Infection of the sleeves of fibrin is overwhelmed by bacteria that arrive via the cutaneous tunnel. Less often, bacteria are deposited in the course of a bacteremia that originates at a distant site. Various factors that act as adhesives facilitate bacterial aggregation in the fibrin-catheter system. Among these are fibronectin, laminin, fibrinogen, and collagen;[145,146] of these, fibronectin is the most important.

Infection of an intravascular device by *S. aureus* requires a specific concentration of the organism within the skin tunnel. Local infection is often apparent before the vascular portion of the catheter is involved. This in not the case when *S. epidermidis* is involved. The site of insertion may appear uninvolved when the distal portion of the catheter is infected with this organism.

Once the barriers of the skin and mucosa have been breached, polymorphonuclear leukocytes become the most important defense against infection by *S. aureus*. Patients whose white blood cells are low in number and quality of function are very susceptible to the development of all types of staphylococcal disease.[143] Individuals with abnormalities of chemotaxis (Job's syndrome) often suffer from bacteremia or infective endocarditis caused by *S. aureus*. Ineffective chemotaxis may be associated with an increase in the incidence of staphylococcal infection in patients with HIV.[144]

Opsonization of *S. aureus* depends on the presence of specific IgA antibodies and the activated subunit of $C3_B$. Complement appears to be most important. Patients with agammaglobulinemia do not have an increased incidence of staphylococcal infections. However, this is not the case in those with a deficiency of complement.[143] Individuals with impaired intracelluar killing (e.g., chronic granulomatous disease) develop severe infections caused by catalase-producing organisms such as *S. aureus*. Five percent of coagulase-positive *S. aureus* remain viable for 30–40 min. in normally functioning leukocytes. *S. epidermidis* is killed completely shortly after being phagocytized. The relatively long survival of *S. aureus* in leukocytes appears to be very important in the pathogenesis of sustained bacteremia and the eventual development of infective endocarditis. This organism may employ white blood cells to spread throughout the body. The concentration of *S. aureus* is reduced more than 1,000-fold within 20 min after it is injected into the vein of an animal. This reduction is related to the activity of circulating phagocytes. Bacteremia may persist because a small fraction of *S. aureus* resists intracellular killing and is eventually released back into the intravascular space. The more organisms entering the bloodstream, the higher the possibility that bacteremia may develop.[146]

Defects in cellular immunity do not appear to play an important role in the development of infections caused by *S. aureus*. Patients with immunological abnormalities do not appear to experience an unusually high incidence of significant staphylococcal disease.[147]

In a review of their experience with staphylococcal bateremia in 55 patients, Wilson and Hamburger[148] noted that 44% had preexisting valvular or congenital cardiac disease, 64% developed infective endocarditis, and 71% died. On the basis of this experience, they suggested that antimicrobial therapy be continued for at least 6 weeks in patients with staphylococcal bacteremia because of the high incidence of unexpected valvular infection and death in untreated patients. A similar experience was reported by Skinner and Keefer[149] prior to the availability of effective antimicrobial agents.

The results of a retrospective study of 28 patients with staphylococcal bacteremia arising from removable foci have been reported by Iannini and Crossley. [143] The patients showed no evidence of underlying cardiac disease or endocarditis when antimicrobial therapy was instituted. An infected intravenous device was removed from 22 patients before treatment was initiated. Although therapy was continued for only 15 days, all patients made an uneventful recovery and developed no problems during the period of follow-up. Nolan and Beaty[142] classified individuals from whose blood *S. aureus* was recovered into two groups: (1) those with primary extracardiac staphylococcal infections and bacteremia (often nosocomial in origin), with no underlying valvular disease or evidence of metastatic infection but often with other medical problems, and (2) those with staphylococcal bacteremia (often community acquired) without a primary infected focus who showed evidence of metastatic infection or cardiac abnormalities. Fifty-five percent of the patients in the first group were considered to have uncomplicated bacteremia and were treated with an antibiotic for a short time; only two patients developed valvular or metastatic infections. However, 24 of the 42 patients in the second group developed endocarditis; metastatic infections occurred in 39.

Watanakunakorn and Baird[150] reported that 38% of patients with staphylococcal bacteremia associated with an infected intravenous device developed endocarditis.[149]

Ehni and Reller[151] have reported a 5–10% incidence of relapse in patients with catheter-associated bacteremia caused by *S. aureus* following a short course (less than 17 days) of antimicrobial therapy. Most of the relapses were secondary to the development of endocarditis.

Although available data are controversial, it is clear that inappropriately treated staphylococcal bacteremia is an important risk factor in the development of endocarditis. This appears to be less common in a nosocomial or transient bacteremia originating in a primary extracardiac focus of infection.[142–148] Failure to initiate appropriate antimicrobial therapy, and to continue it for an adequate period because a murmur is present in the early stage of acute disease, leads to the development of several potentially lethal complications of infective endocarditis.

The precise incidence of infective endocarditis associated with staphylococcal bacteremia cannot be determined with certainty. It is probably in the range of 30–40% because of the very high incidence of valvular infection caused by *S. aureus*. We have treated patients with an effective antimicrobial agent for 4 weeks.

In an attempt to define the risk of infective endocarditis and serious metastatic infections in patients with staphylococcal bacteremia, attention has focused on studies of the role of immunological phenomena. The presence of antibodies active against ribitol teichoic acid, a component of the cell wall of the staphylococcus, has been examined using counterimmunoelectrophoresis,[151,152] passive double agar-gel diffusion, and solid-phase radioimmunoassay for specific antistaphylococcal immunoglobulins.[153,154] The presence of high titers of antibody to teichoic acid or staphylococcal sonicates after about 2 weeks of treatment correlated closely with clinical evidence of infective endocarditis and/or deep-seated metastatic infection.[155–157] The potential value of these studies is illustrated by an individual reported by Bernhardt and colleagues.[158] The patient developed bacteremia with *S. aureus* following insertion of an infected intravenous catheter. After 2 weeks of therapy with parenteral amoxicillin, the patient defervesced. There was no clinical evidence of endocarditis or metastatic infection. All blood cultures were sterile during treatment. Antibodies for teichoic acid, determined by agar-gel diffusion, were initially absent but became detectable in serum in the second week of treatment. Three weeks after discharge from the hospital, the patient was readmitted with vertebral osteomyelitis complicated by a spinal epidural abscess. *S. aureus* (same phage type as the one present in the blood initially) was recovered from both sites.

Knowledge of the sensitivity of the various techniques used to prepare the antigens has permitted investigators to establish criteria for the determination of specific antibodies. Presently, however, the methodology of the test and the specificity of the antigens have not been adequately standardized and cannot be used in clinical studies. Measurement of antibodies to teichoic acid is sensitive (93%) for the detection of endocardial disease in patients with staphylococcal bacteremia. The predictive value of these studies is about 85%. In about 50% of persons with uncomplicated valvulitis, there is a significant increase in the titer of antibody. Presently, we do not recommend the use of serological studies to make important clinical decisions regarding the significance of bacteremia caused by *S. aureus*. Increased experience with these methods may provide a more precise approach to identifying patients with staphylococcal endocarditis, severe extracardiac infections, or bacteremia.

All individuals from who *S. aureus* has been recovered in at least four sets of blood cultures must be investigated for the possibility of infective endocarditis. Antimicrobial agents must then be studied for their effect on the circulating organism. The single antibiotic or combination of antibiotics is chosen on the basis of in vitro sensitivity tests, pharmacokinetics, and other considerations (see Chapter 13).

The experience of Bernhardt and his colleagues,[158] as well as our studies, emphasize the danger of inadequate initial antimicrobial therapy. A young man was admitted to the hospital with fever. Six cultures of his blood grew coagulase-positive staphylococci. Because the portal of entry of the organisms could not be identified, he was treated with an adequate dose of an effective antimicrobial agent for 2 weeks and discharged from the hospital. No cardiac murmurs were detected during his hospitalization. About 4 weeks later, he was readmitted with high fever and intractable congestive cardiac failure. Cardiac examination disclosed free aortic regurgitation. Multiple cultures of his blood grew coagulase-positive staphylococci. His response to antimicrobial therapy was prompt and effective. The congestive failure did not respond to medical management. The patient made a satisfactory recovery after the damaged aortic valve was replaced by a prosthesis. This experience emphasizes the risk of developing acute, destructive infective endocarditis when bacteremia is present but there is no evidence of valvular disease. An approach to the differentiation of uncomplicated staphylococcal bacteremia from endocarditis has been suggested by Thompson[127] (Table 4.3).

Coagulase-Negative *S. aureus* (CONS)

Over the last quarter of a century, CONS has been involved in a variety of infections.[159–164] A major factor contributing to the increase in disease produced by this organism has been its capacity to infect all types of prosthetic devices. This organism belongs in the family Micrococceae and includes 21 species. It is sensitive to novobiocin, produces acid from carbohydrates, and is susceptible to lysostaphin or lysozyme. The most common organisms in this group are *S. epidermidis* and *S. saprophyticus*. These are involved in human disease most often. All species colonize the skin and mucous membranes.[165] There are 11 human commensals, each of which has a unique ability to infect "hardware of all sorts" that has been implanted in humans.

Table 4.3. Factors That Distinguish *S. aureus* Endocarditis from Bacteremia

A. Diagnostic of endocarditis
  1. New pathological or changing heart murmur
  2. Major embolic event (s)
  3. New splenomegaly*
  4. Peripheral microembolic signs*

B. Characteristic of endocarditis
  1. Intravenous drug use (addicts)
  2. Prosthetic valve (late-onset infection only)
  3. Meningitis (de novo)
  4. Severe renal failure, micro-hematuria (especially casts)
  5. Cardiac conduction defects, pericarditis, congestive heart failure
  6. Teichoic acid antibodies (substantial titer)

C. Suggestive of endocarditis
  1. Rheumatic valvular heart disease
  2. community-acquired bacteremia, delayed treatment, no primary site of infection

D. Bacteremia or endocarditis
  1. Disorders of mentation
  2. Metastatic abscesses
  3. Shock
  4. Delayed response to treatment, persistent fever, blood cultures positive on treatment

E. Suggestive of bacteremia only
  1. Hospital-acquired bacteremia
  2. Promptly treated bacteremia related to wounds or use of intravenous devices

*Usually absent, however.
Adapted from Ref. 127.

A number of epidemiological techniques have been developed to track nosocomial infections caused by *S. epidermidis* and to determine whether a new infection is a relapse of a reinfection. Several approaches have been developed to ascertain this.[166,167] Most useful have been phage typing and various molecular techniques, including DNA hybridization and profiling the DNA of the plasmids of an organism. Phage typing has the disadvantage of limited clinical availability, as well as a lack of standardization. Study of the profiles of plasmids is complicated by spontaneous loss of the genetic material present in many organisms. This alters the value of clinical typing more significantly. In addition, various laboratory procedures may lead to the conversion of plasmids during extraction.

The pathogenicity of these organisms was first identified in the 1960s when they were found to infect a number of medical devices, including neonatal umbilical catheters and atrioventricular shunts. *S. epidermidis* has a striking ability to adhere to and proliferate on the surfaces of foreign bodies. This is dependent on nonspecific factors such as electrostatic and hydrophobic forces, as well as on specific extracelluar slime-like substances produced by the organism. The presence of the glycocalyx correlates positively with the ability of *S. epidermidis* to infect prosthetic devices[165] and to protect pathogens from host defenses by interfering with phagocytosis, but it does not impede access to the organism's nutritional support.[165] This extracellular product blocks the synthesis of immunoglobulins.[168,169] The most important factor in the development of infection is breaking of the mucocutaneous barrier. This usually occurs when a medical device in implanted.[170] Exposure to multiple antimicrobial agents puts patients at high risk of developing significant infections with *S. aureus.*

The most common immunological defect that predisposes patients to the development of bacteremia is impairment of effective phagocytosis. Although *S. epidermidis* may produce infective endocarditis in individuals with an underlying cardiac defect, episodes of the disease may be associated with the intravenous use of drugs or the presence of a prosthetic valve.[164] When a normal valve is involved, infection is most often superimposed on the damage produced by rheumatic cardiac disease. Currently, CONS accounts for 5% of all native endocardial diseases in adults and as many as 22% in children.[171] Endocarditis caused by CONS is similar to but longer in duration than that produced by viridans streptococci. One report indicates that CONS may infect normal valves and lead to congestive heart failure.[172] In two patients studied by one of us (L.W.) before prosthetic valves were available, several relapses developed following the discontinuation of antimicrobial therapy. Each relapse was marked by the reappearance of the organisms in the blood isolated initially. Both patients died with intractable cardiac failure; the disease persisted for 9 months in one.

Infective endocarditis caused by CONS is usually acute and is complicated by systemic embolization, abnormal cardiac conduction, and severe congestive heart failure.[172] In the 1980s, most reported cases of endocardial disease caused by CONS involved prosthetic valves.[173,174] The skin appears to be the source of organisms in many patients. Prompt treatment of cutaneous infections in individuals with prosthetic valves prevents this type of endocardial disease. Contamination during cardiopulmonary bypass surgery in CONS has been documented the source of infection of a prosthetic valve.[173]

Despite the very low invasive capacity of CONS, the fatality rate of prosthetic valve endocarditis caused by these organisms is high (29%).[175] This may be related to the complicated nature of the infective process bacause the base of a mechanical valve, rather than its leaflets, is most often involved.[175] The relatively poor therapeutic results are related to the low sensitivity of this organism to a variety of antimicrobial agents. Methicillin-resistant strains are often recovered from prosthetic valves infected less than 12 months after surgery.[176,177]

Most strains of CONS are resistant to all of the common beta-lactam antibiotics. Despite in vitro studies indicating the sensitivity of these organisms to the cephalosporins, such agents are usually ineffective clinically. The results of sensitivity testing are often erroneous because these organisms exhibit heteroresistance. Infection acquired 1 year or more after surgery is often caused by strains of CONS sensitive to most of the penicillins and cephalosporins.[176] In addition, testing the sensitivity of these organisms is difficult because species of CONS exhibit fluctuating responsiveness to various antibiotics due to the unstable nature of the resistance factors they carry. Vancomycin appears to be the drug of choice for management of methicillin-resistant strains of CONS.[178] The quinolones and teicoplanin may be effective against multiresistant strains of CONS.[176,179]

A combination of rifampin, gentamicin, and vancomycin has been found to produce increased activity against CONS.[180] *S. haemolyticus* is the first member of this group of organisms to become resistant to vancomycin[181]. These bacteria are resistant to erythromycin, clindamycin, the tetracyclines, and chloramphenicol.[182,183] Appreciating these limitations of antibiotic therapy has led to the recommendation that all cardiac valves infected by CONS be removed and replaced with an appropriate prosthesis early in the course of the disease.[184]

Micrococci

Micrococci are occasionally involved in the pathogenesis of infective endocarditis. A few cases in which *Micrococcus tetragenus* produced disease have been reported.[185] *M. sedentarius* and *M. mucilaginosus incertae sedia* have also caused infection.[186,187] Most cases have been subacute.

Streptococcus pneumoniae

In 1931, Thayer reported that 15% of all cases of infective endocarditis were caused by the pneumococcus.[188] This decreased to 5–6% after the introduction of penicillin.[6,7,11,18] This decline has been related to the striking decrease in the extrapulmonary complications of pneumococcal pneumonia. Early diagnosis and the early institution of effective antimicrobial therapy lead to a high rate of cure. Endocarditis may develop more frequently in individuals with multilobar infection of the lungs, especially when bacteremia is present and treatment is delayed. This is especially true of type 12 *S. pneumoniae*. Although this strain has been responsible for only 3% of pulmonary infections caused by the pneumococcus, it has been involved in 20% of cases of pneumococcal endocarditis.[189–191]

Valvular infection produced by *S. pneumoniae* resembles disease caused by *S. aureus*. An acute course and intra- and extracardiac complications are common.[189,192,193] In an unpublished study of a large number of patients admitted to a hospital in the preantibiotic era, one of us (L.W.) noted that about one-third of those with pneumococcal pneumonia in whom the clinical course was complicated by the development of pyogenic meningitis had infective endocarditis. A review of pneumococcal endocardial disease in infants has emphasized the difference between the features of the infection in this age group and adults.[194] In infants tachycardia and tachypnea disproportionate to the degree of fever were present. No other focus of pneumococci was identified in 40% of babies. By contrast, another area of infection was always present in adults. Meningitis was infrequent in infants. The mitral valve was involved most often in children; the aortic valve was infected most often in adults.

Gram-Positive Bacilli

Many gram-positive bacilli are insensitive to a number of antibiotics. Only a few cases of infective endocarditis have been caused by facultative anaerobic bacilli. Among the species involved are *Erysipelothrix rhusiopathiae, Listeria monocytogenes,* lactobacilli, aerobic "diphtheroids," *Rothia dentocariosa,* and *Bacillus* species.

Erysipelothrix rhusiopathiae

E. rhusiopathiae, a facultative, anaerobic,[195,196] gram-positive rod, is very important in veterinary medicine. Reservoirs of this bacterium are present in fish, shrimp, birds, soil, rats, domestic and wild decaying animals, and vegetables.[197,198] Among the individuals most likely to be exposed to this organism are veterinarians, fish handlers, butchers, tanners, grocers, and medical students. About one-third of patients are alcoholics. Men are infected more often than women. The portals of entry of the organism are wounds of the hands, buccal cavity, and respiratory tract. In some instances, the initial lesion is a slowly progressive ulcer on the palmar or dorsal surface of the hand and one or more fingers. Infective endocarditis may develop when bacteremia occurs in patients with a localized extravascular site of infection. Endocarditis caused by *E. rhusiopathiae* is usually subacute. The aortic valve is involved most often. Endocardial infection caused by this organism appears to be increasing in frequency. This is underscored by the fact that only 26 cases of infective endocarditis caused by this organism were reported up to 1976. Fifty percent of the patients had normal hearts prior to the onset of the disease. One study[198] pointed out the *E. rhusiopathiae* is involved in the infection of previously damaged native cardiac valves but not prosthetic ones. *E. rhusiopathiae* is resistant to vancomycin. However, like other members of this group of organisms, it is sensitive to penicillin. The rapid identification of *E. rhusiopathiae* and its differentiation from other gram-positive bacteria is very important therapeutically. Mitral and aortic valves are infected most often. In some instances the disease destroys an infected valve, necessitating its replacement by a prosthesis. The fatality rate of endocarditis caused by this organism is about 50%. Thirty-six percent of patients have a characteristic skin lesion, erysipeloid, at the point of entry of the organism into the bloodstream.

Listeria monocytogenes

Although distributed widely in nature, especially among domestic animals and fowl, *L. monocytogenes* is an uncommon cause of human disease. Infection by this organism in adults usually presents as bacteremia or meningoencephalitis. About 50% of patients are immunosuppressed or alcoholics.

L. monocytogenes is a gram-positive bacillus. Because it may appear as a coccobacillus, it has been confused with diphtheroids, streptococci, or *H. influenzae.*[199] Isolation of contaminants from sterile blood or spinal fluid alerts clinicians to the possibility of disease caused by *Listeria.* The most important requirement for identification of the organism is a laboratory staff that considers *L. monocytogenes* a potential cause of disease when a gram-positive bacillus that may be beta-hemolytic is recovered from blood or spinal fluid. "Cold enrichment" permits selective growth of the organism

Listeria produces no toxins. It multiplies in macrophages.[200] The most important defense against this organism is the mononuclear phagocyte.[201] The presence of specific immunoglobulins is required for ingestion of the bacillus by scavenger cells.[202] although transmission from animals to humans occurs, there is no evidence that this takes place in the United States. The infection usually involves city dwellers. Infected dairy products such as milk and cheese are the most common sources of the organism in this country.[203] *Listeria* endocarditis tends to occur in pregnant women and in individuals more than 55 years of age.[204]

L. monocytogenes rarely causes infective endocarditis. The first case was reported in 1978 by Hoeprich and Chernoff.[205] The incidence of endocarditis caused by *Listeria* is increasing. This may be due to an increase in the number of immunodeficient individuals and improved diagnostic methods. However, infective endocarditis due to this organism occurs unusually in immunosuppressed patients.[206–208] The source of *Listeria* is frequently unknown.

Valvalar infection caused by *Listeria* often follow a subacute course. Its clinical presentation resembles that of other organisms, except for a very high incidence of systemic embolization. Although the organism was once thought to infect only the left side of the heart, more recent evidence indicates that this is not the case.[209] Death occurs in 40–50% of patients, and this rate has not changed over the last 10 years. This may be due to a delay in establishing the diagnosis. Many isolates of *L. monocytogenes* are tolerant or relatively resistant to penicillin or ampicillin.[210]

Lactobacillus

Lactobacilli are members of the microflora of the human mouth, intestine, and vagina. Eleven cases of subacute infective endocarditis caused by these organisms have been reported.[211–214] Three species, *Lactobacillus casei*, *L. acidophilus*, and *L. plantarum*, have been involved. Dental procedures are the major predisposing factor in healthy individuals. Eighty-three percent of patients have underlying valvular pathology that is not clinically evident prior to the development of infection. The mitral valve is involved more often that the aortic valve. Rheumatic valvular disease is present in about 80% of patients. Infective endocarditis may develop in the course of acute rheumatic carditis. Systemic embolization occurs in 55% of patients. There is a high incidence of relapse after treatment with as much as 24 million units of penicillin per day. This appears to be due to the large discrepancy between the MIC and the MBC (tolerance) of the organism for penicillin. Limited experience indicates that the use of this antibiotic, (more than 25 million units/day) with gentamicin has achieved optimal results.

Corynebacteria (Diphtheroids)

An increasing number of cases of infective endocarditis caused by aerobic and anaerobic diphtheroids (*Proprionibacterium acnes*) have been reported.[215–219] The term *diphtheroids* includes a heterogeneous group of nondiphtheritic corynebacteria. Among the most common species that cause infective endocarditis are *C. hofmanii*,[220, 223] *C. bovis*,[221] *C. xerosis*,[222] *C. minutissimum*,[224] *C. group G*,[225] and *C. group JK*.[221] *C. group JK* is the most common and clinically the most important of the organisms infecting prosthetic valves; native valves are rarely involved. In 60–70% of patients with a prosthetic valve infected by diphtheroids, the disease becomes clinically obvious within 2 months after cardiac surgery.

A review of diphtheriod endocarditis published in 1977 described 67 cases of valvular disease caused by these organisms. Men were involved almost twice as often as women. Fifty percent of the infections involved prosthetic valves.[226–230] Anaerobic strains of these organisms may occasionally infect normal cardiac valves. Diagnosis of infective endocarditis caused by the diphtheroids may be difficult because both aerobic and anaerobic organisms are normal residents of human skin. This may lead to misinterpretation of a positive blood culture because it fails to distinguish contamination from infection. Evidence supporting the diagnosis of infection by diphtheroids includes (1) five or six cultures of blood, all of which yield the same organism; (2) growth of the bacteria on agar pour plates; and (3) a satisfactory response to treatment with an antimicrobial agent to which the organism is sensitive in vitro.[226]

The antimicrobial sensitivity of organisms recovered from patients with infective endocarditis caused by diphtheroids is quite variable. Many aerobic strains are sensitive to penicillin G in vitro. There is some evidence that penicillin G and gentamicin are synergistic even when the organism is resistant to penicillin alone.[218] Vancomycin, to which all diphtheroids are sensitive, appears to the the drug of choice initially. Proprionibacteria are usually resistant to penicillin but sensitive to erythromycin, chloramphenicol, and clindamycin.

Fewer than 20 cases of endocarditis caused by *C. diphtheriae* have been recorded.[226–233] This organism produced exotoxin in one patient. In others, infecting strains were nontoxigenic. *C. diphtheriae* was not recovered from the pharynx of these patients. One individual with a systolic murmur of the pulmonary valve recovered when treated medically. The clinical course of another was acute and was complicated by destruction of the aortic valve. Despite insertion of a prosthetic valve, the patient died. At autopsy, gram-positive rods were recovered from the valvular vegetations;

a mycotic aneurysm was present in the right iliac artery. A 13-year-old girl, apparently healthy at the onset of infective endocarditis caused by *C. diph-theriae*, had an acute clinical course and failed to respond to the intravenous administration of large doses of penicillin G. However, when treated with erythromycin and trimethoprim-sulfamethoxazole, she recovered despite the fact that she developed mitral regurgitation. Infective endocarditis in a 16-year-old boy with prolapse of the mitral valve was treated successfully with penicillin and valve replacement. Over 50% of patients have survived when treated medically. Endocarditis caused by *C. diphtheriae* may develop in immunized patients. The vaccine protects against the toxic effects but not the tissue invasion of the organism. At present, most instances of diphtheria occur in young people living in the tropics.

Kurthia bessonii

K. bessonii is the only catalase-negative organism in the coryneform group of bacteria.[234] One patient with endocarditis caused by this organism had a long history of intravenous narcotic use. Treatment often requires medical therapy, as well as replacement of the infected valve.

Rothia dentocariosa

R. dentocariosa, an aerobic, gram-positive coccobacillus, is a member of the indigenous microflora of the oral cavity. Various type of oral pathology, including peridontal disease and carious teeth, are the most common sources of the organism. However, it has also been recovered from sputum, operating rooms, and periappendiceal abscesses, as well as in patients older than 50 years. *R. dentocariosa* produces subacute infective endocarditis and is sensitive to penicillin, the drug of choice.[235–238]

Bacillus, *species*

Infective endocarditis is very rarely caused by members of the genus *Bacillus,* which includes a number of gram-positive, facultative, anaerobic, sport-forming bacilli.[239–241] These organisms usually infect cardiac valves previously damaged by rheumatic fever; they may also involve prosthetic valves. Infection of natural and artificial valves is most common in intravenous drug users.[242,243] The tricuspid valve is most often involved. The clinical course of the disease is usually subacute. Valvular infection produced by these organisms is distinctive because of the high incidence of septic pulmonary emboli and/or in situ thrombosis caused by an extracellular toxin produced by *Bacillus* species.

Patients with endocarditis associated with drug use often present with endophthalmitis that usually leads to complete destruction of the involved eye. A similar ocular process may develop following blood transfusion.[244] Endocarditis caused by *Bacillus* species is associated with injury caused by foreign bodies, including pacemakers. The diagnosis is based on multiple positive blood cultures and the clinical picture of infective endocarditis. Gram-positive rods are regularly recovered from blood cultures. Treatment with clindamycin or vancomycin has produced a high rate of cure of endocarditis caused by *Bacillus* species.[245] Medical therapy alone is usually successful.

References

1. Lerner P, Weinstein L: Infective endocarditis in the antibiotic era. *N Engl J Med* 1966; 274:199, 259, 323, 307.
2. King K, Harkness J: Infective endocarditis in the 1980s—Part I, Aetiology and diagnosis. *Med J Aus* 1986;144:536.
3. Parker M, Ball L: Streptococci and serococci associated with systemic infection in man. *J Med Microbiol* 1976;9:275.
4. Gallis H: Viridans and B hemolytic (non group A, B and D) streptococci, in Mandell R, Douglas G, Bennet J(ed): *Principles and Practices of Infectious Disease*, ed 3. New York, Churchill Livingstone, 1990, chap 181.
5. Cherubin C, Neu H: Infective endocarditis at the Presbyterian Hospital in New York City from 1938–1967. *Am J Med* 1971;51:83.
6. Weinstein L: Infective endocarditis: Past, present and future. *J R Coll Phys London*, 1972;6:161.
7. Afrenow M: Review of 202 cases of bacterial endocarditis. *Ill Med J* 1955;107:67.
8. Wilson L: Etiology of bacterial endocarditis: Before and since introduction of antibiotics. *Ann Intern Med* 1963; 58:946.
9. Cates J, Christie R: Subacute bacterial endocarditis: Review of 442 patients treated in 14 centers appointed by Penicillin Trials Committee of Medical Research Council. *Am J Med* 1951;20:93.
10. Geraci J, Martin W: Antibiotic therapy of bacterial endocarditis. VI. Subacute enterococcal endocarditis: Clinical, pathologic and therapeutic consideration of 33 cases. *Circulation* 1954;10:173.
11. Jackson J, Allis F Jr: Bacterial endocarditis. *South Med J* 1961; 54:1331.
12. Morgan W, Bland E: Bacterial endocarditis in the antibiotic era. *Circulation* 1959; 19:753.
13. Friedberg C, Goldman H, Field L: Study of bacterial endocarditis: Comparisons in ninety-five cases. *Arch Intern Med* 1961; 107:6.
14. Wedgewood J: Early diagnosis of subacute bacterial endocarditis. *Lancet* 1955;2:1058.
15. Uwaydah M, Weinberg A: Bacterial endocarditis—A changing pattern. *N Engl J Med* 1965;273:1231.
16. Shinebourne E, Cripps C, Hayward G, et al: Bacterial endocarditis 1956–1965: Analysis of clinical features and treatment in relation to prognosis and mortality. *Br Heart J* 1969; 31:536.
17. Blount J: Bacterial endocarditis. *Am J Med* 1965;38:909.
18. Tompsett R: Bacterial endocarditis: Changes in the clinical spectrum. *Arch Intern Med* 1967;119:329.
19. Levin R, Pulliam L, Mondry C, et al: Penicillin-resistant *Streptococcus constellatus* as a cause of endocarditis. *Am J Dis Child* 1982;136:42.
20. Hosea S: Virulent *Streptococcus viridans* bacterial endocarditis. *Am Heart J* 1981;101:174.
21. Colman G, Williams R: Taxonomy of some human viridans streptococci. In Wannamaker C, Matsen J (eds): *Streptococci and Streptococcal Disease: Recognition, Understanding and Management*. New York, Academic Press, 1972, p 281.
22. Scheld W, Valone J, Sande M: Bacterial adherence in the pathogenesis of endocarditis. Interaction of bacterial dextrose, platelets and fibrin. *J Clin Invest* 1978;61:1394.
23. Tuazon C, Gill V, Gill T: Streptococcal endocarditis—single vs. combination antibiotic therapy and the role of various species. *Rev Infect Dis* 1986;857:60.

24. Sussman J, Baron E, Tenenbaum M, et al: Viridans streptococcal endocarditis: Clinical, neurological and echocardiographic correlations. *J Infect Dis* 1989;101:579.

25. Roberts R, Krieger D, Cullen S, et al: Viridans streptococcal endocarditis: The role of various species including pyndoxal-dependent streptococci. *Rev Infect Dis* 1975; 1955:65.

26. Parker M, Ball L: Streptococci and aerococci associated with systemic infection in man. *J Med Microbiol* 1976;9:275.

27. Naiman R, Barrow J: Penicillin-resistant bacteria in mouths and throats of children receiving continuous prophylaxis abainst rheumatic fever. *Ann Intern Med* 1963;58:768.

28. Doyle E, Spagnulo M, Taranta A, et al: The risk of bacterial endocarditis during antirheumatic prophylaxis. *JAMA* 1967;201:807.

29. Parillo J, Borst G, Mazar M, et al: Endocarditis due to resistant viridans streptococci during oral penicillin chemoprophylaxis. *N Engl Med* 1979;300:290.

30. Brennan R, Durack D: Therapeutic significance of penicillin tolerance in experimental streptococcal endocarditis. *Antimicrob Agents Chemother* 1983;23:253.

31. Holloway Y, Dankert J, Hess J: Penicillin tolerance and bacterial endocarditis. Letter. *Lancet,* 1980;1:592.

32. Dormer A: Bacterial endocarditis: Survey of patients treated between 1945–1956. *Br Med J* 1958:1:63.

33. Davies J: Subacute bacterial endocarditis. *Br Med J* 1957;1:821.

34. Cameron I: Subacute bacterial endocarditis in an edentulous patient: A case report. *Br Dent J* 1971;130:404.

35. Croxson M, Altmann M, O'Brien K: Dental status and recurrence of *Streptococcus viridans* endocarditis. *Lancet* 1971;1:1205.

36. Simon D, Goodwin J: Should good teeth be extracted to prevent *Streptococcus viridans* endocarditis? *Lancet* 1971:1:1207.

37. Hobson F, Jeul-Jensen B: Teeth, *Streptococcus viridans* and subacute bacterial endocarditis. *Br Med J* 1956;2:1501.

38. Beeley L: Teeth, *Streptococcus viridans* and subacute bacterial endocarditis. *Br Dent J* 1969; 127:424.

39. Shales D, Lerner P, Nolonsky D, et al: Infections due to Lancefield group F and related streptococci (*S. milleri, S. angiosus*). *Medicine* 1981;60:197.

40. Bart I, Walter R: Pathogenesis of anaerobic gram-positive cocci. *Infect Immunol* 1984; 15:320.

41. Murray H, Gross K, Mazur H, et al: Serious infections caused by *Streptococcus milleri. Am J Med* 1970;64:759.

42. Stein D, Nelson K: Endocarditis due to nutritionally-deficient streptococci: A therapeutic dilemma. *Rev Infect Dis* 1987;9:1908.

43. Roberts KB, Sidlak MJ: Satellite streptococci. A major cause of "negative" blood cultures in bacterial endocarditis? *JAMA* 1979;241:2293.

44. Narasimhan S, Weinstein A: Infective endocarditis due to a nutritionally-deficient streptococcus. *J Pediat* 1980;96:61.

45. McCarthy L, Bottone E: Bacteremia and endocarditis caused by satelliting streptococci. *Am J Clin Pathol* 1974;61:585.

46. Corey R, Gross K, Roberts R: Vitamin B_6 dependent *S. mitior* (*mitis*) isolated from patients with systemic infection. *J Infect Dis* 1975;117:722.

47. Levine J, Hummer B, Pollock A, et al: Penicillin-sensitive nutritionally variant streptococcal endocarditis: Relapse after penicillin therapy. *Am J Med Sci* 1983;31:202.

48. Gisenberg F, Forbes B, Singh A, et al: Case report: Prosthetic valve endocarditis due to a nutritionally variant streptococcus. *Am J Med Sci* 1988;289:299.

49. Kaipainen W, Seppala K: Endocarditis lenta: Review of 118 patients treated during ten year period 1945–1954. *Acta Med Scand* 1956;155:71.

50. Toh C, Ball K: Natural history of *Streptococcus faecalis* endocarditis. *Br Med J* 1958;1:61.

51. Wilkowske C: Enterococcal endocarditis. *Mayo Clin Proc* 1982;57:101.

52. Karchmer A, Moellering R Jr, Maki D, et al: Unpublished data.

53. Scheld W, Mandel G: Enigmatic enterococcal endocarditis. *Ann Intern Med* 1984;100:816.

54. Megram D: Enterococcal endocarditis. *Clin Infect Dis* 1992;15:63.
55. Mandell G, Kaye D, Levin C, et al: Enterococcal endocarditis: An analysis of 38 patients observed at the New York Hospital–Cornell Medical Center. *Arch Intern Med* 1970; 125:250.
56. Mosher D: in Mandell G, Douglas R, Bennet J (eds): (*Enterococcus species and group D streptococci*). *Principles and Practice of Infectious Disease,* ed 3. New York, Churchill Livingstone, 19, p 1550.
57. Shales D, Levy J: Enterococcal bacteremia without endocarditis. *Arch Intern Med* 1981;141:570.
58. Garrison R, Frye O, Polk H, et al: Enterococcal bacteremia: Clinical implications and determinants of death. *Ann Surg* 1982;196:45.
59. Berk S, Verghele A, Holksclaw S: Enterococcal pneumonia occurrence in patients receiving broad spectrum antibiotic regimens and enteric feeding. *Am J Med* 1983; 711:133.
60. Bryant J, Washington J II: Polymicrobial septicemia. *Lab Med* 1988;9:15.
61. Levi D, Reiner N, Gopa L, et al: Enterococcal endocarditis in heroin addicts. *JAMA* 1976; 235:1861.
62. Maki D, Gazi N: Enterococcal bacteremia clinical features: The risk of endocarditis and management. *Medicine* 1988;67:243.
63. Malone D, Wagner R, Myers J, et al: Enterococcal bacteremia in two large community teaching hospitals. *Am J Med* 1986;81:601.
64. Moellering R, Watson B, Junz L: Endocarditis due to group D streptococci. *Am J Med* 1974;57:239.
65. Ravreby W, Bottone E, Keusch G: Group D streptococcal bacteremia with emphasis on the incidence and presentation of infections due to *Streptococcus bovis. N Engl J Med* 1973; 289:1400.
66. Garvey G, Neu H: Infective endocarditis—an evolving disease. A review of endocarditis at the Columbia-Presbyterian Medical Center 1968–1973. *Medicine* 1978;57:105.
67. Karchmer A, Moellering R Jr, Maki D, et al: Single antibiotic therapy for streptococcal endocarditis. *JAMA* 1979;241:1801.
68. Wilson W, Gerace K, Wilkowski C, et al: Short-term intramuscular therapy with procaine penicillin plus streptomycin for infective endocarditis due to viridans streptococci. *Circulation* 1978;57:1158.
69. Matthai N, Weibel C, McDermott A, et al: *Streptococcus bovis* endocarditis presenting as acute vertebral osteomyelitis. *Arthritis Rheum* 1989;24:1211.
70. Diebel R: The group D streptococci. *Bacteriol Rev* 1964;28:330.
71. Facklam R: Recognition of group D streptococcal species of human origin by biochemical and physiological tests. *Appl Microbiol* 1972;23:1131.
72. Wellstood A: Rapid and effective identification of group A streptococci and enterococci S. pyrrolidoxyl beta napthylamine hydrolysis. *J Clin Microbiol* 1987;25:1805.
73. Gould H, Ramirez-Rouch C, Holmes P, et al: Adherence of bacteria to heart valves in vitro. *J Clin Invest* 1975;56:1364.
74. Drake T, Rodgers C, Sande M: Tissue factor is a major structure for vegetation formation in endocarditis in rabbits. *J. Clin Invest* 1984;73:1750.
75. Murray H, Roberts R: *Streptococcus bovis* bacteremia and underlying gastrointestinal disease. *Arch Intern Med* 1974;81:588.
76. Klein R, Catalano M, Edberg S, et al: *Streptococcus bovis* septicemia and carcinoma of the colon. *Ann Intern Med* 1979;91:560.
77. Hoppes W, Lerner P: Non-enterococcal group D streptococcal endocarditis caused by *Streptococcus bovis. Ann Intern Med* 1974;81:588.
78. Klein R, Recco R, Catalano M, et al: Association of *Streptococcus bovis* with carcinoma of the colon. *N Engl J Med* 1977;297:800.
79. Rose D, Richman H, Localio S: Bacterial endocarditis associated with colorectal carcinoma. *Ann Surg* 1974;179:190.
80. McCoy W, Mason J: Enterococcal endocarditis associated with carcinoma of the sigmoid: Report of case. *J Med Assoc State Ala* 1951;21:162.

81. Haldone E, Haldone J, Digout G, et al: *Streptococcus bovis* endocarditis. *Can Med Assoc J* 1974;111:678.

82. Reid T: Group D streptococcal endocarditis. *Scott Med J* 1977;22:13.

83. Savitch C, Barry A, Hoeprich P: Infective endocarditis caused by *Streptococcus bovis* resistant to the lethal effect of penicillin G. *Arch Intern Med* 1978;138:931.

84. Enzler M, Rouse M, Henry N, et al: In vitro and in vivo studies of streptomycin-resistant penicillin susceptible streptococci in patients with infective endocarditis. *J Infect Dis* 1987;155:951.

85. Finegold J, George M, Mulligan E: Anaerobic Infections. *Dis. Month* 1985;8:31.

86. Gray A: Beta-hemolytic streptococcal bacteremia. *MMWR* 1990;39:2.

87. Savage D, Brown J: Endocarditis caused by group A streptococcus. *Am J Med Sci* 1991;202:921.

88. Barz N, Kish M, Kaufman C, et al: Streptococcal bacteremia in intravenous drug abusers. *Am J Med* 1985;785:569.

89. Ramirez C, Narage S, McCullen D: Group A beta-hemolytic streptococcus endocarditis. *Am Heart J* 1989;108:1383.

90. Keefer C, Ingelfengt F, Spink W: Significance of hemolytic streptococcic bacteremia: A study of two hundred and forty-six patients. *Arch Intern Med* 1937;60:1084.

91. Blair D, Martin D: Beta hemolytic streptococcal endocarditis: Predominance of non–group A organisms. *Am J Med Sci* 1978;276:269.

92. Moody M: Old and new techniques for rapid identification of group A streptococci. In Wannamaker L, Matsen J (eds): *Streptococci and Streptococcal Diseases. Recognition, Understanding and Management.* New York, Academic Press, 1972, p 177.

93. Feingold D, Stagg N, Junz L: Extrarespiratory streptococcal infections. Importance of the various serologic group. *N Engl J Med* 1966;275:356.

94. Pollock H, Dahlgren B: Distribution of streptococal groups in clinical specimens with evaluation of bacitracin screening. *Appl Microbiol* 1974;27:141.

95. Chitwood L, Jennings M, Riley H: Time, cost and efficacy study of indentifying group A streptococci with commercially available reagents. *Appl Microbiol* 1969;18:193.

96. Backer R, Wilson W, Geraci J, et al: Streptococcal infective endocarditis. *Arch Intern Med* 1982;145:899.

97. Gallagher P, Natanakunakora C: Group B streptococcal endocarditis: Reprint of seven cases and review of the literature 1962–1985. *Rev Infect Dis* 1986;8:175.

98. Lerner P, Gopalakrishna K, Wolinsky E, et al: Group B streptococcus (*S. agalactiae*) bacteremia in adults: Analysis of 32 cases and review of the literature. *Medicine* 1977;56:457.

99. Bayer A, Chow A, Anthony B, et al: Serious infections in adults due to group B streptococci. *Am J Med* 1976;61:498.

100. Hager W, Speck E, Puthenpurakel K, et al: Endocarditis with myocardial abscesses and pericarditis in an adult. *Arch Intern Med* 1977;137:1725.

101. Murcia A, Lyons R: Group B streptococcus endocarditis in a prosthetic valve (to the editor). *Arch Intern Med* 1978;138:1304.

102. Mohr D, Feist D, Washington J II, et al: Infections due to group C streptococci in man. *Am J Med* 1979;66:450.

103. Stein B, Panualker A: Group C streptococcal endocarditis. Case report and review of literature. *Infection* 1985;13:282.

104. Davies M, Ireland M, Clark D: Infective endocarditis from group C streptococci causing stenosis of both the aortic and mitral valves. *Thorax* 1981;36:69.

105. Portnoy D, Wink K, Richards G, et al: Bacterial endocarditis due to penicillin-tolerant group C streptococcus. *Can Med Assoc J* 1980;122:69.

106. Mohr D, Feist B, Washington J, et al: Meningitis due to group C streptococci in an adult. *Mayo Clin Proc* 1978;53:529.

107. Harder D, Wilkowske C, Washington J II, et al: *Streptococcus mutans* endocarditis. *Ann Intern Med* 1974;80:364.

108. Wilson A, Wilkowske C, Wright G, et al. Treatment of streptomycin-susceptible and streptomycin-resistant enterococcal endocarditis. *Ann Intern Med* 1984;100:816.

109. Neefe L, Chretien J, Delaha E, et al: *Streptococcus mutans* endocarditis. Confusion with enterococcal endocarditis by routine laboratory testing. *JAMA* 1974;230:1298.
110. Bourgault A, Wilson W, Washington J II: Antimicrobial susceptibilities of species of *viridans* streptococci. *J Infect Dis* 1979;140:316.
111. Robbins N, Szilagyi G, Tanowitz H, et al: Infective endocarditis caused by *Streptococcus mutans*. *Arch Intern Med* 1977;137:1171.
112. Tiverton C, Herman P, Washington J: Beta-hemolytic group F streptococcal bacteremia, a study and review of the literature. *Rev Infect Dis* 1985;7:498.
113. Shlaes P, Lerner P, Wolinsky E, et al: Infection due to Lancefield group F and related streptococci (*S. milleri, S. anginosus. Medicine* 1981;60:197.
114. Bouza E, Meyer RD, Busch DF: Group G streptococcal endocarditis. *Am J Clin Pathol* 1978;70:108.
115. Smyth E, Pallett A, Davidson R: Group G streptococcal endocarditis: Two case reports, a review of the literature and recommendations for treatment. *J Infection* 1988;16:169.
116. Varran C, Lerner P, Shlaes D, et al: Infection due to Lancefield group G streptococci. *Medicine* 1985;64:75.
117. Ralston K, Chandrasekar P, Lefrock J: Clinical features and antimicrobial therapy of infection caused by group G streptococci. *Infection* 1985;13:203.
118. Venezio F, Gullberg R, Nessenfelder G, et al: Group B streptococcal endocarditis and bacteremia. *Am J Med* 1989;81:29.
119. Bevanger L, Stamnes T: Group L streptococci as the cause of bacteremia and endocarditis. *Acta Pathol Microbiol Scand (Sect B)* 1979;87:301.
120. Dismukes W, Karchmer A, Buckley M, et al: Prosthetic valve endocarditis. *Circulation* 1973;48:365.
121. Pein E, Wilson W, Kunz K, et al: *Aerococcus viridans* endocarditis. *Mayo Clin Proc* 1984;59:47.
122. Ferraro M: *Stomatococcus mucilaginosus* endocarditis in a heroin addict. Letter. *J Infect Dis* 1980;155:1787.
123. Bun-Joi A, Rupoesa H, Brager C, et al: Antimicrobial susceptibility of *Gerella haemolysis* isolated from patients with infective endocarditis. *Am J Clin Microbiol* 1982;1:102.
124. Mylotte J, McDermott C, Spooner J: Prospective study of 114 consecutive cases of *Staphylococcus aceria* bacteremia. *Rev Infect Dis* 1987;9:891.
125. Sanagria J, Alport J, Goldberg R, et al: Increasing frequency of staphylococcal infective endocarditis: Experience at a university hospital 1981–1988. *Arch Intern Med* 1990;150:1305.
126. Pankey G: Acute bacterial endocarditis at University of Minnesota hospitals, 1939–1959. *Am J Med* 1962;64:583.
127. Thompson R: Staphylococcal infective endocarditis. *Mayo Clin Proc* 1982;57:106.
128. Finland M, Barnes M: Changing etiology of bacterial endocarditis in the antibacterial era: Experience at Boston City Hospital 1933–1965. *Ann Intern Med* 1970;72:341.
129. Wilson L: Etiology of bacterial endocarditis: Before and since introduction of antibiotics. *Ann Intern Med* 1963;58:946.
130. Aly R, Shinefield H, Litz C, et al: Role of teichoric acid in the binding of *Staphylococcus aureus* to normal epithelial cells. *J Infect Dis* 1980;141:463.
131. Fausten V, Marke V, Cosre J: Bacterial adherence to pharyngeal cells during viral infections. *J Infect Dis* 1980;141:172.
132. Vann J, Hamill J, Albrecht R, et al: Immunoelectron microscopic localization of fibronectin in adherence of *Staphylococcus aureus* to cultured bovine endothelial cells. *J. Infect Dis* 1989;160:538.
133. Beille M: Vascular endothelial immunology and infectious disease. *Rev Infect Dis* 1989;11:273.
134. Sheagren J: *Staphylococcus aureus*, the persistent pathogen. *N Engl J Med* 1984;310:1368.
135. Mandell G: Catalase superoxide dismutase and virulence of *Staphylococcal aureus*, in vitro and in vivo: Studies with emphasis on staphylococcal–leukocyte interaction. *J Clin Invest* 1975;55:561.
136. Rogolsky M: Non-enteric toxins of *Staphylococcus aureus*. *Danish Med Bull* 1979;43:320.

137. Wilkinson B: Staphylococcal capsules and slime. In Easmone C (ed): Staphylococci and Staphylococcal Disease. New York, Academic Press, 1983, p 20.
138. Hawinger J, Timmons S, Strong D, et al: Identification of a region of human fibrinogen interacting with staphylococcal clumping frictor. *Biochemistry* 1982;21:1407.
139. Hackbarth C, Chambers H: Methicillin-resistant staphylococci: Detection methods and treatment of infection. *Antimicrob Agents Chemother* 1989;33:995.
140. Sabath L, Wheeler N, Lauerdiere M, et al: A new type of penicillin resistance of *Staphylococcus aureus. Lancet* 1977;1:445.
141. Faville R Jr, Zaske D, Kaplan E, et al: *Staphylococcus aureus* endocarditis. Combined therapy with vancomycin and rifampin. *JAMA* 1978;240:1963.
142. Nolan C, Beaty H: *Staphylococcus aureus* bacteremia: Current clinical patterns. *Am J Med* 1976;60:495.
143. Iannini P, Crossley K: Therapy of *Staphylococcus aureus* bacteremia associated with a removable focus of infection. *Ann Intern Med* 1976:81:558.
144. Drake T: *Staphylococcus aureus* induced tissue factor expression in cultured human valve endothelium. *J Infect Dis* 1980;157:749.
145. Linares J, Siges-Serra A, Garan J, et al: Pathogenesis of catheter sepsis: A prospective study with quantitative and semi-quantitative cultures of catheter hub and segments. *J Clin Microbiol* 1985;21:357.
146. Cheung A, Fuchetti L: The role of fibrinogen in staphylococcal adherence to catheter in vitro. *J Infect Dis* 1990;161:1177.
147. Creger W, Coggins C, Hancock E: *Annual Review of Medicine,*Vol 32. Palo Alto, CA, *American Reviews,* 1981, p 624.
148. Wilson R, Hamburger M: Fifteen years' experience with staphylococcus septicemia in a large city hospital: Analysis of fifty-five cases in Cincinnati General Hospital 1940–1954. *Am J Med* 1957;22:437.
149. Skinner D, Keefer S: Significance of bacteremia caused by *Staphylococcus aureus. Arch Intern Med* 1942;68:851.
150. Watanakunakorn C, Baird IM: *Staphylococcus aureus* bacteremia and endocarditis associated with a removable infected intravenous device. *Am J Med* 1977;63:253.
151. Ehni W, Reller B: Short course therapy for catheter-associated *Staphylococcus aureus* bacteremia. *Arch Intern Med* 1989;149:533.
152. Nagel J, Tuazon C, Cardella T, et al: Teichoic acid serologic diagnosis of staphylococcal endocarditis. *Ann Intern Med* 1975;82:13.
153. Jackson L, Sottile M, Aguilar-Torres F, et al: Correlation of antistaphylococcal antibody titers with severity of staphylococcal disease. *Am J Med* 1978;64:629.
154. Wheat L, Kohler R, White A: Solid-phase radioimmunoassay for immunoglobulin G *Staphylococcus aureus* antibody in serious staphylococcal infection. *Ann Intern Med* 1978;89:467.
155. Tuazon C, Sheagren J: Teichoic acid antibodies in the diagnosis of serious infections with *Staphylococcus aureus. Ann Intern Med* 1976;84:543.
156. Thisyukorn U, Shelton S, Tzai Y, et al: Detection of teichoic acid antibodies in children with staphylococcal infection. *Pediatr Infect Dis* 1984;13:22.
157. Wheat L, Luft F, Tabbarah Z: Serologic diagnosis of access device–related staphylococcal bacteremia. *Am J Med* 1979;67:603.
158. Bernhardt L, Antopol S, Simberkoff M: Association of teichoic acid antibody with metastatic sequelae of catheter-associated *Staphylococcus aureus* bacteremia. *Am J Med* 1979;67:603.
159. Tuazon C, Sheagren J, Choa M, et al: *Staphylococcus aureus* bacteremia: Relationship between formation of antibodies to teichoic acid and development of metastatic abscesses. *J Infect Dis* 1978;137:57.
160. Quinn E, Cox J Jr: *Staphylococcus albus (epidermidis)* endocarditis: Report of 16 cases seen between 1953–1962. *Antimicrob Agents Chemother* 1963;3:635.
161. Geraci J, Hanson K, Giuliani E: Endocarditis cuased by coagulase-negative staphylococci. *Mayo Clin Proc* 1968;43:420.

162. Baker G, Stewart G: Primary *Staphylococcus albus* endocarditis. *Guys Hospital Rep* 1961;110:299.

163. Brandt L, Swahn B: Subacute bacterial endocarditis due to coagulase-negative *Staphylococcus albus*. *Acta Med Scand* 1960;166:125.

164. Williams D, Peterson P, Verhoef J, et al: Endocarditis caused by coagulase-negative staphylococci. *Infection* 1979;7:5.

165. Kloss W: Coagulase-negative staphylococci. *Clin Microbiol Newlett* 1982;4:75.

166. Archer G, Karchmer H, Vishniavsky N, et al: Plasmid pattern dialysis for the differentiation of infecting from non-infecting *Staphylococcal epidermidis*. *J Infect Dis* 1984; 149:903.

167. Parisi J: Coagulase-negative staphylococcus in epidemiological typing of *Staphylococcus epidermidis*. *Microbiol Rev* 1985;49:126.

168. Patrick C: Coagulase-negative staphylococci: Pathogen with increasing clinical significance. *J Pediatr* 1990;116:497.

169. Venditti M, Santini C, Serra P, et al: Comparative in vitro activities of new fluoroquinolones and other antibiotics against coagulase-negative staphylococcus blood isolates from neutrogenic patients and relationship between susceptibility and slime production. *Antimicrob Agents Chemother* 1989;33:209.

170. Nade J, Schimpff S, Newman K, et al: *Staphylococcus epidermidis*—an increasing cause of infection in patients with granulocytopenia. *Ann Intern Med* 1982;97:503.

171. Johnson C, Rhodes R: Pediatric endocarditis. *Mayo Clin J* 1982:57:89.

172. Kirby W: Vancomycin therapy in severe staphylococcal infection. *Rev Infect Dis* 1981; 3 (Suppl):286.

173. Low D, McGeer A, Poon R: Activities of claptomycin and teicoplanin against *Staphylococcus heamolyticus* and *Staphylococcus epidermidis,* including valuation of susceptibility testing recommendations. *Antimicrob Agents Chemother* 1983;23:932.

174. Calderwood S, Swinski L, Watenaux C, et al: Risk factor for the development of a prosthetic valve endocarditis. *Circulation* 1988;72:37.

175. Calderwood S, Swinski L, Karchmer A, et al: Prosthetic valve endocarditis: Analysis of factors affecting outcome of therapy. *J Thorac Cardiovasc Surg* 1986;92:770.

176. Karchmer A, Archer G, Dismukec G: *Staphylococcus epidermidis* causing prosthetic valve endocarditis: Microbiologic and clinical observations as guides to therapy. *Ann Intern Med* 1983;98:447.

177. Christensen G, Bisno A, Paresi J, et al: Nosocomial septicemia due to multiple antibiotic-resistant *Staphylococcus epidermidis*. *Ann Intern Med* 1982;96:1.

178. Kirby W: Vancomycin therapy in severe staphylococcal infection. *Rev Infect Dis* Suppl, 1981; 286.

179. Law D, McGeer A, Poor N: Activities of claptomycin and teicoplanin against *Staphylococcus haemolyticus* and *Staphylococcus epidermidis* including evaluation of susceptibility testing. *Antimicrob Agents Chemother* 1989;33:522.

180. Long F, Chang D, Lash P: Synergy of combinations of vancomycin, gentamicin and rifampin against methicillin-resistant coagulase-negative staphylococci. *Antimicrob Agents Chemother* 1983;23:932.

181. Laverdiere M, Peterson P, Verhoef J, et al: In vitro activity of cephalosporins against methicillin-resistant coagulase-negative staphylococci: Minimal effect of beta-lactamases. *Antimicrob Agents Chemother* 1980;17:179.

182. Dannerman T, Nadiuk D, Kloos W: Susceptibility of staphylococcus species and subspecies to teicuplanin. *Antimicrob Agents Chemother* 1991;35:1919.

183. Arditi M, Yogel R: In vitro interaction between rifampin and clindamycin against pathogenic coagulase-negative staphylococci. *Antimicrob Agents Chemother* 1989;33:245.

184. Okies J, Viroslav J, Williams T: Endocarditis after valvular replacement. *Chest* 1972; 59:198.

185. Lewisohn M: *Micrococcus tetragenus* septicemia: Report of case including subacute bacterial endocarditis of pulmonic valve and mycotic aneurysm, with autopsy findings and review of the literature. *Arch Intern Med* 1957;99:824.

186. Old D, McNeill G: Endocarditis due to *Micrococcus sedentarius incertae sedis. J Clin Pathol* 1979;32:951.
187. Rubin S, Lyons R, Murcia A: Endocarditis associated with cardiac catheterization due to a gram-positive coccus designated *Micrococcus mucilaginosus incertae sedis. J Clin Microbiol* 1978;7:546.
188. Thayer W: Bacterial or infective endocarditis. *Edinburgh Med J* 1931;38:237.
189. Straus A, Hamburger M: Pneumococcal endocarditis in the penicillin era. *Arch Intern Med* 1966;118:190.
190. Bullowa J, Wilcox C: Incidence of bacteremia in the pneumonias and its relation to mortality. *Arch Intern Med* 1935;55:558.
191. Ruegsegger J: Pneumococcal endocarditis. *Am Heart J* 1958;56:867.
192. Austrian R: Pneumococcal endocarditis, meningitis and rupture of the aortic valve. *Arch Intern Med* 1957;99:539.
193. Preble H: Pneumococcus endocarditis. *Am J Med Sci* 1904;128:782.
194. Polaymat A, Rhatigan R, Levin S: Pneumococcal endocarditis in infants. *South Med J* 1979;72:448.
195. Morris C, Schwabacher H, Lynch P, et al: Two fatal cases of septicemia due to *Erysipelothrix insidiosa. J Clin Pathol* 1965;18:614.
196. Woodbine M: *Erysipelothrix rhusiopathiae:* Bacteriology and chemotherapy. *Bacteriol Rev* 1950;14:161.
197. Rucha M, Fontoura P, Azevedo S, et al: Erysipelothrix endocarditis with previous cutaneous lesion: Report of case and review of the literature. *Rev Inst Med Trop (São Paulo)* 1989;31(4):286.
198. Gorby Peacock J: *Erysipelothrix rhusiopathiae* endocarditis: Microbiologic, epidemiologic and clinical fetures of an occupational disease. *Rev Infect Dis* 1950;10(2):317.
199. Bille J, Doyle M: *Listeria* and *Erysipelothrix,* in Balows, N, Hausler K, Herrmann N, et al (eds): *Manual of Clinical Microbiology,* ed 50. Washington DC, American Society of Microbiology, 1991, chap 32, p 287.
200. Niemann R, Forbes B: Listeriosis in adults: A changing pattern. Report of eight cases and review of the literature 1968–1978. *Rev Infect Dis* 1980;2:207.
201. Hoff H, Rocouch J, Marget W: *Listeria* and listeriosis. *Infection* 1988;16(Suppl 2): S174.
202. Sem P, Farina D: Human listeriosis. *Infect Med* 1982;3:204.
203. Linnan M, Veda F: Epidemic listeriosis associated with Mexican-style cheese. *N Engl J Med* 1988;319:823.
204. Ganz N, Myerowitz R, Medeiros H, et al: Listeriosis in immunocompromised patients: A cluster of eight cases. *Am J Med* 1975;58:637.
205. Hoeprich P, Chernoff H: Subacute bacterial endocarditis due to *Listeria monocytogenes* endocarditis in hypertrophic cardiomyopathy. *Br Med J* 1978;15:181.
206. Joiner C: *Listeria monocytogenes* endocarditis in hypertrophic cardiomyopathy. *Br Med J* 1978;15:192.
207. Saravolatz L, Burch K, Madhavan T, et al: Listerial prosthetic valve endocarditis: Successful medical therapy. *JAMAS* 1978;240:2186.
208. Breyer R, Arnett E, Spray L, et al: Prosthetic valve endocarditis due to *Listeria monocytogenes. Am J Clin Pathol* 1978;69:186.
209. Carvagal A, Fredericksen W: Fatal endocarditis due to *Listeria monocytogenes. Rev Infect Dis* 1988;10:616.
210. Bayer A, Char H, Guze L: *Listeria monocytogenes* endocarditis: Report of a case and review of the literature. *Am J Med Sci* 1977;273:319.
211. Axelrod J, Keusch G, Bottone E, et al: Endocarditis caused by *Lactobacillus plantarum. Ann Intern Med* 1973;78:33.
212. Dupont B, Lapreste C: Malaide d'Osler a Lactobacille. *Nouv Presse Med* 1977;6:3627.
213. Griffiths J, Daly J, Dodge R: Two cases of endocarditis due to *Lactobacillus* species: Antimicrobial susceptibility—review and discussion on therapy. *Clin Infect Dis* 1992;15:250.
214. Sussman J, Baron E, Goldberg S, et al: Clinical manifestation of lactobacillus endocarditis: Reveiw of a case and review of the literature. *Rev Infect Dis* 1986;8:771.

215. Kaplan K, Weinstein L: Diphtheroid infections in man. *Ann Intern Med* 1969;70:919.
216. Boyce J: A case of prosthetic valve endocarditis caused by *Corynebacterium hofmanni* and *Candida albicans*. *Br Heart J* 1975;37:1195.
217. Gerry J, Greenough W III: Diphtheriod endocarditis: Report of nine cases and review of the literature. *Johns Hopkins Hosp Bull* 1976;139:61.
218. Morris A, Guild I: Endocarditis due to *Corynebacterium* pseudo-diphtherium: Five case reports, review and antibiotic susceptibilities of nine strains. *Rev Infect Dis* 1991; 13:887.
219. Lewis J, Abramson J: Endocarditis due to *Proprionbacterium acnes*. *Am J Clin Pathol* 1980;74:690.
220. Van Scoy R, Cohen S, Geraci J, et al: Coryneform bacterial endocarditis. *May Clin Proc* 1977;52:216.
221. Murray B, Karchmer A, Moellering R Jr: Diphtheroid prosthetic valve endocarditis: A study of clinical features and infecting organisms. *Am J Med* 1980;69:838.
222. Lipsky B, Goldherzer H, Tompkins L, et al: Infections caused by nondiphtheria corynebacterium. *Rev Infect Dis* 1982;4:1200.
223. Vale J, Scotch G: *Corynebacterium bovis* as a cause of human disease. *Lancet* 1977;2:682.
224. Herschorn B, Brucher H: Embolic retinopathy due to *Corynebacterium minutissimum* endocarditis. *Br J Ophthalmol* 1985;69:29.
225. Austin G, Hill E: Endocarditis due to *corynebacterium;* CDC (Group G-2). *J Infect Dis* 1903;147:1106.
226. Kudo P, Nishiwaki Y, Susuki J: Bacteremia due to diphtheria bacilli and followed by diphtheria symptoms. *Hirosaki Med J* 1973;25:130.
227. Davidson S, Rotem Y, Bogkowski B, et al: *Corynebacterium diphtheriae* endocarditis. *Am J Med Sci* 1976;271:351.
228. Guard R: Non-toxigenic *Corynebacterium diphtheriae* causing subacute bacterial endocarditis: Case report. *Pathology* 1979;11:533.
229. Love J, Medina D, Anderson S, et al: Infective endocarditis due to *Corynebacterium diphtheriae:* Report of a case and review of the literature. *Johns Hopkins Med J,* 1981;148:41.
230. Jootar P, Gherunpong V, Saitanu K: *Corynebacterium pyogenes* endocarditis—Report of a case with necropsy and review of the literature. *J Med Assoc Thailand* 1978; 61:596.
231. Howard W: Acute ulcerative endocarditis due to the bacillus diphtheria. *Johns Hopkins Hosp Bull,* 1983;4:32.
232. Trepeta R, Edberg S: *Corynebacterium diphtheriae* endocarditis: Sustained potential of a classical pathogen. *Am J Clin Pathol* 1987;8:679.
233. Surinavin S, Suthea N, Ayuthaya P: Diphtheriae septicaemia and possible endocarditis: A case report and review of the literature. *Eur J Pediatr* 1988;144:395.
234. Rasmussen V, Bremmelgaard A, Korner B, et al: Case report: Acute *Corynebacterium* endocarditis causing aortic valve destruction: Successful treatment with antibiotics and valve replacement. *Scand J Infect Dis* 1979;11:89.
235. Pancoast S, Ellner P, Jahre J, et al: Endocarditis due to *Kurthia bessonii*. *Ann Intern Med* 1979;90:936.
236. Sudduth E, Rozich J, Farrar W: Rothia dentocariosa endocarditits complicated by perivalvular abscess. *Clin Infect Dis* 1993;17:772.
237. Pape J, Singer C, Kiehn T, et al: Infective endocarditis caused by *Rothia dentocariosa*. *Ann Intern Med* 1979;91:746.
238. Shands J: *Rothia dentocariosa* endocarditis. *Am J Med* 1988;85:280.
239. Reeler L: Endocarditis caused by *Bacillus subtilis*. *Am J Clin Pathol* 1973;60:714.
240. Wanvarie S, Rochanawatanon M: *Bacillus cereus* endocarditis. *J Med Assoc Thailand* 1979;62:34.
241. Block C, Levy M, Fritz V: *Bacillus cereus* endocarditis: A case report. *S Afr Med J* 1978;53:556.
242. Sliman R, Rehm S, Shlaes D: Serious infections caused by *Bacillus* species. *Medicine* 1987;66:218.

243. Steen M, Bruno-Murtha F, Chaux G, et al: *Bacillus cereus* endocarditis: Report of a case and review. *Clin Infect Dis* 1992;14:945.
244. Turazon C, Hill R, Shaegreen J: Microbiologic study of street heroin and injection paraphernalia. *J Infect Dis* 1979;129:3271.
245. Weber D, Javiteer S, Rinfalen W, et al: In vitro susceptibility of *Bacillus cereus* to selected antimicrobial agents.*Antimicrob Agents Chemother* 1988:32:6412.

5

Microbiology of Infective Endocarditis and Clinical Correlates: Gram-Negative and Other Organisms

In an extensive review of infective endocarditis caused by gram-negative bacteria, Cohen and his colleagues[1] called attention to a number of microbiological, pathological, and clinical features of this type of endocardial disease. They emphasized the following points:

> In sharp contrast to the relatively high frequency with which gram-positive cocci are involved in the pathogenesis of endocarditis has been the paucity of reports of this disease in which gram-negative bacilli are involved. This difference becomes striking when one considers the high incidence of bacteremia associated with infection or manipulation of the gneitourinary and intestinal tracts (areas in which these species are numerous), and is especially notable because they involve primarily older individuals, many of who have underlying atherosclerotic valvular disease but very few of whom develop infective endocarditis. The rarity of this disease in complicating typhoid fever, in which bacteremia is universally present, or salmonella gastroenteritis, during which invasion of the blood stream is not uncommon in the young and the elderly, emphasizes this point. Although there has been a recent increase in the incidence of infective endocarditis caused by gram-negative bacteria in individuals addicted to the intravenous use of drugs and in those with cardiac prostheses, this remains a relatively uncommon type of disease.

Gram-negative bacilli have been responsible for about 3% of all cases of endocarditis.[1-4] This proportion has increased recently, which may be related to several factors. Among these are (1) an increase in the use of invasive diagnostic procedures; (2) suprainfection related to the indiscriminate use of antibiotics; (3) placement of valvular prostheses; (4) extensive and complicated surgical and other manipulations of the gastrointestinal and genitourinary tracts; and (5) widespread addiction to intravenous drugs. These, together with improvements in diagnostic microbiology, explain most of the growth in the frequency of infective endocarditis caused by gram-negative organisms. Patients with hepatic cirrhosis may have a striking susceptibility to the development of endocardial infection caused by these bacteria. The infection rate is three times higher than in patients with normal hepatic functions.[3]

Currently, endocarditis produced by gram-negative organisms is much less frequent that endocarditis caused by gram-positive bacteria. Streptococi, staphylococci, and *Pseudomonas aeruginosa* adhere, to a much higher degree, to valvular endothelium than *Escherichia coli* or *Klebsiella pneumoniae*, the gram-negative strains most often involved in bacteremia. Infection of native valves occurs less often than when gram-positive bacteria are involved. This is not the case in patients with prosthetic valves or those addicted to intravenous drug use.[1]

Experience with infective endocarditis at the Mayo Clinic reveals a progressive increase in the disease due to gram-negative bacteria.[4] A total of fifty-six cases of valvulor infection were studied over 21 years (1958–1979). Over the last ten years of this study, ten percent of the cases were caused by gram-negative organisms.

The importance of antimicrobial therapy in the pathogenesis of gram-negative, infective endocarditis was pointed out by Finland and Barnes.[5] Of 400 new cases of endocarditis at Boston City Hospital, 42 were caused by gram-negative bacilli. About two-thirds of these cases were associated with or followed by infections in which gram-positive organisms were initially involved. This raised the possibility that the endocardial process represented suprainfection.

In 44 patients with endocarditis caused by gram-negative bacteria other than *Salmonella* species, *E. coli* was the most common organism (17 patients). This was followed by *Serratia marcescens, Klebsiella-Enterobacter* (9 patients), *Proteus,* and *Providencia.*[4,6]

The intravenous use of narcotics and other drugs has been responsible, in great part, for the sharp increase in the incidence of infective endocarditis caused by gram-negative organisms.[7] Although *S. aureus* remains the agent most often involved in endocardial infection in narcotic addicts, gram-negative bacilli have been responsible for about 13% of the cases. *Ps. aeruginosa* has been the causative agent in about 60%.[8] Some strains of gram-negative organisms have been more prevalent than others in some areas of the United States. Two-thirds of reported instances of addict-associated endocarditis caused by *Ps. aeruginosa* were identified in the Detroit area; two-thirds of patients infected by *Ser. marscescens* were reported from San Francisco; and 80% of patients infected by *Ps. cepacia* lived in New York City. The reason for the geographic distribution is not clear. However, it has been suggested that this may be related to the habitat (tapwater sinks or soil) in which these organisms are acquired. Currently, MRSA is the agent most often recovered from addicts in Detroit. The mode of distribution does not necessarily reflect microbial contamination of the illicit drug.[9]

Polymicrobial infection with gram-positive or gram-negative organisms has been identified in about 30% of drug addicts with infective endocarditis. This is in sharp contrast to an incidence of 2% in nonaddicts. [7,10] It has been suggested that a new valvular infection produced by virulent gram-positive cocci, especially *S. aureus,* may injure a valve and set the stage for secondary invasion by garm-negative bacteria.[11] It is also likely that polymicrobial infection may, in fact, be a suprainfection induced by therapy with broad-spectrum antimicrobial agents.

The mean age of patients with infective endocarditis caused by gram-negative organisms is 39 years.[1] It is significantly lower in individuals with disease caused by *S. viridans.* Abnormal valves are involved in most cases. Twenty-five percent of patients with valvular infection caused by *Ps. aeruginosa* or *S. marcescens* have had previously normal hearts; most have abused drugs intravenously. Cardiac failure occurs in about 50% of patients with endocardial disease caused by gram-negative bacteria but in only 14% when the disease is caused by *Ps. aeruginosa.* Congestive heart failure develops most often in patients with gram-negative endocarditis that involves a prosthetic valve; this is most common with an aortic prosthesis. Cardiac decompensation develops in 37% of addicts with infection of the left side of the heart but in only 3% of those with infection of the right side of the heart. Systemic and pulmonary embolization occurs in 50% of patients with endocarditis caused by gram-negative organisms. Despite vigorous medical and surgical treatment, the fatality rate of aerobic, gram-negative endocarditis ranges from 38% to 83%.[4]

Enteric Bacteria

For the purpose of this discussion, only *E. coli, Enterobacter* species, *Klebsiella* species, and indole-negative and -positive strains of *Proteus* species are defined as enteric organisms. These bacteria are members of the normal intestinal microflora. Some species of *Pseudomonas* and *Salmonella* are excluded from this discussion because the first is present in the intestinal tract of about 10% of healthy individuals and the second occurs only occasionally in the bowel.

Escherichia coli

Endocarditis, caused by *E. coli,* is uncommon in patients who are not immunosuppressed, addicted to narcotics, or carry a prosthetic valve[12–29] (Table 5.1). In many instances, a murmur or underlying cardiac disease is often not recognized before infective endocarditis develops. This disease has been identified in about 50% of patients. Cardiac surgery is required to establish the diagnosis in about 20% of individuals. Disease caused by the organism progresses rapidly. The mean duration of symptoms prior to hospitalization is about 2 weeks. The mitral valve is infected most often. Severe infections produced by *E. coli* are commonly associated with bacteremia. It is often difficult to determine whether the recovery of an organism represents an uncomplicated bloodstream infection or reflects the pres-

Table 5.1. Clinical Features of Patients with *Escherichia coli* Endocarditis ($n = 14$)

Mean age	51 yr (range, 2–72 yr)
Male:female ratio	5:2
Previous heart disease	57%
Predisposing conditions	
GU infection*	57%
Other†	36%
No source	7%
Duration of symptoms prior to admission (median)	2 wk
Peripheral stigmata	50%
Congestive heart failure	43%
New or changing murmur	89%
Arterial embolization	36%
Shock	14%
Site of involvement	
Aortic valve	7%
Mitral valve	57%
VSC	14%
Others‡	22%
Mortality	57%

*Acute pyelonephritis was present in four of the eight patients with GU infection.

†Pneumonia, cholecystitis, cardiac surgery.

‡Infected left ventricular mural thrombus, aortic and mitral prosthetic valvular infection.

Source: Adapted from Ref. 1.

ence of infective endocarditis. The possibility that this disease is present must be given serious attention in the following situations: (1) bacteremia persists despite the absence of physical evidence of cardiac involvement; (2) a recognized extracardiac source of bacteremia is poorly controlled by appropriate antimicrobial therapy; or (3) in the absence of shock, the organism is recovered from the blood over a long time, despite adequate therapy. Echocardiography may be helpful because *E. coli* often produces proliferative or destructive valvular lesions. The fatality rate is 57%; the male:female ratio is 5:1.

Enterobacter *Species*

Enterobacter species are an increasingly important cause of nosocomial infections. However, these organisms are involved in only a few instances of infective endocarditis.[30–38] About 50% follow manipulation of the genitourinary tract. In most instances, the valvular infection is acquired during hospitalization for an unrelated disorder. Infection of prosthetic valves usually develops shortly after cardiac surgery. Patients treated with potentially effective antibiotics may die despite the fact that the infecting organism is sensitive in vitro to the drugs being administered. Cure often requires prolonged treatment with antimicrobial agents and replacement of the infected valve.

Klebsiella *Species*

Only a few cases of infective endocarditis caused by *K. pneumoniae* have been reported.[31,32] Infection of the urinary tract has been the primary source of bacteremia and endocardial disease. The clinical signs of infective endocarditis appear to be more common in this disease than in infection caused by *E. coli*. Treatment of *Klebsiella*-induced endocarditis with antimicrobial agents often fails to alter the clinical course. Survival is more common when the infected valve is replaced.

Proteus *Species*

Although various species of *Proteus* are involved in a large variety of infections, especially of the urinary tract, they have caused very few cases of infective endocarditis.[13–19] Disease produced by *Proteus*, usually affects the elderly (in the sixth decade of life) and occurs most often in individuals with infection of the urinary tract. Underlying mitral valve disease is usually present. Large cardiac vegetations may develop. Focal embolic glomerulonephritis has been reported. Most patients die despite adequate therapy.

Pseudomonas aeruginosa

Most infections caused by *Ps. aeruginosa* involve intravenous drug addicts.[39–41] This organism has been involved in 88% of polymicrobial endocardial infections in drug abusers. However, disease produced by *Ps. aeruginosa* may also involve nonaddicted individuals with no historical or physical evidence of a predisposing cardiac disorder[42–76] (Table 5.2).

The pathogenesis of the disease caused by *Ps. aeruginosa* is multifactorial. The organism elaborates numerous factors that determine its virulence. It invades the trachea, where it produces several toxins,[77,78] and it is responsible for a number of syndromes associated with infection. *Ps. aeruginosa* produces five types of extracellular proteases, including elastase and alkaline protease. These are responsible for the necrosis of tissues, especially the elastic layer of the lamina propria of blood vessels, and are involved in the development of the classical lesion, ecthyma gangrenosum, a feature of septicemic pseudomonal infection. The proteases interfere with the normal function of polymorphonuclear leukocytes, monocytes, and K and T cells. They also cleave complement and IgG. Cytotoxin, previously known as *leukocydin*, produced by the organism, injures white blood cells and other eukaryotic cells by injuring their membranes. Hemolysins destroy various glycolipids and contribute to the potential for invasion of the bloodstream

Table 5.2. Clinical Features of Patients with *P. aeruginosa* Endocarditis ($n = 101$)

Mean age	31.8 yr (range, 11 mo–81 yr)
Male:female ratio	3.4:1
Previous heart disease*	36%
Predisposing conditions	
Drug addiction	64%
Recent heart surgery	15%
Cardiac angiography	5%
Urinary tract infection	
or instrumentation	4%
Infections at various sites[†]	9%
Polymicrobial bacteremia	24%
Splenomegaly	13%
Peripheral stigmata	18%
Congestive heart failure	14%
Embolization	
Pulmonary	49%
Arterial[‡]	20%
Myocardial abscesses	9%
Central nervous system	
involvement[§]	23%
Valve involved	
Tricuspid	41%
Pulmonic	3%
Aortic	11%
Mitral	14%
Aortic and mitral	10%
Mixed right- and left-sided	7%
Ventricular septal defect (VSD)	9%
Other or not determined	5%
Deaths	51%

*Underlying heart disease was present in 13/65 addicts and 23/36 nonaddicts (4 addicts had cellulitis at sites of infection).

[†] Cholangitis, septic abortion, endometritis, gunshot wound, lung abscess, infected burns, infected dialysis site, fistula.

[‡] Most commonly to central nervous system, kidneys, and spleen.

[§] Mycotic aneurysm, meningitis, abscess, coma not due to drug overdose, abnormal spinal fluid.

Source: Adapted from Ref. 1.

and metastatic activity of the organism.[79] Exotoxin A[80] interferes with protein synthesis and produces dermatonecrosis when injected into the skin of animals. Pseudomonal keratitis follows the application of exotoxin to the cornea. Exoenzyme destroys tissue and produces toxicity.[81] The ability of exotoxin A to produce systemic toxicity and death in most animals is better established that that ascribed to exoenzyme S. The administration of antibodies active against toxin A confers protection when given early in the course of pseudomonal bacteremia.

Many strains of *Ps. aeruginosa* are resistant to the bactericidal activity of normal serum.[82] Phagocytosis is critical for clearance of the organism from the bloodstream. The polysaccharide capsule, the glycocalyx, permits bacteria to adhere to normal mucosal surfaces; blocks phagocytosis by leukocytes, monocytes, and macrophages;[83] and interferes with opsonization. It may decrease the antimicrobial activity of the aminoglycosides.

Endotoxin produced by *Ps. aeruginosa* is a key factor in the development of septic shock similar to that produced by other gram-negative bacteria. It appears to stimulate the production and release of a variety of cytokines, especially tumor necrosis factor.[84]

Endocarditis caused by *Ps. aeruginosa* is found primarily in narcotic addicts, in those who have recently undergone cardiac surgery, and in those who have developed bacteremia from an extracardiac source.[85] Given that the organism attacks normal as well as damaged cardiac valves, it is remarkable that the endocardial disease it produces has not been more common, especially in immunosuppressed hosts and those with a primary extracardiac infection. Many nonaddicts with infective endocarditis caused by this organism develop the disease during or after antimicrobial therapy for an unrelated infection. The most common illicit drug currently used by patients with pseudomonal endocarditis is a combination of pentazocine and tripelennamine ("T's and blues"). The source of *Ps. aeruginosa* in drug addicts appears to be contaminated needles, rather than the drugs themselves or the skin of the patient.[86]

There are some pathognomonic signs and symptoms that suggest the presence of infective valvulitis caused by *Ps. aeruginosa*. Histological examination of areas of embolization discloses characteristic necrosis of the walls of small arteries and veins. Ecthyma gangrenosum is the cutaneous manifestation of this pathological process. Meningitis and cerebral infarction are present in some patients. The tricuspid valve is involved most often (70% of cases). When the right side of the heart is infected, the clinical course is usually subacute, but it may be acute and complicated by septic pulmonary emboli. Valvular infection of the left side of the heart may be complicated by refractory congestive cardiac failure and large systemic emboli. Less often, but not unusually, multiple valves and the mural endocardium may be infected.

The duration of symptoms prior to the diagnosis of infective endocarditis caused by *Ps. aeruginosa* ranges from 1 day to more than 1 year. In more than 50% of patients, the diagnosis may be established within several weeks of the onset of symptoms. Some individuals, especially drug addicts with involvement of the left side of the heart, exhibit a prolonged and ultimately fatal course despite aggressive therapy with appropriate antimicrobial agents. Twenty-seven of 64 patients (42%) with pseudomonal infective endocarditis treated with antimicrobial agents alone have been cured.[1] Twenty-four of 37 patients (65%) whose valves were replaced with prostheses, in addition to therapy with antibiotics, survived. Finally, 40% and 69% of individuals with disease of both the left and right sides of the heart, respectively, recovered.

Although *Pseudomonas maltophilia* is essentially nonpathogenic for humans, it has caused nosocomial infections of wounds, the eyes, the urinary tract, and the lungs and may be a transient member of the microflora of hospitalized patients. It has been suggested the *Ps. maltophilia* be included in the genus *Xanthomonas* as a distinct species, *X. maltophilia*. Bacteremia is a fairly common complication of disease caused by this organism. Most instances of endocarditis caused by this agent involve prosthetic valves.[87–92] Infection develops within 2 weeks following cardiac surgery in 50% of patients. One individual being treated for infective endocarditis caused by viridans streptococci developed suprainfection caused by *Ps. maltophilia*. Arterial embolization is recognized as a complication. Antimicrobial therapy alone appears to be insufficient to achieve a cure. Replacement of the involved valve is mandatory. The sources of infection include contaminated venipuncture tubes and cardiac bypass pumps. The organism is usually sensitive to chloramphenicol and trimethoprim-sulfamethoxazole; it is resistant to the aminoglycosides and cephalosporins.

In contrast to other species of *Pseudomonas*, the clinical course of disease produced by *Pseudomonas cepacia* is generally indolent and is characterized primarily by loss of weight, fever, and fatigue[93–103] (Table 5.3). Ecthyma gangrenosum often develops in this type of infective endocarditis. Patients

Table 5.3. Clinical Features of *P. cepacia* Endocarditis ($n = 15$)

Mean age	34.3 yr (range, 23–66 yr)
Male:female ratio	13:1
Underlying disease*	53%
Predisposing events†	100%
Mean duration of symptoms prior to diagnosis	27 days (range, 3–90 days)
Polymicrobial bacteremia‡	20%
Peripheral stigmata	33%
Splenomegaly	20%
Congestive heart failure	40%
Embolization§	47%
Myocardial abscess	27%
Site of involvement	
Aortic valve	40%
Mitral valve	13%
Aortic and mitral prostheses	27%
Tricuspid valve	20%
Deaths	60%

*Prosthetic valves, four (two drug addicts); calcific aortic stenosis, one; prior endocarditis, three; rheumatic heart disease, one.

†Drug addiction, 11; prostatitis, 2; recent cardiac surgery, 2.

‡*Candida S. aureus, S. viridans.*

§Pulmonary, three; peripheral arterial, four.

Source: Adapted from Ref. 1.

with infected prosthetic valves develop symptoms within 10 days after surgery. Embolization followed by pulmonary infarction may occur after microbial seeding of the tricuspid valve. Cardiac failure and arterial embolization are comon when the mitral or aortic valves are involved. About 75% of patients with infective endocarditis caused by *Ps. cepacia* are intravenous drugs abusers. Seven of 11 individuals were cured when treated with antimicrobial agents alone; 5 required replacement of the infected valves. *Ps. cepacia* is sensitive to chloramphenicol and trimethoprim-sulfamethoxazole, third-generation cephalosporins, aztreonam, and imipenen. Although valvular infection caused by this organism is associated primarily with narcotic abuse, it also follows the insertion of an intracardiac prosthesis in patients with postoperative infections. The sources of the organism are heparin-flushing solutions and disinfectants.

Several species of *Pseudomonas*, including *Ps. stutzeri*, *Ps. fluorescens*, and *Ps. putida,* produce bacteremia and/or endocarditis. These organisms are ubiquitous members of the hospital environment and infect primarily patients undergoing chemotherapy for lymphomas and leukemias. *Ps. stutzeri* is involved in the pathogenesis of infective endocarditis in patients with prosthetic valves.[92]

Salmonella *Species*

Patients with infective endocarditis caused by various serotypes of *Salmonella* are usually older than 50 years[104-124] (Table 5.4). Infection produced by these organisms is not associated with the intravenous use of drugs. The disease may involve prosthetic valves. The mural endocardium is frequently the site of microbial invasion. *Salmonella* is usually acquired outside the hospital environment. One-third of individuals with salmonella bacteremia have some type of immunosuppressive disorder. Underlying cardiac abnormalities exist in most patients with endocardial disease due to these organisms.

The clinical course of salmonella valvular infection may be complicated by atrial thrombosis, extensive valvular perforation and destruction, pericarditis, and myocardial abscesses. New or progressive congestive cardiac failure, peripheral manifestations including Osler's nodes, petechiae, and subungual hemorrhages; and new or changing murmurs have been described. Congestive heart failure usually develops within 4 weeks after the diagnosis of endocarditis. Previously damaged mitral and aortic valves are the sites on which salmonella is deposited. The presence of valvular infection produced by this organism is often cryptic. Cardiac surgery or autopsy may be required to establish the presence of the disease in about 75% of patients. The fatality rate is about 75% despite therapy with effective antimicrobial agents. Removal of an infected valve and replacement with a prosthesis fails to prevent a fatal outcome in some patients. Treatment with large doses of chloramphenicol or ampicillin has led to a cure in an appreciable number of patients.

Salmonella species adhere strongly to damaged endothelium.[125] This may

Table 5.4. Clinical Features of Patients with *Salmonella* Endocarditis (n = 25)

Mean age	48 yr (range, 12–76 yr)
Male:female ratio	14:11
Previous heart disease	80%
Predisposing conditions	
Gastroenteritis	42%
Immunosuppression	4%
Nosocomial infection	4%
Duration of symptoms prior to admission (median)	6 wk
Peripheral stigmata	68%
Congestive heart failure	63%
New or changing murmur	76%
Arterial embolization	21%
Abscesses	25%
Site of involvement	
Aortic valve	24%
Mitral valve	32%
Aortic and mitral valves	12%
Left atrium	16%
Left and right ventricles	8%
Prosthetic mitral valve	4%
Prosthetic aortic valve	4%
Deaths	68%

Source: Adapted from Ref. 1.

explain the observation that, of all the gram-negative organisms, salmonellae are most often involved in the pathogenesis of infective endocarditis and arterial mycotic aneurysms. Early reports indicated that *S. choleraesuis* and *S. typhimurium* were the serotypes most often responsible for the disease. However, 12 other species, including *S. typhi,* have been identified as causes of salmonellosis.

Although a number of gram-negative organisms are involved in the pathogenesis of infection of the intestinal tract, fewer than half of the reported cases of infective endocarditis have caused gastroenteritis. Physical signs consistent with endocardial infection have been identified in about 90% of these cases. Failure of an intestinal infection caused by salmonellae to respond after 7 to 10 days of treatment with an appropriate antibiotic suggests that infective endocarditis or mycotic aneurysms may be present even in the absence of clinical findings.

Haemophilus *Species*

Less that 1% of cases of infective endocarditis are caused by members of the genus *Haemophilus.* These organisms, together with *Actinobaccillus acti-*

nomycetemcomitans, Cardiobacterium hominis, Eikenella corrodens, and *Kingella kingii,* constitute the HACEK group.[126] *H. parainfluenzae* and *H. aphrophilus* are responsible for most infections[127–133] (Table 5.5). Only seven cases of valvular disease caused by *H. influenzae* have been reported. The mean age of the patients was 25 years (range, 1–37 years); four had underlying rheumatic heart disease and two had no identifiable cardiac disease. Symptoms were present for 2 weeks in one patient, 2–3 months in four, and more than 1 year in one. The peripheral stigmata of infective endocarditis and splenomegaly were present in four individuals. The mitral or aortic valves were involved in five individuals and the tricuspid valve in one of four who survived. All patients were treated with penicillin and streptomycin. One, who eventually died, received penicillin and a sulfonamide; pulmonary infarction and encephalitis were identified at post mortem. A 1-year-old boy in whom the endocarditis was complicated by metastatic meningitis died despite therapy with chloramphenicol and ampicillin. Necropsy disclosed perforation of the mitral valve. Considering the frequency with which infections caused by *H. influenzae* are associated with bacteremia, especially in young children, it is striking that infective endocarditis is relatively uncommon.

Table 5.5. Clinical Features of Patients with *H. parainfluenzae* Endocarditis (*n* = 29)

Mean age	30.9 yr (range, 9–57 yr)
Male:female ratio	1.07:1
Previous heart disease*	52%
Predisposing conditions	
Dental procedure or poor dentition	45%
Drug abuse	3%
Ear or sinus infections	10%
Mean duration of symptoms prior to diagnosis	5 wk (range, 1 day–6 mo)
Splenomegaly	31%
Peripheral stigmata	59%
Congestive heart failure	10%
Arterial embolization†	55%
Sites of involvement	
Aortic valve	17%
Mitral valve	67%
other‡	17%
Deaths	10%

*Rheumatic heart disease, eight; congenital heart disease, four; previous endocarditis, three; mitral prostheses, one; history of murmur, two.
†Nine to the central nervous system and seven to large vessels such as the femoral or brachial artery.
‡Pulmonic, one; tricuspid, two; mitral prosthesis, one.
Source: Adapted from Ref. 1.

H. parainfluenzae is a member of the indigenous flora of the oro- and nasopharynx. Endocarditis caused by this organism has been increasing in frequency.[132-153] It is most common in young adults. Both normal and diseased valves may be involved. The clinical course is subacute in most patients. Murmurs develop late in the course of the disease, despite frequent involvement of the aortic and especially the mitral valve; cardiac failure is uncommon. Multiple episodes of arterial embolization by fragments of giant valvular vegetations are common, and large vessels may be occluded. This may be related to an intrinsic property of the genus *Haemophilus* or may reflect the duration of disease prior to diagnosis. Delay in recovery of *H. parainfluenzae* from the blood is common. This may be related to the strict requirement of some strains for the V factor.

The fatality rate from infection caused by *H. parainfluenzae* is about 10%. This is so despite the widespread availability of effective antimicrobial drugs. There is no consensus concerning optimum therapy of endocarditis caused by *H. parainfluenzae*. Large doses of ampicillin together with gentamicin or streptomycin have been employed. Most of the problems with therapy are probably related to the difficulty in identifying the organism.

Both *H. aphrophilus* and *H. paraphrophilus* are involved in the pathogenesis of infective endocarditis. Most patients from whom these organisms have been recovered were less than 50 years of age[155-180] (Table 5.6). None used illicit drugs.

The diagnosis is usually not established until the disease has been present for more than a month. Eighty percent of patients have had previously damaged valves. In some instances, evidence of endocarditis was identified only at autospy or in the course of cardiac surgery. In others, it was based on the presence of Osler's nodes, Janeway lesions, Roth's spots, subungual hemorrhages, or petechiae. An increase in the level of preexisting cardiac failure is characteristic. Despite antimicrobial therapy, unremitting active infection persists and leads to death.

Brucella *Species*

Brucella species rarely produce endocarditis[181-192] (Table 5.7). Most patients who acquire the disease are younger than 50 years of age. Sheep herders, meat cutters, and individuals who drink unpasteurized milk are most likely to develop brucellosis. The strains of the organism commonly involved are *Br. abortus, Br. melitensis,* and *Br. suis.* Episodes of infective endocarditis caused by these organisms may be superimposed on underlying rheumatic valvular disease or may involve prosthetic valves. Native mitral valves are infected most often. The disease is usually subacute and is characterized by an insidious onset with low-grade fever and a prolonged clinical course before the diagnosis is established, often more than 3 months after the development of symptoms. However, brucellosis may be acute and complicated by perforation of valves, embolic phenomena, and congestive cardiac failure. Extracardiac manifestations are present in all patients. The vegetations produced by this organism have been described as bulky, ul-

Table 5.6. Clinical Features of Patients with *H. aphrophilus* Endocarditis (*n* = 27) (Includes One Case of *H. paraphrophilus*)

Mean age	43 yr (range, 24–74 yr)
Male:female ratio	20.7:1
Previous heart disease	88%
Predisposing conditions	
Dental disease/procedures	33%
Upper respiratory infection	19%
Duration of symptoms prior to admission	4 wk
Peripheral stigmata	63%
Congestive heart failure	50%
New or changing murmurs	37%
Arterial embolization	31%
Abscesses	15%
Site of involvement*	
Mitral valve	56%
Aortic valve	33%
Tricuspid valve	5.5%
Prosthetic mitral valve	5.5%
Deaths	41%

*The site of the valvular leasion was undetermined in eight cases.
Source: Adapted from Ref. 1.

cerative, destructive, fibrosing, nodular, and calcific. The aortic valve is often infected in individuals with fulminating disease. Mycotic, aneurysmal dilation of the aortic sinus, myocarditis, diffuse myocardial abscesses, and granulomas have been present in some patients. The incidence of infective endocarditis caused by *Brucella* is less than 1% worldwide. However, it may be as high as 8–10% in areas where brucellosis is endemic. Endocardial infection occurs in fewer than 2% of patients with brucellosis. It is associated with a high incidence of death, especially in untreated individuals.

Pasteurella *Species*

Pasteurella is rarely involved in the pathogenesis of infective endocarditis. Most infections follow bites by animals. Patients usually develop cellulitis within 24 hr. Sixty-five percent of these are produced by cats and 35% by dogs.[193,194] The next most common portal of entry into the circulation is the pharynx.

Pasteurella are nonsporulating, gram-negative, nonmotile, facultatively anaerobic cocobacilli that grow on many common media at 37°C. These organisms may be confused with *H. influenzae*, *Acinetobacter*, and other gram-negative bacteria. Two patients with disease caused by a *P. multocida*–like organism were not bitten or scratched by animals.[194] Despite claims

Table 5.7. Clinical Features of Patients with *Brucella* Endocarditis ($n = 12$)

Mean age	41 yr (range, 23–63 yr)
Male:female ratio	All male
Previous heart disease	88%
Predisposing conditions	
Exposure to unpasteurized milk	25%
Meat cutting	17%
Exposure to diseased sheep	17%
Duration of symptoms prior to admission (median)*	28 wk
Peripheral stigmata	75%
Congestive heart failure	91%
New or changing murmurs	75%
Arterial embolization	88%
Site of involvement	
Aortic valve	75%
Mitral valve	8.3%
Aortic and mitral valves	8.3%
Prosthetic mitral valve	8.3%
Deaths[†]	83%

*Differentiation between symptoms of brucellosis with and without endocarditis was impossible.
[†]Both survivors were treated surgically and medically.
Source: Adapted from Ref. 1.

that this bacterium may cause infective endocarditis, the organism recovered from the blood did not have the biological characteristics of *Pasteurella*. Infection in one patient involved an abnormal mitral valve. Both individuals were febrile and exhibited the classical peripheral signs of infective endocarditis. Symptoms had been present for more than 3 months in one individual and for 6 months in the other before the etiology of the disease was defined. Although both patients responded to antimicrobial therapy over 3 months, one died of an unknown cause shortly after discharge from the hospital. The other required replacement of the aortic valve after the infection was eradicated because intractable congestive heart failure had developed.

In addition two other species of *Pasteurella*, *P. pneumotropica* and *P. hemolytica,* may produce infective endocarditis. Prior valvular disease is usually present. One individual had been bitten by a cat; the other had contact with a household pet. Although treatment with penicillin G cured the infection in both patients, one died following the development of nephritis and cardiac failure. The other succumbed to cerebral embolization and congestive cardiac failure.[195,196]

Available data indicate that *Pasteurella* infects previously damaged valves preferentially.[197] Congestive cardiac failure is a common complication. Surgical removal and replacement of the involved valve is required in most cases. Penicillin is the drug of choice for infections caused by these organisms. Ampicillin and ciprofloxacin inhibit the growth of *P. multocida*. The cephalosporins are often active in vitro but are less effective clinically.

Acinetobacter *Species*

The natural habitats of *Acinetobacter* are soil and water. This organism may often be recovered from sink traps, skin, the upper respiratory tract, the feces of some healthy individuals, and the hospital environment.

Three syndromes of infective endocarditis are produced by *Acinetobacter*[198–207] (Table 5.8). In the first, all patients have underlying rheumatic or congential cardiac disease. A pelvic abscess was the source of the organism in one individual and dental manipulation in another; symptoms were present for 1 month before the diagnosis was established. Cardiac failure and embolization have complicated the clinical course of the disease in more than half of the patients; 50% died shortly after the onset of the illness. The second syndrome is characterized by the manifestations of acute infective endocarditis and involves chiefly individuals with previously normal hearts. Many of these patients are addicted to the intravenous use of heroin. Embolization is common. The fatality rate in this group is 75%. In the third syndrome, the diagnosis is uncertain because of the possibility of an extracardiac source of a bacteremia in patients with recent valvular replacement. Most individuals have been treated successfully with an-

Table 5.8. Clinical Features of Patients with *Acinetobacter* Endocarditis ($n = 9$)

Mean age	31.1 yr (range, 18–52 yr)
Male:female ratio	1.5:1
Previous heart disease	56%
Predisposing events*	56%
Duration of symptoms prior to diagnosis	26 days (range, 1 day–4.5 mo)
Peripheral stigmata	67%
Splenomegaly	44%
Congestive heart failure	33%
Arterial embolization	67%
Site of involvement	
Aortic valve	67%
Mitral valve	22%
Prosthetic aortic and mitral valves	11%
Deaths	56%

*One case of heroin addiction, recent dental work, prostatitis, acute poliomyelitis with tubo-ovarian abscess.

Source: Adapted from Ref. 1.

timicrobial agents alone, despite the fact that many had prosthetic valves in place.

Infection caused by *Acinetobacter anitratum* followed a stab wound that occurred 2 weeks prior to the onset of infective endocarditis.[198] *Acinetobacter calcoaceticus* includes two subspecies, *A. anitratus* and *A. iwoffi*. The former produces acid from dextrose. These organisms are rods during rapid growth; they appear to be coccoid during the stationary phase. They are encapsulated, nonmotile, aerobic, gram-negative bacteria and often resist decolorization. Thus, they may appear to be gram-positive. *Acinetobacter* possesses no known virulence factors. It is the most common gram-negative organism that may persist on the skin of health care workers.[199] *Acinetobacter* has been a leading cause of pseudobacteremia caused by improper techniques used to culture blood.[200]

In general, subspecies of *Acinectobacter* are resistant to the penicillins, third-generation cephalosporins, and gentamicin. Resistance to tobramycin and amikacin is less common. Imipenem and the quinolones are effective. The combination of carbenicillin and gentamicin produces synergism even when mild resistance to the aminoglycosides is present.[201]

Serratia

Infections produced by the opportunistic organism *S. marcescens* occur primarily among hospitalized patients and abusers of intravenous drugs (75%)[208–226] (Table 5.9). It is responsible for about 4% of nosocomial bacteremias. The sources of this bacterium are intravenous catheters and respirators. Irradiation appears to increase the risk of invasion by this organism. Involvement of prosthetic valves is common. An interesting epidemiological phenomenon has been the relatively high incidence of this type of infective endocarditis on the West Coast of the United States, especially in San Francisco.

The clinical course of endocarditis caused by *Serratia* is most often subacute. Macroembolization, a reflection of the presence of large, friable vegetations, is common. In about one-half of the patients in whom prosthetic valves are involved, cultures of blood become positive within 3 weeks after cardiac surgery. In others, the valvular infection has been present for more than a month before the diagnosis is established. The organisms may be recovered from the bloodstream continuously over a period of 4 weeks before therapy is initiated. A new or changing murmur, progressive cardiac failure, or the appearance of peripheral manifestations of infective endocarditis are present in most patients. Endocardial infection produced by this organism has been identified only at autospy in about 30% of patients and in 15% during cardiac surgery. The disease may be complicated by valvular destruction and/or the development of contiguous myocardial abscesses. About 30% of individuals treated intravenously with single or multiple antibiotics for about 6 weeks have been cured. The combined use of carbenicillin and gentamicin is presently regarded as standard therapy for infection produced by *Serratia*.

Table 5.9. Clinical Features of Patients with *Serratia* Endocarditis (*n* = 19)

Mean age	41 yr (range, 24–72 yr)
Male:female ratio	9:10
Previous heart disease	73%
Predisposing conditions	
Drug use	37%
Prosthetic valve surgery	37%
Preceding urinary tract infection	26%
Preceding antibiotic use	47%
Others*	20%
Duration of symptoms prior to admission (medial)	2 wk
Peripheral stigmata	26%
Congestive heart failure	53%
New or changing murmur	63%
Arterial embolization	53%
Abscesses	26%
Site of involvement	
Aortic valve	11%
Mitral valve	22%
Tricuspid valve	27%
Prosthetic valves†	37%
Deaths	63%

*Infected intravenous or intra-arterial line, pneumonia, abdominal surgery, debility.
†Aortic, four; mitral, four; tricuspid, one; pulmonic, one.
Source: Adapted from Ref. 1.

Campylobacter fetus

C. fetus causes septic abortion in sheep and cattle. The organism was first recognized as a human pathogen in 1947. Since then, a few cases of infective endocarditis caused by this organism have been described.[227–231] Most involved middle-aged men with apparently normal hearts. A minority had a murmur or a history of cardiac disease. Factors that may predispose to invasion of the cardiac valves by *C. fetus* are (1) manipulation of the teeth, including extraction; (2) systemic lupus erythematosus; and (3) alcoholism. The aortic valve is usually involved. Most patients have one or more of the peripheral manifestations of endocarditis. Only a minority have significant contact with animals.

    C. fetus is a gram-negative, motile, comma-shaped rod. In contrast to *C. jejuni,* this organism produces a primary systemic illness. Both species appear to have a predilection for necrosis of vascular sites. Bacteremia with *C. fetus* is associated with a high incidence of phlebitis. Cattle and sheep are the reservoirs of this bacterium.

Streptobacillus moniliformis

The gram-negative bacillus *S. moniliformis* causes rat bite fever. Infection of the endocardium by this organism is never primary.[232–236] It usually occurs as a complication of systemic disease produced by *S. moniliformis,* which is present in the nasopharynx of rats. Haverhill fever, a type of rat bite fever, is acquired by the ingestion of milk or other food contaminated by *S. moniliformis,* a facultative, anaerobic, pleomorphic, gram-negative rod. When cultured in blood, this organism is easily identified by the presence of "puff balls" that collect at the bottom of the flask; this often requires incubation for 2 to 6 days. Hamburger and Knowles[235] have described an interesting case of infective endocarditis caused by this organism. The patient was a physician who, after being bitten by a rat, rapidly developed a cardiac murmur, arthritis, and a rash. The classical rash, mainly on the arms and legs, appeared 4 days after he was bitten. About 50% of patients develop septic arthritis or periarthritis that usually involves the knees; this resolves in a few days but may recur.

Spirillum minus

Sp. minus is an anaerobic, gram-negative, spiral organism. It also causes rat bite fever (called *sodoku* in Japan). One case of infective endocarditis produced by this organism has been reported.[236] In contrast to infection by *S. moniliformis,* arthritis is uncommon. Generalized lymphadenopathy is usually present. Fever is most often relapsing. up to 50% of patients have a false-positive reagin test for syphilis. Previously injured valves are usually the sites of infective endocarditis.

HACEK Group Organisms

The HACEK group of organisms includes *H. aphrophilus, A. actinomycetemcomitans, Cardiobacterium hominis, E. corrodens,* and *K. kingii.* These bacteria require incubation in an atmosphere rich in carbon dioxide and tend to infect human cardiac valves. All inhabit the human oropharynx.

Cardiobacterium hominis is a slowly growing (2–3 weeks), pleomorphic, gram-negative bacillus that requires carbon dioxide for multiplication[237–250] (Table 5.10). It is present in the pharnyx of 77% of healthy persons. It is part of the normal flora of the large bowel of many individuals. Most patients with infective endocarditis caused by *C. hominis* experience an indolent clinical course featured by low-grade fever. *C. hominis* usually attacks previously injured valves. Patients with this disease have had severe periodontal disease and have undergone a number of dental procedures. The characteristic features of this type of endocardial infection are nonspecific and include loss of weight, anemia, a normal sedimentation rate, and a slightly elevated peripheral white blood count. The aortic and mitral valves are equally involved. Embolization has been a significant prob-

Table 5.10. Clinical Features of Patients with *C. hominis* Endocarditis (*n* = 17)

Mean age	49.2 yr (range, 29–62 yr)
Male:female ratio	1.8:1
Previous heart disease	75%
Predisposing events	
Dental work or infection	35%
Upper respiratory infection	18%
Mean duration of symptoms	
prior to diagnosis	5.5 mo (range, 2 wk–18 mo)
Temperature > 100.5°C	94%
Peripheral stigmata	81%
Splenomegaly	62%
Congestive heart failure	62%
Arterial embolization	38%
Mycotic aneurysm	9%
Sites of involvement	
Mitral valve	43%
Aortic valve	36%
Aortic and mitral valves	7%
Other*	14%
Deaths	24%

*VSD in one, pulmonic valve in one.
Source: Adapted from Ref. 1.

lem in about 50% of patients. Medical therapy alone usually cures the disease. *C. hominis* recovered from the blood requires incubation for 5–7 days. Subculture on agar containing yeast extract yields noncorroding colonies of gram-negative bacilli.[249] *C. hominis* is distinguished from other slowly growing members of the HACEK group by a positive oxidase test and the fermentation of sugars. The organism is pleomorphic, with bulbous swelling at both ends, and forms chains, clusters, or rosettes. *C. hominis* is usually sensitive to penicillin, chloramphenicol, and the tetracyclines. Susceptibility to other antimicrobial agents varies.

Valvular disease produced by *A. actinomycetemcomitans* occurs more often in middle-aged and older men[251–266] (Table 5.11). Abnormal aortic and mitral valves are involved in about two-thirds of patients. Oral infections and dental manipulation are the predisposing factors in most cases. The clinical course of infective endocarditis is subacute and insidious. The outstanding clinical features are fever, generalized malaise, and loss of weight. The onset of the disease is rarely acute. Congestive cardiac failure and embolization may supervene. The slow multiplication of the organism in the presence of carbon dioxide delays the diagnosis. Incubation for at least 48 hr is required for growth to become visible. Successful incubation may require as long as 25 days. The bacterium is a coccobacillus and resembles various strains of *Haemophilus*. *A. actinomycetencomitans* is sensitive to third-

Table 5.11. Clinical Features of Patients with *A. antinomycetem-comitans* Endocarditis ($n = 14$)

Mean age	47.4 yr (range, 27–68 yr)
Male:female ratio	13.1:1
Previous heart disease*	86%
Predisposing conditions	
Dental procedure or	
poor dentition	43%
Recent thoracotomy	7%
Recent trauma	14%
Mean duration of symptoms	
prior to diagnosis	3.5 mo (range, 3 days–10 mo)
Oral antibiotics administered	
prior to diagnosis	57%
Fever	100%
Murmur (new or changing)	100%
Splenomegaly	71%
Peripheral stigmata	50%
Congestive heart failure	57%
Arterial embolization	43%
Site of infection	
Aortic valve	46%
Mitral valve	31%
VSD	8%
Prosthetic aortic valve	15%
Deaths	36%

*Rheumatic or congenital heart disease in 10, prosthetic aortic valve in 2.
Source: Adapted from Ref. 1.

generation cephalosporins, trimethoprim-sulfamethoxazole, aminoglycosides, chloramphenicol, quinolones, and tetracycline. The effectiveness of the penicillins varies among isolates. Erythromycin is usually of little benefit. The fatality rate due to infection caused by this organism is about 36% in patients with either native or prosthetic valves.

E. corrodens is a member of the normal microflora of the oropharynx. It is probably responsible for the frequent infections associated with dental manipulation.[267-269] Infection is also due to the intravenous or oral use of illicit drugs, especially the amphetamines. *E. corrodens* is a slowly growing, gram-negative, facultative anaerobe. The strict anaerobic strains have been assigned to the genus *Eikenella*.

All patients with infective endocarditis caused by *E. corrodens* have been more than 50 years of age and have had a prior episode of respiratory infection or dental extraction. Underlying cardiac disease has been present in all individuals. Infection of both the tricuspid and aortic valves has been found in a patient at necropsy. Prosthetic valves have been involved. Macroemboli may complicate the course of the disease. The beta-lactam antibiotics vancomycin and gentamicin are quite active against this organism.

Kingella species[270,271] are small, gram-negative rods that may be pleomorphic. An atmosphere of 5–10% carbon dioxide is required for multiplication of these organisms. Pitting of agar is characteristic. *Kingella* is a newly described genus and includes three species—*K. kingae*, *K. denitrificans*, and *K. indologenes*. These organisms were considered to be *Moraxella*-like in the past. Most cases of infective endocarditis are caused by *K. kingae*. Embolic stroke is a complication in about 25% of patients with valvular disease produced by various species of *Kingella*. All strains of the organism are senstitive to the penicillins, cephalosporins, aminoglycosides, tetracyclines, trimethoprim-sulfamethoxazole, erythromycin, and chloramphenicol.

Flavobacterium

Members of the genus *Flavobacterium* are present in water and produce orange, red, or brown pigment.[272,273] *F. meningosepticum* does not produce pigmented colonies. This strain infects patients most often, possibly due to the presence of a capsule. It has been recovered from various fluids used in hospitals (e.g., disinfectants used to flush vascular catheters). Most instances of infective endocarditis caused by this organism have been nosocomial in origin. Both prosthetic and native valves have been infected. Most isolates are sensitive to penicillin and other beta-lactam, drugs, aminoglycosides, erythromycin, tetracycline, vancomycin, clindamycin, and trimethoprim-sulfamethoxazole. Rifampin and imipenem may also be effective.

Edwardsiella tarda

E. tarda produces a gastroenteritis resembling that caused by salmonellae.[274] Bacteremia is unusual. The first case of disease caused by this organism was reported in 1976. It appears to be susceptible to most antimicrobial agents.

Citrobacter

Citrobacter species were previously included in the genus *Salmonella*. This group of organisms has been responsible for a significant number of nosocomial infections, especially in debilitated patients.[275] Among the various species in this genus, *C. diversus* appears to be the most invasive because it possesses an outer membrane. It usually causes acute aortic valvulitis. Organisms recovered from patients with infective endocarditis are sensitive to cephalothin and the aminoglycosides.

Moraxella Species

M. kingae has been assigned to the genus *Kingella*. The organisms included in this group are *M. nonliquefaciens* and *M. osloensis*.[276–286] Patients infected by these agents range in age from 4 to 77 years. Abnormal cardiac valves, ventricular septal defects, prolapsed mitral valves, and a history of a murmur are present in most patients; some do not have an underlying cardiac disorder. Congestive cardiac failure, splenic emboli, and myocardial abscesses may complicate infections produced by these organisms. This type of valvular disease has rarely been diagnosed because the organism involved is confused with other pleomorphic, gram-negative bacteria. The usual clinical course has been described as stormy. Most species of *Moraxella* are sensitive to penicillin and many other antimicrobial agents. Individual susceptibility tests are required for each isolate thought to be of clinical importance.

Aeromonas hydrophila

Endocarditis caused by *A. hydrophila* is rare.[281–283] A typical patient was a 62-year-old woman with hepatic cirrhosis who was undergoing chronic hemodialysis. She had had recent contact with flood water, a common type of exposure for infection caused by this organism. This case history emphasized the role of the reticuloendothelial system of the liver in clearing bacteremia. *Aeromonas* may produce ecthyma gangrenosum because of its pathogenicity for muscle. Members of this genus are facultative anaerobic rods that produce beta hemolysis on blood agar. Most strains are resistant to all of the penicillins but are susceptible to the third-generation cephalosporins. All are sensitive to chloramphenicol, trimethoprim-sulfamethoxazole, aztreonam, quinolones, and most of the aminoglycosides.[282]

Bordetella bronchiseptica

B. bronchiseptica is a common inhabitant of the respiratory tract and middle ear of a number of animals. It is an uncommon member of the indigenous human microflora and is usually not pathogenic for humans. This organism has rarely been involved in the pathogenesis of infective endocarditis. A published case was that of a 60-year-old man with underlying valvular disease who developed endocarditis involving two organisms, *B. bronchiseptica* and a microaerophilic staphylococcus.[283] He recovered after treatment with a combination of penicillin, streptomycin, and tetracycline.

Bacteroides and *Fusobacterium*

Various species of *Bacteroides*—nonsporulating, gram-negative, anaerobic organisms—have been involved in the pathogenesis of infective endocarditis[284-296] (Table 5.12). When anaerobic streptococci are excluded, other anaerobes account for about 1.3% of all cases of valvular disease; most common is *B. fragilis*. Other species of *Bacteroides, Fusobacterium, Clostridium,* and *Propionibacterium acnes* may be involved. Sixteen percent of the anaerobes responsible for valvular insufficiency are unclassified. Most are thought to be *B. fragilis.*

Underlying cardiac disease is present in most patients infected by *Bacteroides* or *Fusobacterium.* The clinical course is most often subacute. The fatality rate has been approximately 60%. Arterial embolization has occurred in about two-thirds of patients, possibily related to the production of heparinase by *Bacteroides.* Twenty-five percent of cases of infective endocarditis are presently caused by gram-negative anaerobes. *B. fragilis* often enters the bloodstream from the gastrointestinal tract. *B. oralis* and other species of *Bacteroides* are present in the upper respiratory tract.

Endocarditis caused by *Fusobacterium* is unusual. The clinical course of the infection is acute, in sharp contrast to infection with gram-negative anaerobes. Fusobacteria are very common inhabitants of human gingival crevices and the oropharynx. Infection of these areas, as well as the lungs, are the most frequent means by which these organisms invade the bloodstream and produce infective endocarditis.

The paucity of infective endocarditis caused by gram-negative, anaerobic, nonsporulating organisms may be related to an inappropriate oxidation-reduction potential at the intravascular sites or to the relative inability of the organism to adhere to a valvular surface. Endocarditis caused by anaerobic bacteria is fatal in 21–46% of cases. The exact incidence of infection by these bacteria is hard to ascertain because of the difficulty in culturing the more fastidious anaerobes. Except for species of *Bacteroides,* most organisms are sensitive to the penicillins.

Table 5.12. Clinical Features of Patients with *Bacteroides* Endocarditis ($n = 11$)

Mean age	42 yr (range, 18–56 yr)
Male:female ratio	7:3
Previous heart disease	78%
Predisposing conditions*	46%
Duration of symptoms prior to admission (median)	8 wk
Peripheral stigmata	91%
Congestive heart failure	36%
Arterial embolization	64%
Site of involvement	
Aortic valve	64%
Mitral valve	36%
Deaths	64%

*Periodontal disease, appendicitis, gastroenteritis, pregnancy, alcoholism.
Source: Adapted from Ref. 1.

Alcaligenes Species

Various species of *Alcaligenes* are normal inhabitants of the human respiratory and gastrointestinal tracts. Endocarditis is rarely caused by these organisms.[297,298] The most common isolate has been *A. faecalis*. The aortic valve has been involved in all reported cases. The fatality rate has been 100%. Strains of these organisms are distinguished from *Flavobacterium* and *Eikenella* by their ability to grow on MacConkey agar. They are often sensitive to trimethoprim-sulfamethoxazole and are variably sensitive to the aminoglycosides, penicillins, chephalosporins, and quinolones.

Providencia

Endocarditis caused by *Providencia* is rare.[299] Most patients have infection of the unrinary tract and noninfectious renal disease. Diabetes mellitus is often an associated illness. The fatality rate is high.

Capnocytophaga canimorsus

C. canimorsus, formerly DF-1, is a dysgonic fermenter. It is a gram-negative bacillus that grows well in blood cultures but not on MacConkey agar.[300–302] This organism usually infects splenectomized or other impaired hosts following a dog bite. Endocarditis caused by these organisms is subacute. An important clinical sign of the disease is the development of symmetrical peripheral gangrene. The antibiotic of choice for treatment is penicillin.

Gram-Negative Cocci

Megasphaera elsdenii has produced infective endocarditis.[303] The organism is a gram-negative, anaerobic coccus and is a normal inhabitant of the human gastrointestinal tract. The aortic valve has usually been involved. One report has documented the need for replacement of the infected valve with a prosthesis; this led to a cure.

Neisseria gonorrhoeae

This gonococcus was involved in 5–10% of all cases of infective endocarditis prior to the availability of effective antimicrobial therapy.[185,304] Despite the presently high prevalence of the organism, the incidence of infective endocarditis has been strikingly low even in cases in which bacteremia has complicated the genital disease. Fewer than 100 documented cases of gonococcal endocarditis have been reported in the English literature since the introduction of penicillin in 1942.[305–318] The rarity of cardiac involvement has been clearly related to the effective management of the primary gonococcal infection, even when this has been complicated by the presence of bacteremia. Currently, infective endocarditis complicates about 1–2% of cases of disseminated gonococcal infection.

Over 50% of patients with gonococcal endocarditis are men. It is striking that not all of those who developed clinical cardiac involvement suffered from genital infection. However, in most instances, involvement of the heart occurs about 3 weeks after the onset of the genital infection. The duration of symptoms prior to hospitalization has varied from 5 days to 8 weeks (average, 30 days). Gonococcal arthritis has developed in about 50% of patients; it has been the primary problem in 25%. Polyarthralgia has been less common. Most patients younger than 30 years of age have preexisting cardiac disease. The aortic valve is involved in about 50% of all patients.

The clinical course of infective endocarditis caused by *N. gonorrhoeae* is most often acute, is marked by intra- and extracardiac complications, and in many ways resembles the disease caused by *S. aureus*. One report has pointed out that the course of gonococcal endocarditis may be subacute.[317] Involvment of the right side of the heart may be relatively comon in patients with gonococcal endocarditis. A daily double spike of fever has been characteristic of the disease in about 50% of patients. Neither of these characteristics is presently considered a marker for the disease. Circulating immune complexes have been detected during active infection.

Strains of *N. gonorrhoeae* that cause disseminated disease are resistant to the bactericidal activity of human serum.[318] The organism is the AHU auxotype and is very sensitive to penicillin.

Neisseria meningitidis

This organism is presently an uncommon cause of infective endocarditis.[319] Disease produced by this organism is now easily cured even when meningococcemia, meningitis, or metastatic disease is present. In untreated patients the disease is acute in onset and progresses rapidly to death due to profound vascular collapse. In resembles infection caused by *S. aureus* and may lead to the development of several types of cardiac complications, including myocardial abscesses, myocarditis, pericarditis, and myopericarditis. These appear to be produced by immunological processes. The meningococcus may also infect prosthetic valves.[319]

"*Nonpathogenic*" Neisseria

Among the "nonpathogenic" species *Neisseria* that may be involved in the pathogenesis of endocarditis are *N. flava, N. mucosa, N. pharyngis,* and *N. sicca; Barnhamella catarrhalis* may also be involved.[320] Three patients with endocarditis caused by *N. mucosa* have been reported; in two cases, disease followed dental extraction with penicillin prophylaxis.[321,322] Endocardial disease caused by *N. sicca* has been identified in seven patients 14–27 years of age.[323–329] Four had no underlying cardiac disorders; two had rheumatic heart disease; and the third had had a mitral valvular prosthesis. The onset of infective endocarditis is always acute. Embolic phenomena were almost universal. In general, infections involved prosthetic valves or previously damaged native valves. All the organisms were sensitive to penicillin.

Branhamella catarrhalis

B. catarrhalis has been an uncommon cause of infective endocarditis.[320] This organism was initially sensitive to all the beta-lactam antibiotics. However, it now produces lactamases that destroy the activity of the penicillins. The endocardial disease caused by *B. catarrhalis* requires treatment with a cephalosporin or a combination of a penicillin and clavulanic acid or sulbactam inhibitors of beta-lactamase.

Yeasts and Fungi

In 1950, Zimmerman predicted an increase in the incidence of infections caused by *Aspergillus* and other fungi because of the widespread use of antimicrobial and cytotoxic agents.[330] Experience over the past 45 years has confirmed this statement. Among the factors that lead to disease produced by these organisms are (1) prolonged exposure to antimicrobial agents and corticosteroids; (2) cardiac surgery; (3) addiction to the intravenous use of narcotics; (4) tracheal intubation; (5) abortion; (6) gynecological procedures; (7) urethral and dental manipulations; and (8) burns.[331] Various species of *Candida* and *Histoplasma* have been responsible for most instances of endocardial disease.[331] However, other yeasts and fungi, *Blastomyces, Coccidioides, Aspergillus, Cryptococcus,* and *Mucor* have also been involved in the pathogenesis of endocarditis.[332–357]

Various species of *Candida* have been involved most often in infection of natural and prosthetic cardiac valves. Prior to 1945, only three patients with candidal valvular disease had been reported; two were addicted to narcotics. Since 1958, *C. albicans* has been the organism most often involved.[331,346] This is probably related to an increase in both drug addiction and cardiac surgery.

C. parapsilosis, C. guilliermondii, C. krusei, C. stellatodiae, and *C. tropicalis* cause disseminated disease.[338–340] One-third of all episodes of infective endocarditis produced by these organisms has followed open heart surgery. About 25% of patients develop suprainfections during antibiotic treatment. The mitral valve has been involved most often.[358] A left atrial myxoma infected by *Candida* has been reported.[359]

Endocardial disease caused by *Candida* is usually diagnosed during life. These organisms have been recovered from cultures of blood in about 75% of patients. Vascular trauma induced by intravenous lines establishes a portal of entry for the organism. Low-grade infection may persist for as long as 5–10 weeks before the infection is identified. Embolic occlusion of intracranial vessels develops in about 50% of patients.[357] Myocardial microabscesses are common and cause disturbances in electrical conduction.[358]

The presence of candidal disease must be considered when individuals with known systemic fungal infections exhibit the clinical manifestations of infective endocarditis. This is especially the case when a cardiac murmur is audible, when embolization of large vessels has occurred, or when manifestations suggesting valvular disease are present but cultures of the blood are sterile. Because the valvular vegetations invaded by *Candida* are large, emboli (average diameter, 1.5–5 cm) often occlude arteries, especially those in the legs. Yeasts and hyphal elements have been identified in emboli removed from blood vessels and infarcted organs. In some instances, this is the only basis on which the diagnosis of endocarditis is established.

Infective endocarditis caused by true fungi rarely involves normal native valves. In most instances, valvular prostheses have been infected. Various species of *Aspergillus* have produced disease in about one-third of individuals with infected prosthetic valves. *A. fumigatus* is involved most often. *C. albicans* accounts for one-third of the cases of fungal endocarditis following cardiac surgery. Nine cases of mural endocarditis caused by *Aspergillus* have been reported.[360–363] This disease has also occurred in immunosuppressed individuals and in those with severe debilitating disorders. All had been treated with broad-spectrum antimicrobial drugs, cytotoxic agents, or corticosteroids, or had undergone endotracheal intubation or repeated surgical procedures. Other factors that predispose patients to invasion by *Aspergillus* are uremia and gram-negative bacterial sepsis. The most likely source of the fungi that invade the heart during open cardiac surgery appears to be the air in the operating room. The presence of a foreign body, such as a prosthetic valve, may interfere with the ability of the normal defense mechanisms to clear the organisms before they multiply, invade, and produce infection.[363] The classical peripheral manifestations of infective endocarditis or large embolic occlusions have not been observed in these individuals. The presence of myocardial abscesses may lead to the development of cardiac arrhythmias.[364] Cultures of the blood of patients with aspergillotic valvular infection are almost always sterile. The clinical course of this disease is usually subacute and always fatal.

Individuals with infective endocarditis caused by *Histoplasma capsulatum* live in the eastern United States or the Mississippi Valley. Splenomegaly is present in 50% and anemia in 75% of these cases. Leukopenia is a problem in 10% and microscopic hematuria in 50%. A study of 22 individuals infected by this organism[365] disclosed that the aortic valve alone was involved in 10 and the mitral valve in 5 patients; both valves were infected in 2 patients. The presence of cardiac disease is not a prerequisite for valvular infection in elderly patients. Embolic occlusion of large arteries is an important marker for infective endocarditis caused by *H. capsulatum*.

Most patients with disease caused by *H. capsulatum* were described prior to the availability of amphotericin and the surgical replacement of infected valves. The results of recent studies have indicated that five patients with infection caused by this organism recovered when they were treated with amphotericin.[366,367]

Among other fungi involved in the pathogenesis of infective endocarditis are *Penicillium, Phialophora, Hormodendium, Pacilomyces, Curbiluca, Saccharomyces, Mucor, Torulopsis glabrata, Cryptococcus,* and *Trichosporon cutaneum.*[329–332,368–371]

Mycobacteria

Mycobacteria rarely cause infective endocarditis. However, these organisms may invade normal or prosthetic valves and valvular homografts. Three species—*Mycobacterium chelonei, M. fortuitum,* and *M. gordonae*—are known to cause infective endocarditis.[372–377] Eight of 16 porcine valves cultured by Laskowski et al.[373] before they were implanted in patients grew *M. chelonei.* The authors suggested that the organism was present prior to removal of the valve or was contaminated after it was removed and placed in 2% glutaraldehyde, a nonmycobactericidal solution. In a similar study, Tyras et al.[374] retrieved the tubercle bacillus from 8 of 20 porcine xenografts that had been inserted in patients. Isolation of the organism required 2 to 3 weeks of incubation in thioglycolate broth. Clinical evidence of infection in patients developed 5 months after insertion of the porcine graft. Tubercle bacilli were recovered from the pericardium and pericardial fluid. It has been suggested that porcine grafts be cultured for at least 3 weeks prior to placement.[373,374] Appropriate antimicrobial therapy should be initiated only when there is clear-cut evidence of infective endocarditis.

Endocarditis caused by *M. tuberculosis* is very rare and involves only native valves. It usually develops as a complication of disseminated tuberculosis, or it may spread from initial sites of infection such as pericarditis or myocardial abscess.[378–380] Studies at autospy have disclosed endocardial miliary tubercles and tuberculomas on a cavitated valve.

It has been reported that *M. tuberculosis* may invade homograft valves.[381] Of 800 patients who received these grafts, *M. tuberculosis* was identified in the lesions of 6. This was probably a complication of disseminated (miliary) tuberculosis. Symptoms of the disease may appear within a few weeks or as long as 1 year postoperatively.

Rickettsiae

Marmion et al.[382] suggested in 1953 that *Coxiella burnetii,* the causative agent of Q fever, may produce a chronic form of infective endocarditis in patients with underlying cardiac disease. Valvular infections caused by this organism were first described 6 years later.[383] Since then, more than 200 cases of the disease have been reported.[384–397] All have been associated with complications characteristic of systemic disease. Most patients with this form of endocarditis have lived in Australia, New Zealand, and Great Britain. The disease also occurs in the United States.[393]

The clinical presentation of infective endocarditis caused by *C. burnetii* has been remarkably uniform.[384,385] The patients involved have ranged in age from 27 to 70 years; most have been men in the fifth decade of life. The male:female ratio is 6:1; this may be related to the occupations of the patients. The duration of fever prior to the establishment of the diagnosis of infective endocarditis has been as short as 1 year and as long as 20 years. Infected animals, parturient cats, and unpasteurized milk have been the sources of the organism. The most common underlying cardiac disorders are rheumatic fever and congestive cardiac failure. The aortic valve is involved in about 80%, the mitral valve in 25%, and both in 6% of patients.[385] Infection of prosthetic valves by *C. burnetii* has been reported.[394–397] The onset of illness has usually been insidious. Nonspecific symptoms of infection are present before the manifestations of infective endocarditis become apparent. The infected valves are often calcified and the vegetations necrotic. Aneurysms of the aortic wall at the base of the leaflets are common. The clinical course of infection involving prosthetic valves has been characterized by varying degrees of fever, malaise, clubbing of the fingers, petechiae, congestive cardiac failure, changing cardiac murmurs, and embolic phenomena. Hematuria, hepatosplenomegaly, and hepatitis are uncommon in endocarditis of prosthetic valves.

The diagnosis of this disease is established either by isolation of *C. burnetii* from valvular vegtations or by a significantly high titer of phase 1, complement-fixing antibody. Specific immunofluorescent antibody staining of tissue obtained by biopsy may be of diagnostic value.

Actinomyces

Infective endocarditis caused by *Actinomyces* is rare. The species involved are *A. israelii (bovis)*, *Nocardia israelii,* and *N. asteroides.*[398–401] Most cases of nocardial valvular infection involve patients with cardiac prostheses.

Less than 2% of cases of actinomycosis involve the heart. The incidence of cardiac infection in patients with underlying thoracic disease is 75%. The pericardium is involved most often (79%) and is the site from which the disease spreads to the endocardium and aortic valves (35%). This organism seldom invades the valves. The bloodstream is rarely the source of valvular infection.

Chlamydia Species

In 1974, Ward and Ward[402] suggested that the organism responsible for psittacosis might cause infective endocarditis. They studied seven patients with valvular infection who had had documented contact with birds. Although they identified circulating antibody to *Chlamydia psittaci,* they failed to isolate the organism. Stains of an endocardial biopsy specimen with fluorescein-labeled specific antibody produced a positive reaction in the aortic valve in two patients but only in the left atrium in five. Regan et al.[403] reported a case of valvular disease in which serological studies suggested the presence of chlamydial disease. However, the organism was not recovered and an endocardial biopsy was not obtained. Jariwalla et al.[404] studied a patient with infective endocarditis involving the aortic valve in which *C. psittaci* was identified by electron microscopy. A positive reaction developed when the infected valve was stained with antibody specific for *C. psittaci*.

Most cases of psittacosis follow contact with psittacine birds. Other vectors, including cats, have been proposed. The organism usually invades previously damaged valves and runs a subacute course. The fatality rate remains high (40%) despite appropriate antimicrobial therapy and replacement of the infected valve.[405] The diagnosis of psittacosis is established most often by the detection of specific complement-fixing antibodies.

A patient with infective endocarditis caused by *Chlamydia trachomatis*, in which the left coronary cusp of the aoritc valve and pericardium were involved, has been reported.[406] *Chlamydia pneumoniae* (TWAR agent) has been reported to cause endocardial disease.[407]

Cell Wall–Deficient Organisms

The possibility that cell wall–deficient organisms (protoplasts, spheroplasts, L-forms) may play an important role in human disease has been suggested for may years.[408–410] Four criteria for their identification and their relation to specific infections have been suggested by Charache:[411] (1) typical morphology in stained preparations; (2) failure to grow on routine media; (3) reversion to classical morphology; and (4) consistency of the isolate with the patient's disease. Several cases of infective endocarditis thought to be caused by cell wall–deficient organisms (*persisters*) have been described.[412–418] These have been characterized by persistent fever in the absence of bacteremia during and after treatment with penicillin. This antibiotic has been thought to convert normal to cell wall–deficient organisms. Whether or not these microbes are responsible for negative routine blood cultures in patients with prolonged fever is still not clear.

Electron microscopy of the valvular vegetations in four patients with endocarditis disclosed not only morphologically normal organisms but also cell wall–deficient forms. The latter predominated in three patients.[411]

Viruses

The role of viral infection in the pathogenesis of infective endocarditis has been the subject of investigation for years.[419] Experimental studies by Burch and colleagues have indicated that coxsackie B virus and adenoviruses can produce endocarditis in mice.[420–423] The role of these agents in the pathogenesis of infective endocarditis in human has not been proved.

HIV viruses may produce a number of cardiac abnormalities, including pericarditis and pericardial effusion. Right ventricular or biventricular dysfunction of unknown etiology has been reported.[424] Marasmic valvular vegetations are very common in patients with AIDS.[425]

Polymicrobial Endocarditis

Polymicrobial infections of cardiac valves have been reported by a number of investigators.[426,427] In 86 patients with subacute endocarditis studied by Pankey from 1939 to 1959, 5.4% had disease in which at least two organisms were involved; a streptococcus was present in every case.[428] In contrast, mixed bacterial valvulitis was present in only 1 of 250 individuals who came to the attention of Dale and Geraci over a period of 10 years.[284]

Saravolatz and his colleagues reviewed 203 cases of infective endocarditis admitted to the Henry Ford Hospital between 1953 and 1969.[429] From 1976 to 1978, nine individuals were found to have valvular infection caused by multiple organisms. All the patients were men and were 24 to 39 years old (mean, 28 years). Heroin addiction was a problem in all but one. Eight individuals had no previous history of cardiac disease; two had undergone surgery, one for the repair of an atrial septal defect and the other for replacement of an aortic valve. The average duration of symptoms prior to diagnosis was 16 days (range, 3–35 days). Septic pulmonary emboli were present in two individuals. Murmurs were present in seven patients when they entered the hospital; the others developed this in the first 24 hr after admission. Few had any of the peripheral stigmata of endocarditis. Insufficiency of the tricuspid and mitral valves was common. Aortic regurgitation was present in one case, and combined tricuspid and mitral insufficiency in another.

Ps. aeruginosa has been the organism most often involved in the pathogenesis of polymicrobial endocarditis.[427] Other bacteria—*S. faecalis, S. aureus, H. influenzae, H. parainfluenzae,* and *S. epidermidis*—are less common. Four species of streptococci were involved in one patient. The most comon combination of organisms has been *S. faecalis* and *Ps. aeruginosa* (two cases). In a review of 31 instances of polymicrobial endocarditis, Saravolatz and his colleagues[429] noted that 81% occurred in heroin addicts and 14% in patients who had undergone cardiac surgery. The organisms involved most often were *S. aureus* (about 50%), *Candida,* non–group D. streptococci, *Ps. aeruginosa,* and *Serratia.*

The incidence of polymicrobial infective endocarditis increased sharply during the 1980s.[426] The disease involved young individuals most often and was about twice as common in men as in women. Fifty percent of drug addicts had infections of the tricuspid value; one-third developed septic pulmonary emboli. Patients with bacteremia caused by multiple organisms were twice as likely to die as those infected by a single agent.

Fifty-two percent of all patients with polymicrocial infective endocarditis have required cardiac surgery dispite aggressive medical treatment; the fatality rate has been 32%. The increasing incidence of polymicrobial valvulitis appears to be related to the increasingly frequency of cardiac surgery and the intravenous use of narcotics and other drugs.

Microbiology of Infected Prosthetic Valves

Many microbial genera and species have been involved in the pathogenesis of infection of prosthetic cardiac valves.[428,430] Most of the organisms have been identical to those that invade native valves; some have infected only valvular prostheses. For example, *S. aureus, S. epidermidis,* various streptococci, *Haemophilus, Brucella,* and *Candida* species may invade natural and prosthetic valves. Among the gram-negative bacteria that infect valvular prostheses are *Serratia, Acinetobacter caloaceticus, Ps. cepacia, Ps. aeruginosa, Ps. malthophila, Flavobacterium, Bacteroides, Ed. tarda* and *E. corrodens.* Coagulase-negative staphylococci (CONS) infect prosthetic valves more often than natural ones and cause infection early in the postoperative period. Endocarditis of prosthetic valves caused by staphylococci develops most often within 60 days after surgery, followed by disease due to nonenterococcal streptococci (19%) and *S. aureus* (10%). Both staphylococci and streptococci have been involved more often in patients in whom infection occurred late in the course of the disease. CONS are involved more frequently in the early stage of prosthetic valve endocarditis; streptococci are more common in the late stage of the disease. Gram-negative organisms and fungi produce infection at the same rate in early and late disease.

A study of prosthetic valve endocarditis (PVE) by Karchmer et al.[431] indicated that methicillin resistance was present in 87% of CONS recovered from prosthetic valves within a year after surgery; this decreased to 22% after 1 year. They suggested that 1 year was the period that separates early from late PVE.

Most instances of valvular infection caused by *Propionibacterium acnes, Bacteroides* species, and *E. corrodens* have occurred in patients with cardiac prostheses. Endocarditis caused by atypical mycobacteria, such as *M. chelonei* and *M. gordonae,* has involved only valvular prostheses.[372–374,377]

The documented increase in the incidence of infective endocarditis caused by yeast and fungi appears to be limited to valvular prostheses and patients addicted to intravenous drugs.[331,334] *Candida* and *Aspergillus* are involved most often. Among the species of *Candida* recovered from infected prostheses have been *C. albicans, C. parapsilosis, C. tropicalis, C. stellatoidea, C. krusei,* and *Torulopsis glabrata.* More than 40 cases of aspergillotic prosthetic valvulitis have been reported. Among the species involved have been *A. fumigatus, A. flavus, A. niger, A. austus, A. terrai, A. glaucus,* and *A. sydowi.*[344] Cultures of blood have been sterile in more than 95% of patients.

Other fungi recovered from infected cardiac prostheses have been *Paecilomyces variota, Penicillium, Philophlora mutabilis, Cryptococcus, Hormodendrum, Mucor, Histoplasma, Curvilacea,* and *Acremonium.*[432,433] Many infections of prosthetic valves, especially those caused by uncommon bacteria, yeasts, and fungi, are suprainfections that develop in the course of antimicrobial chemoprophylaxis and/or chemotherapy.[332] Introduction of organisms into the bloodstream during the intravenous use of narcotics is another important factor.

Culture-Negative Infective Endocarditis

Almost from the time infective endocarditis was recognized as a clinical entity,[434] persistent sterile blood cultures of patients have been a problem. Blood cultures presently fail to detect organisms in about 7.5% of presumed infective endocarditis. A better term for this disease may be *apparent culture-negative endocarditis.* The reasons for apparently sterile cultures of blood are (1) treatment prior to diagnosis; (2) the presence of fastidious, slow-growing organisms; (3) infection by agents other than bacteria; (4) right-sided endocarditis; (5) mural endocardial infection in patients with a ventricular septal defect; (6) postmyocardial infarction; (7) the presence of pacemaker wires; (8) the presence of uremia; and (9) blood cultures obtained 3 months after the onset of symptoms (Table 5.13). Antigen–antibody complexes may make it difficult to culture organisms.[435–437] Among noninfectious diseases that may involve the endocardium are atrial myxoma, rheumatic fever, marantic endocarditis, endocardial fibroelastosis, fibroplastic endocarditis (Loeffler's endocarditis), carcinoid syndrome, neoplasms, and Libman-Sacks disease (Table 5.14).

Pasanti and Smith[436] have pointed out that many patients with sterile cultures of the blood may experience significant embolic episodes and congestive cardiac failure. This binding may be of great concern in individuals

Table 5.13. Categories of Apparent Culture-Negative Endocarditis

1.	Noninfective endocarditis
2.	Prior antimicrobial treatment
3.	"Fastidious" bacteria
4.	Q fever
5.	Fungi
6.	Acid-fast bacteria
7.	Chlamydia
8.	? L forms of bacteria
9.	? Virus
10.	Right-sided endocarditis
11.	Uremia

Source: Adapted from Van Scoy RE: Culture-negative endocarditis. *Mayo Clin Proc* 1982; 57:150.

Table 5.14. Noninfective Endocardial Diseases

1. Myxoma
2. Rheumatic fever
3. Lupus nonbacterial verrucous endocarditis
   4. Marantic endocarditis
5. Endocardial fibroelastosis
6. Fibroplastic endocarditis (Loeffler's disease)
   7. Carcinoid

Source: Adapted from Van Scoy RE: Culture-negative endocarditis. *Mayo Clin Proc* 1982;57:150.

with a sterile prosthetic valve. Its importance has been emphasized by the results of a study of two individuals with prolonged fever and many "sterile" cultures of the blood. When it was thought that the clinical course was not consistent with the postpericardiotomy syndrome, the patients were treated with corticosteroids. Although they defervesced and improved clinically, cultures of the blood grew *S. epidermidis* after treatment was initiated. It is clear that the use of anti-inflammatory agents in patients with a prosthetic valve, may mask symptoms and signs and interfere with critical host responses.[438]

References

1. Cohen P, Maguire J, Weinstein L: Infective endocarditis caused by gram-negative bacteria: A review of the literature, 1945–1977. *Prog Cardiovasc Dis* 1980;22:205.
2. Cherubin C, Neu H: Infective endocarditis at the Presbyterian Hospital in New York City from 1938–1967. *Am J Med* 1977;51:83.
3. Snyder N, Allerbury C, Correira J, et al: Increased occurrence of cirrhosis and bacterial endocarditis. *Gastroenterology* 1977;73:1107.
4. Geraci J, Wilson W: Endocarditis due to gram-negative bacteria: Report of 56 cases. *Mayo Clin Proc* 1982;57:145.
5. Finland M, Barnes M: Changing etiology of bacterial endocarditis in the antibacterial era: Experience at Boston City Hospital 1933–1965. *Ann Intern Med* 1972;72:341.
6. Carruthers M: Endocarditis due to entericbacilli other than salmonellae: Case reports and literature review. *Am J Med Sci* 1977;273:203.
7. Pelletier L, Petersdorf R: Infective endocarditis: A review of 125 cases from the University of Washington Hospitals, 1963–1972. *Medicine* 1977;56:287.
8. Reisberg B: Infective endocarditis in the narcotic addict. *Prog Cardiovasc Dis* 1979;22:193.
9. Neufeld G, Branson C, Marshall A, et al: Infective endocarditis as a complication of heroin use. *South Med J* 1976;69:1148.
10. Thadepalli H, Francis CK: Diagnostic clues in metastatic lesions of endocarditis in addicts. *West J Med* 1978;128:1.
11. Archer G, Fekety F, Supena R: *Pseudomonas aeruginosa* endocarditis in drug addicts. *Am Heart J* 1974;88:570.
12. Fowle A. Zorab P: *Escherichia coli* endocarditis successfully treated with oral trimethoprim and sulfamethoxazole. *Br Heart J* 1970;32:127.

13. Rosen P, Armstrong D: Infective endocarditis in patients treated for malignant neoplastic diseases: A post-mortem study. *Am J Clin Pathol* 1973;59:241.
14. Griffin R Jr, Jones G, Cobbs C: Aortic insufficiency in bacterial endocarditis. *Ann Intern Med* 1972;76:23.
15. Fletcher D: *Bacillus coli* endocarditis: Review of the literature with report of a case. *Am Heart J* 1947;34:743.
16. Hansing C, Allen V, Cherry J: *Escherichia coli* endocarditis: A review of the literature and a case study. *Arch Intern Med* 1967;120:472.
17. Love J, Powell C, Strunk W, et al: Acute bacterial endocarditis of *Escherichia coli* origin: Streptomycin treatment. *Naval Med Bull* 1949;49:1070.
18. Meneely J Jr: Bacterial endocarditis following urethral manipulation: Report of two cases. *N Engl J Med* 1948;239:708.
19. Hoffman M, Wellman W, Sayre G: *Escherichia coli* endocarditis: Report of a case. *Mayo Clin Proc* 1951;26:1.
20. Ross C, Wheeler J, Hagemann P: *Escherichia coli* endocarditis: Report of a case presenting a difficult problem in chemotherapy. *Arch Intern Med* 1952;90:258.
21. Smith A: Endocarditis due to *Escherichia coli*. *N Engl J Med* 1950;243:129.
22. Castleman B, McNeely B: Case 45-1970: Presentation of a case. *N Engl J Med* 1970;283:982.
23. Castleman B, McNeely B: Case 29-1971: Presentation of a case. *N Engl J Med* 1971;285:220.
24. Stanton R, Lindesmith G, Meyer B: *Escherichia coli* endocarditis after repair of ventricular septal defects. *N Engl J Med* 1968;279:737.
25. Taniguchi T, Murphy F: Clinical notes, suggestions and new instruments. *JAMA* 1950;143:427.
26. Satterwhite T, McGee Z, Schaffner W, et al: Infection of an avulsed papillary muscle tip simulating bacterial endocarditis. *Am Heart J* 1973;86:107.
27. Wallace A, Young W Jr, Osterhout S: Treatment of acute bacterial endocarditis by valve excision and replacement. *Circulation* 1965;31:450.
28. Robertston T: Paracolon bacillus endocarditis of the pulmonic valve secondary to infected polycystic kidneys. *Arch Pathol* 1947;43:318.
29. Friedman I, Goldin M: Paracolon endocarditis. *Am J Clin Pathol* 1949;19:840.
30. Simberkoff M, Isom W, Smithivas T, et al: Two-stage tricuspid valve replacement for mixed bacterial endocarditis. *Arch Intern Med* 1974;133:212.
31. Corliss R: Gram-negative septicemia, including a case of acute endocarditis. *Wisc Med J* 1964;63:144.
32. Sussman L, Cohen I, Freund A: Acute *Aerobacter aerogenes* endocarditis complicating genitourinary tract infection. *NY State Med J* 1950;50:583.
33. Stringer P: Bacterial endocarditis and urology. *Br Med J* 1965;1:1072.
34. Wallace CS: Case reports: Bacterial endocarditis with emphasis on the *Escherichia-Aerobacter* group as the causative agent: Report of a fatal case. *Ann Intern Med* 1951; 34:1563.
35. Bashour F, Winchell C: Right-sided bacterial endocarditis. *Am J Med Sci* 1960;240: 411.
36. Iannani P, Huff S, Quintiliani R: Severe sepsis from *Enterobacter*. *Arch Surg* 1960; 107:854.
37. Lerer R: Postoperative endocarditis due to *Enterobacter cloacae*. *Am J Dis Child* 1973;126:352.
38. Weinstein L, Rubin R: Infective endocarditis—1973. *Prog Cardiovasc Dis* 1973;16: 239.
39. Menda K, Borbach S: Favorable experience with bacterial endocarditis in heroin addicts. *Ann Intern Med* 1973;78:25.
40. Banks T, Fletcher R, Ali N: Infective endocarditis in heroin addicts. *Am J Med* 1973;55:444.
41. Lutgens W: Endocarditis in "main line" opium addicts. *Arch Intern Med* 1949;83: 653.

42. Reyes M, Brown W, Lerner A: Treatment of patients with *Pseudomonas* endocarditis with high dose aminoglycoside and carbenicillin therapy. *Medicine* 1978;57:57.

43. Arbulu A, Thoms N, Wilson R: Valvulectomy without prosthetic replacement: A life-saving operation for tricuspid *Pseudomonas* endocarditis. *J Thorac Cardiovasc Surg* 1972;64:103.

44. Bryan C, Marney S, Alford R, et al: Gram-negative bacillary endocarditis: Interpretation of the serum bactericidal test. *Am J Med* 1975;58:209.

45. Diaz C, Fossieck B, Parker R: *Pseudomonas* endocarditis: Cure with carbenicillin and polymyxin B. *South Med J* 1977;60:869.

46. Cooper R, Leach R, Noble R: *Pseudomonas* endocarditis in a heroin addict. *J KY Med Assoc* 1976;74:135.

47. Yoshikawa T, Bayer A, Guze L: Endocarditis due to *Pseudomonas aeruginosa* in a heroin addict: Successful treatment with trimethoprim-sulfamethoxazole mixture plus colistin. *Chest* 1977;794:796.

48. Black S, L'Rourke R, Karliner J: Role of surgery in the treatment of primary infective endocarditis. *Am J Med* 1975;56:357.

49. Sparagana M, Rubnitz M, Grieble H, et al: Fever, heart murmur and hemiparesis in heroin addict. *Postgrad Med* 1984;55:193.

50. Pazin G, Peterson K, Griff F, et al: Determination of site of infection in endocarditis. *Ann Intern Med* 1975;82:746.

51. Kramer N, Gill S, Patel R, et al: Pulmonary valve vegetations detected with echocardiography. *Am J Cardiol* 1987;39:1064.

52. Robinson O, Hoopers E, Conn J, et al: Acute bacterial endocarditis in a burned patient. *Ann Surg,* 1964;30:617.

53. Teitel M, Florman A: Postoperative endocarditis due to *Pseudomonas aeruginosa. JAMA* 1960;172:329.

54. Brunsdon D, Entricknap J, Milstein B: A case of bacterial endocarditis due to *Pseudomonas pyocyanea* complicating valvulotomy for advanced mitral stenosis. *Guy Hosp Rep* 1953; 102:303.

55. Uthman S, Uwaydah M: A successfully treated case of *Pseudomonas* endocarditis with review of the literature. *Lab Med J* 1967;20:245.

56. Stanley M: *Bacillus pyocyaneus* infections: A review and report of cases and discussion of newer therapy, including streptomycin. *Am J Med* 1947;2:253.

57. Demuth W, Rawson A: *Pseudomonas* septicemia and endocarditis. *Am J Med Sci* 1948; 216:195.

58. Coller F, Dyer D: Acute bacterial endocarditis due to *Pseudomonas aeruginosa*—Report of a case. *AMA Arch Pathol* 1981;51:179.

59. Littlefield J, Muller W, Damman J: Successful treatment of *Pseudomonas aeruginosa* septicemia following total aortic valve replacement. *Circulation* 1965;31–32(Suppl 1): 103.

60. Carruthers M, Kanokvechayant R: *Pseudomonas aeruginosa* endocarditis: Report of a case, with review of the literature. *Medicine* 1973;55:811.

61. Hunter T: Use of streptomycin in the treatment of bacterial endocarditis. *Am J Med* 1947;2:436.

62. Waisbren B, Hastings E: Bacterial endocarditis due to *Pseudomonas aeruginosa. Arch Pathol* 1953;55:218.

63. Hodges R, Alvarez R: Puerperal septicemia and endocarditis caused by *Pseudomonas aeruginosa. JAMA* 1960;173:1081.

64. Pressman R, Geczy M, Maranhao V, et al: Successful treatment of bacterial endocarditis due to *Pseudomonas aeruginosa. Am J Cardiol* 1966;17:97.

65. Linde L, Heins H: Bacterial endocarditis following surgery for congenital heart disease. *N Engl J Med* 1960;263:65.

66. Curtin J, Petersdorf R, Bennett I: Acquired arteriovenous fistula complicated by *Pseudomonas aeruginosa* endarteritis and endocarditis. *Bull Johns Hopkins Hosp* 1957; 101:140.

67. Witchitz S, Gilbert C, Witchitz J, et al: *Pseudomonas aeruginosa* endocarditis: A report of nine cases. *Eur J Cardiol* 1976;4:91.
68. Lloyd K, Gordon J: Bacterial endocarditis due to *Pseudomonas aeruginosa. Ann Intern Med* 1961;55:814.
69. Uman S, Johnson C, Beirne G, et al: *Pseudomonas aeruginosa* bacteremia in a dialysis unit. I. Recognition of cases, epidemiologic studies and attempts at control. *Am J Med* 1977;62:667.
70. Beckwith J, Wood J, Muller W: Postoperative endoauriculitis due to *Pseudomonas aeruginosa* cured by a second operation. *Trans Am Clin Climatol Assoc* 1960;72:1.
71. Geraci J: The antibiotic therapy of bacterial endocarditis. *Med Clin North Am,* 1958;42:1101.
72. Geraci J, Dale A, McGoon D: Bacterial endocarditis and endarteritis following cardiac operations. *Wisc Med J* 1963;62:302.
73. Kenoyer W, Stone C, Levin W: Bacterial endocarditis due to *Pseudomonas aeruginosa* treated with neomycin. *Am J Med* 1952;13:108.
74. Firor W: Infection following open-heart surgery with special reference to the role of prophylactic antibiotics. *J Thorac Cardiovasc Surg* 1967;53:371.
75. Sykes C, Beckwith J, Wood J: Postoperative endoauriculitis due to *Pseudomonas aeruginosa* cured by a second operation. *Arch Intern Med* 1966;110:151.
76. Weiland M, Federman M, Kline-King C, et al: Left-sided endocarditis due to *Pseudomonas aeruginosa:* A report of 10 cases and review of the literature. *Medicine* 1986;65:180.
77. Stratton C: *Pseudomonas aeruginosa* revisited: 1990 Infection control. *Hosp Epidemiol* 101:190.
78. Woods D, Iglewski B: Toxins of *Pseudomonas aeruginosa:* New perspectives. *Rev Infect Dis* 1983;5:8715.
79. Liu P: Extracellular toxins of *Pseudomanas aeruginosa. J Infect Dis* 1974;130(Suppl 1):197.
80. Doring J, Maier M, Muller E, et al: Virulence factors of *Pseudomonas aeruginosa. Antimicrob Agents Chemother* 1987;39:136.
81. Nicas J, Bradley J, Forkner J, et al: The role of exoenzymes in infection with *Pseudomonas aeruginosa. J Infect Dis* 1905;152:716.
82. Young F: Human immunity to *Pseudomonas aeruginosa*— I. In vitro interaction of bacterial, polymorphonuclear leukocytes and serum factors. *J Infect Dis* 1972;126:257.
83. Schwartzmann S, Boring J III: Antiphagocytic effect of slime from a mucoid strain of *Pseudomonas aeruginosa. Infect Immunol* 1971;3:762.
84. Daggett R, Harrison G, Carter J: Mucoid *Pseudomonas aeruginosa* in patients with chronic illnesses. *Lancet* 1971;1:236.
85. Levine D, Crane L, Zemos N: Bacteremia in narcotic addicts at a Detroit medical center: II. Infective endocarditis: A prospective comparative study. *Rev Infect Dis* 1986;8:371.
86. Tuazon C, Sheagren J: Staphylococcal endocarditis in parenteral drug abusers: Source of the organism. *Ann Intern Med* 1975;82:788.
87. Yu V, Rumans L, Wing E, et al: *Pseudomonas maltophilia* causing heroin-associated infective endocarditis. *Arch Intern Med* 1978;138:1667.
88. Yeh T, Anabtawi I, Cornett V, et al: Bacterial endocarditis following open-heart surgery. *Ann Thorac Surg* 1967;3:29.
89. Buckely M: Late prosthetic valve endocarditis: Clinical features influencing therapy. *Am J Med* 1978;64:199.
90. Dismukes W, Karchmer A, Buckley M, et al: Prosthetic valve endocarditis: Analysis of 38 cases. *Circulation* 1973;48:365.
91. Fischer J: *Pseudomonas maltophilia* endocarditis after replacement of the mitral valve: A case study. *J Infect Dis* 1985;10(Suppl 1):S721.
92. Senel J: *Pseudomonas maltophilia* pseudosepticemia. *Am J Med* 1978;64:403.
93. Hamilton J, Burch W, Grimmett G, et al: Successful treatment of *Pseudomonas cepacia* endocarditis with trimethoprim-sulfamethoxazole. *Antimicrob Ag Chemother* 1973;4:551.

94. Neu H, Garvey G, Beach M: Successful treatment of *Pseudomonas cepacia* endocarditis in a heroin addict with trimethoprim-sulfamethoxazole. *J Infect Dis* 1973;128:768.
95. Mandell I, Feiner H, Prince N, et al: *Pseudomonas cepacia* endocarditis and ecthyma gangrenosum. *Arch Dermatol* 1977;113:199.
96. Seligman S, Madhavan T, Alcid D: Trimethoprim-sulfamethoxazole in the treatment of bacterial endocarditis. *J Infect Dis* 1973;128:757.
97. Noriega E, Rubinstein E, Simberkoff M, et al: Subacute and acute endocarditis due to *Pseudomonas cepacia* in heroin addicts. *Am J Med* 1975;59:29.
98. Graber C, Jervey L, Ostrander W, et al: Endocarditis due to a lanthanic, unclassified gram-negative bacterium (group IVd). *J Clin Pathol* 1968;49:220.
99. Rahal J, Simberkoff M, Hyams P: *Pseudomonas cepacia* tricuspid endocarditis: Treatment with trimethoprim, sulfonamide and polymyxin B. *Rev Infect Dis* 1973;128:762.
100. Speller D, Stephens M, Viant A: Hospital infection by *Pseudomonas cepacia. Lancet* 1971;1:798.
101. Street A, Durach D: Experience with trimethoprim-sulfamethoxazole in treating infective endocarditis. *Rev Infect Dis* 1988;10:915.
102. Hadry P, Ederer G, Matsen J: Contamination of commercially-packaged urinary catheter kits with the pseudomonad EO-1. *N Engl J Med* 1970;282:33.
103. Gilarch G: *Pseudomonas* and related genera, in Bulows A, Hauscherr W, Herrmann K, et al (eds): *Microbiology,* ed 5. Washington, DC, American Society for Microbiologists, 1991, chap 41.
104. Gill G: Endocarditis caused by *Salmonella enteritidis. Br Heart J* 1979;42:353.
105. Doraiswami S, Friedman S, Kagan A, et al: *Salmonella* endocarditis complicated by a myocardial abscess. *Am J Cardiol* 1970;26:102.
106. Swiet J: Medical memorandum: Subacute bacterial endocarditis due to *Salmonella typhimurium. Br Med J* 1949;2:1155.
107. Langaker O, Svanes K: Myocardial abscess due to *Salmonella typhimurium. Br Med J* 1973;35:871.
108. Thomas M: A case of acute infective endocarditis caused by *Salmonella dublin. AMA Arch Pathol* 1952;53:408.
109. Nushan H, Sawyer C, Rogers R, et al: Bacterial endocarditis due to *Salmonella typhimurium. Am J Cardiol* 1961;7:608.
110. Shilkin K: Case reports: *Salmonella typhimurium* pancarditis. *Postgrad Med J* 1969;45:40.
111. Wall N, Hobbs R: Acute ulcerative endocarditis with overwhelming septicemia due to *Salmonella choleraesuis. PA Med J* 1953;56:892.
112. Kuzman W: Recurrent bacterial endocarditis due to *Salmonella newport* and diphtheroid bacillus: Report of a case with cure. *Dis Chest* 1967;51:654.
113. Geraci J, Dearing W: *Salmonella panama* endocarditis cured with kanamycin therapy: Report of a case. *Mayo Clin Proc* 1962;37:352.
114. Rich M, St Mary E: Case reports: *Salmonella* subacute bacterial endocarditis. *Ann Intern Med* 1956;44:162.
115. Kulpati D, Bhargava S, Gupta G, et al: *Salmonella* endocarditis. *J Assoc Phys India* 1968;16:535.
116. Yamamoto N, Magidson O, Posner C, et al: Probable *Salmonella* endocarditis treated with prosthetic valve replacement: A case report. *Surgery* 1974;76:678.
117. Fraser R, Rossall R, Dvorkin J: Bacterial endocarditis occurring after open-heart surgery. *Can Med Assoc* 1967;196:1551.
118. Levin S: Endocarditis due to *Salmonella enteritidis:* A case report. *Cuthrie Clin Bull* 1960;30:46.
119. Schneider P, Nernoff J III, Gold J: Acute *Salmonella* endocarditis: Report of a case and review. *Arch Intern Med* 1967;120:478.
120. Decker J, Clancy C: *Salmonella* endocarditis: Report of three cases, including one of mural endocarditis. *Bull Ayer Clin Lab* 1959;4:1.
121. Kurz E, Crehan E, Thomson C: Case reports: *Salmonella* endocarditis with streptomycin failure. *Ann Intern Med* 1949;31:497.
122. Sakurai M, Bloodworth J Jr: Acute bacterial endocarditis due to *Salmonella:* A case report. *Ohio State Med J* 1963;59:391.

123. McFadzean A, Chi-To H: Bacterial endocarditis due to *Salmonella* sp. (type *sendai*) with recovery. *Arch Intern Med* 1952;90:858.

124. Stumpe A, Baroody N Jr: Case reports: *Salmonella* endocarditis. *Arch Intern Med* 1951;88:679.

125. Cohen P, O'Brien T, Schoenbaum S, et al: Risk of endothelial infection in adults with *Salmonella* bacteremia. *Ann Intern Med* 1978;89:931.

126. Meyer G, Gerding G: Favorable prognosis of patients with prosthetic valve endocarditis cured gram-negative bacilli of the HACEK group. *Am J Med* 1988;85:104.

127. Middleton W: Streptomycin therapy of *Hemophilus* endocarditis lenta. *Am J Med* 1945;93:511.

128. Ree G, Mundodi B, Martin M: *Haemophilus* endocarditis. *Lancet* 1977;2:305.

129. Martin W, Spink W: Endocarditis due to type B *Hemophilus influenzae* involving only the tricuspid valve. *Am J Med Sci* 1947;214:139.

130. Goetz F, Peterson E: Endocarditis due to *Hemophilus influenzae*. *Am J Med* 1949;7: 274.

131. Laird W, Nelson J, Weinberg A, et al: Fatal *Haemophilus influenzae* endocarditis diagnosed by echocardiography in an infant. *Pediatrics* 1979;64:292.

132. Lynn D, Kane J, Parker R: *Haemophilus parainfluenzae* and *H. influenzae* endocarditis: A review of forty cases. *Medicine* 1977;56:115.

133. Geraci J, Wilkowske C, Wilson W, et al: *Haemophilus* endocarditis: Report of 14 patients. *Mayo Clin Proc* 1977;52:209.

134. Emmerson A, Perinpanayagam R, Barnado D: *Haemophilus* endocarditis. *Postgrad Med J* 1981;57:117.

135. McGee C, Priest W: Subacute bacterial endocarditis due to *Hemophilus parainfluenzae*. *JAMA* 1948;137:1315.

136. Bland E, Finland M: Medical Grand Rounds—Subacute bacterial endocarditis. *Am Pract* 1947;1:498.

137. Zeman F: Subacute bacterial endocarditis in the aged. *Am J Med* 1945;29:661.

138. Hodge J, Bremner D: *Haemophilus* endocarditis and the isolation of haemophilic bacteria in blood culture: Case report *NZ Med* 1974;79:824.

139. Blair D, Walker W, Doseman T, et al: Bacterial endocarditis due to *Haemophilus parainfluenzae*. *Chest* 1977;71:146.

140. Raucher B, Tobkin J, Mandel L: Occult polymicrobial endocarditis with *Haemophilus parainfluenzae* in intravenous drug abusers. *Am J Med* 1983;143:18.

141. Dahlgren J, Tally F, Brothers G, et al: *Haemophilus parainfluenzae* endocarditis. *Am J Clin Pathol* 1974;62:607.

142. Olinger M: Mixed infection in subacute bacterial endocarditis. *Arch Intern Med* 1948;8:334.

143. Chunn C, Jones S, McCutchan J, et al: *Haemophilus parainfluenzae* infective endocarditis. *Medicine* 1977;56:99.

144. Gordon A, Love W: Endocarditis due to *Haemophilus parainfluenzae*. *J Med Microbiol* 1970;3:550.

145. Boughton C: Subacute bacterial endocarditis due to *Haemophilus parainfluenzae*. *Med J Aust* 1965;1:804.

146. Hunter T, Duane R: Subacute bacterial endocarditis due to gram-negative organisms. *JAMA* 1946;132:209.

147. Goudie J, Lowther C: Subacute bacterial endocarditis due to *Haemophilus parainfluenzae* and *Strep. viridans*. *Br Med J* 1951;1:217.

148. Massell B, Zeller J, Dow J, et al: Streptomycin treatment of bacterial endocarditis. *N Engl J Med* 1948;238:464.

149. Smith P, Chambers W, Walker C: Case report: Ampicillin-resistant *Haemophilus parainfluenzae* endocarditis. *Am J Med Sci* 1979;278:173.

150. Julander I, Lindberg A, Svanbom M: *Haemophilus parainfluenzae*—an uncommon cause of septicemia and endocarditis. *Scand J Infect Dis* 1980;12:85.

151. Blair D, Weiner L: Prosthetic valve endocarditis due to *Haemophilus parainfluenzae* biotype II. *Am J Dis Child* 1979;133:617.

152. Jemsek J, Greenberg S, Gentry L, et al: *Haemophilus parainfluenzae* endocarditis: Two cases and review of the literature in the past decade. *Am J Med* 1979;66:51.

153. Cole R, Winickoff R: *Haemophilus parainfluenzae* endocarditis. *South Med J* 1979;72:516.

154. Greenspan J, Noble J, Tennenbaum M: Cure of *Haemophilus parainfluenzae* endocarditis with chloramphenicol. *Arch Intern Med* 1981;141:1222.

155. Sutter V, Finegold S: *Haemophilus aphrophilus* infections: Clinical and bacteriologic studies. *Ann NY Acad Sci* 1970;74:468.

156. Johnson R, Kennedy R, Marton K, et al: *Haemophilus* endocarditis: New cases, literature review and recommendations for management. *South Med J* 1977;70:1098.

157. Gullott R: Aortic insufficiency due to *Haemophilus aphrophilus* with prosthetic valve replacement. *Chest,* 1973;63:476.

158. Goldsweig H, Matsen J, Castaneda A: *Haemophilus aphrophilus* endocarditis in a patient with a mitral valve prosthesis: Case report and review of the literature. *Thorac Cardiovasc Surg* 1972;63:408.

159. Spicer A, Mitchell E: Subacute bacterial endocarditis due to *Haemophilus aphrophilus.* *J Irish Med Assoc* 1970;73:57.

160. Faris H, Cathcart R, Graber C, et al: Tricuspid endocarditis caused by *Haemophilus aphrophilus.* *J SC Med Assoc* 1970;66:409.

161. Witorsch P, Gorden P: *Hemophilus aphrophilus* endocarditis: Report of three cases. *Ann Intern Med* 1964;60:957.

162. Elster S, Mattes L, Meyers B, et al: *Hemophilus aphrophilus* endocarditis: Review of 23 cases. *Amer J Cardiol* 1975;35:72.

163. Fortune R, Bell F: *Hemophilus aphrophilus* endocarditis, with cerebral embolism, in an Alaskan Eskimo. *Ann Intern Med* 1966;64:873.

164. Russell J: The identification of gram-negative pleomorphic bacilli with special reference to a case of *Hemophilus aphrophilus* endocarditis. *Am J Clin Pathol* 1965;44:86.

165. McClung O, Menk K, Carr I: *Haemophilus aphrophilus* endocarditis. *VA Med Month* 1966;93:193.

166. Goldberg L, Cecil R: *Hemophilus aphrophilus* endocarditis treated with ampicillin. *VA Med Month* 1966;93:73.

167. Anand C, Mackay A, Evans J: *Haemophilus aphrophilus* endocarditis in pregnancy. *J Clin Pathol* 1976;29:812.

168. Keith T, Lyon S: *Hemophilus aphrophilus* endocarditis. *Am J Med* 1963;34:535.

169. Quinn E, Cox F, Jones D, et al: Clinical experience with parenteral ampicillin. *Antimicrob Agents Chemother,* 1964;4:226.

170. Dung W, Lin T: Subacute bacterial endocarditis due to *Hemophilus aphrophilus.* *Am Heart J* 1966;71:251.

171. Bauer CL, Walker WJ: *Hemophilus aphrophilus* endocarditis successfully treated with ampicillin and streptomycin. *Calif Med* 1966;104:475.

172. Pine R, Ballard H: *Hemophilus aphrophilus* endocarditis. *Br Med J* 1970;2:344.

173. Farrand R, MacCabe A, Jordan O: *Haemophilus aphrophilus* endocarditis. *J Clin Pathol* 1969;22:486.

174. Dorff B, Kilian M: *Haemophilus aphrophilus* endocarditis. *Scand J Infect Dis* 1974;6:291.

175. Raper A, Kemp V: Use of steroids in penicillin-sensitive patients with bacterial endocarditis. *N Engl J Med* 1965;273:297.

176. Toshach S, Bain G: Acquired aortic sinus aneurysm caused by *Hemophilus aphrophilus.* *Am J Clin Pathol* 1958;30:328.

177. Silva M, Rubin S, Lyons R, et al: *Haemophilus paraphrophilus* endocarditis in a prolapsed mitral valve. *Am J Clin Pathol* 1976;66:922.

178. Csukas Z, Ban E: *Haemophilus paraphrophilus* isolated from endocarditis. *Acta Microbiol Acad Sci Hung* 1978;25:179.

179. Hammond G, Richardson H, Lian C, et al: Two cases of *Hemophilus* endocarditis or prolapsed mitral valves—*Hemophilus paraphrophilus* or *parainfluenzae*? *Am J Med* 1978;65:537.

180. Root T, Silva E, Edwards L, et al: *Hemophilus aphrophilus* endocarditis with a probable dental focus or infection. *Chest* 1981;80:109.

181. Cleveland J, Suchor R, Dague J: Destructive aortic valve endocarditis from *Brucella abortus:* Survival with emergency aortic valve replacement. *Thorax* 1978;33:616.

182. Peery T, Belter L: Brucellosis and heart disease. II. Fatal brucellosis—A review of the literature and report of new cases. *J Pathol* 1960;36:673.

183. Pratt D, Tenney J, Bjork C, et al: Successful treatment of *Brucella melitensis* endocarditis. *Am J Med* 1978;64:897.

184. O'Meara J, Eykyn S, Jenkins B, et al: *Brucella melitensis* endocarditis: Successful treatment of an infected prostehtic valve. *Thorax* 1974;29:377.

185. Quintin T, Stalker M: Case reports: Endocarditis due to *Brucella abortus. Can Med Assoc* 1946;55:50.

186. Wanderman K, Yarom R: Brucellosis with endocarditis. Report of an unusual case with observations on the relationship to aortic stenosis and on treatment. *Isr J Med Sci* 1970;6:273.

187. Lalliatth J. Shrhaiber H, Kinan Y, et al: Brucella endocarditis. *J Cardiovasc Surg* 1989;30:782.

188. Fulu A, Araj G, Khateeb M, et al: Human brucellosis in Kuwait: A prospective study of 400 cases. *Q J Med* 1988;249:39.

189. Jenredi M, Halim M, Hardera J, et al: Brucella endocarditis. *Br Heart J* 1987;58: 279.

190. Spink W, Hall W, Shaffer J, et al: Human brucellosis: Its specific treatment with a combination of streptomycin and sulfadiazine. *JAMA* 1948;136:382.

191. Beebe R, Meneely J: *Brucella melitensis* endocarditis: Report of a case. *Am Heart J* 1949;38:788.

192. Voth H: *Brucella* bacteremia with endocarditis. *J Kansas Med Soc* 1949;50:330.

193. Lehmann V, Knutsen S, Ragnhildstveit E, et al: Endocarditis caused by *Pasteurella multocida. Scand J Infect Dis* 1977;9:247.

194. Phillips I, Midgley J, Lapage S: Endocarditis due to a *Pasteurella multocida*-like organism. *E Afr Med J* 1970;47:440.

195. Raffi F, Bamer J, Bacon P, et al: *Pasteurella multocida* bacteremia: Report of thirteen cases over twelve years and renewing of the literature. *Scand J Infect Dis* 1987;19: 385.

196. Weber P, Wolfson J, Swarz M, et al: *Pasteurella multocida* infections: Report of 34 cases and review of the literature. *Medicine* 1989;63:133.

197. Raz R, Ahoy G, Sobel J: Nosocomial bacteremia due to *Acinetobacter calcoaceticus. Infection* 1982;10:168.

198. Altman K, Sacks F: Bronchopneumonia and endocarditis: Caused by *Acinetobacter anitratum (Herellae vaginicola). NY State J Med* 1979;79:1434.

199. Retailliau H, Hightower A, Dixon R, et al: *Acinetobacter calcoaceticus:* A nosocomial pathogen with an unusual seasonal pattern. *J Infect Dis* 1979;139:371.

200. Ristuccia P, Cunha B: *Acinetobacter. Infect Cont* 1983;4:226.

201. Shalit I, Dan M, Gutman R, et al: Cross resistance to ciprofloxam and other antimicrobial agents among clincal isolates of *Actinetobacter calcoaceticus* biovar antiratus. *Antimicrob Agents Chemother,* 1990;34:494.

202. Carlson D: Endocarditis caused by *Herellea:* Report of a case, with postmortem observations. *Am J Clin Pathol* 1963;40:54.

203. Buchanan TM: *Mina polymorpha* endocarditis: A patient with two artificial heart valves. *South Med J* 1972;65:693.

204. Almog C, Sompolinsky D, Itzchak I, et al: Bacterial endocarditis due to *Mina morpha. Isr J Med Sci* 1967;3:875.

205. King O, Copeland G, Berton W: Cardiovascular lesions of the *Mimeae* organism. *Am J Med* 1963;35:241.

206. Phillips J: *Mimeae* endocarditis: A clinical syndrome. *Am J Med Sci* 1966;252:101.

207. Block P, DeSanctis R, Weinberg A, et al: Prosthetic valve endocarditis. *J Thorac Cardiovasc Surg* 1970;60:541.

208. Yu V: *Serratia marcescens:* Historical perspective and clinical review. *N Engl J Med* 1979;300:887.

209. Alexander R, Holloway A, Honsinger R: Surgical debridement for resistant bacterial endocarditis. A case of antibiotic-refractory *Serratia marcescens* infection on the tricuspid valve cured by operative excision. *JAMA* 1969;210:1757.

210. Farhoudi H, Banks T, Ali N: A case report of *Serratia* endocarditis with review of the literature. *Med Ann DC* 1974;43:401.

211. Reisell P, Jansson E: *Serratia marcescens* endocarditis. *Ann Intern Med* 1973;79:454.

212. Khan F, Khan A: *Serratia marcescens* endocarditis. *Ann Intern Med* 1973;79:454.

213. Sands M, Sanders C: *Serratia marcescens* endocarditis. *Ann Intern Med* 1976;85: 397.

214. Suri R, Selby D, Hawks G, et al: *Serratia marcescens* endocarditis: A report of a case involving Cross-Jones mitral valve prosthesis, with a review of the literature. *Can Med Assoc J* 1971;104:1013.

215. Richards N, Levitsky S: Outbreak of *Serratia marcescens* infections in a cardiothoracic surgical intensive care unit. *Ann Thorac Surg* 1975;19:503.

216. Davis J, Foltz E, Blakemore W: *Serratia marcescens:* A pathogen of increasing clinical importance. *JAMA* 1970;214:2190.

217. Alexander R, Reichenbach D, Merendino K: *Serratia marcescens* endocarditis: A review of the literature and report of a case involving a homograft replacement of the aortic valve. *Arch Surg* 1969;98:287.

218. Denney J, Kaye D, Hagstrom J: Medical intelligence: Brief recording: Endocarditis due to *Serratia marcescens. N Engl J Med* 1967;276:1362.

219. Quintiliani R, Gifford R: Endocarditis from *Serratia marcescens. JAMA* 1969;208: 2055.

220. Amoury R, Bowman F Jr, Malm J: Endocarditis associated with intracardiac prostheses: Diagnosis, management and prophylaxis. *J Thorac Cardiovasc Surg*1966;51:36.

221. Wilkowske C, Washington J II, Martin W, et al: *Serratia marcescens:* Biochemical characteristics, antibiotic susceptibility, patterns and clinical significance. *JAMA* 1970; 214:2157.

222. Howe A, Huges M: Bacterial endocarditis due to *Chromobacterium prodigiosum. Br Med J* 1954;1:968.

223. Williams J Jr, Johnson J III: *Serratia marcescens* endocarditis. *Arch Intern Med* 1970; 125:1038.

224. Wheat R, Zuckerman A, Rantz L: Infection due to chromobacteria: Report of eleven cases. *Arch Intern Med* 1951;88:461.

225. Mills J, Drew D: *Serratia marcescens* endocarditis: a regional illness associated with intravenous drug abuse. *Ann Intern Med* 1976;84:29.

226. Cooper R, Mills J: *Serratia* endocarditis: A follow-up report. *Arch Intern Med* 1980;140:99.

227. Franklin B, Ulmer D: Human infection with *Vibrio fetus. West J Med* 1979;120:200.

228. Loeb H, Bettag J, Young N, et al: *Vibrio fetus* endocarditis: Report. *Am Heart J* 1966;71:381.

229. Lee M, Ludwig J, Geraci J, et al: Fatal *Vibrio fetus* endocarditis: Report of one case and review of the literature. *Virchows Arch Pathol Anat* 1970;350:87.

230. Dzau V, Shur P, Weinstein L: *Vibrio fetus* endocarditis in a patient with systemic lupus erythematosus. *Am J Med Sci* 1976;272:331.

231. Schmidt U, Chmel H, Kaminski Z, et al: The clinical spectrum of *Campylobacter fetus* infections: Report of five cases and review of the literature. *Q J Med* 1980;49: 431.

232. Peterson E, McCulbugh N, Eisele C, et al: Subacute bacterial endocarditis due to *Streptobacillus moniliformis. JAMA* 1950;144:621.

233. McCormack R, Kaye D, Hook E: Endocarditis due to *Streptobacillus moniliformis:* A report of two cases and review of the literature. *JAMA* 1967;200:183.

234. Simon M, Nilson D: *Streptobacillus moniliformis* endocarditis: A case report. *Clin Pediatr* 1985;25:110.

235. Hamburger M, Knowles H: *Streptobacillus moniliformis* infection complicated by acute bacterial endocarditis. *Arch Intern Med* 1953;92:216.
236. McIntosh C, Vickers P, Isaacs A: Spirillum endocarditis. *Postgrad Med J* 1975;51:675.
237. Geraci J, Greipp P, Wilkowske C, et al: *Cardiobacterium hominis* endocarditis: Four cases with clinical and laboratory observations. *Mayo Clin Proc* 1978;53:49.
238. Laguna J, Derby B, Chase R: *Cardiobacterium hominis* endocarditis with cerebral mycotic aneurysm. *Arch Neurol* 1975;32:638.
239. Applebaum E, Galfand M: A case of bacteremia due to an unidentified gram-negative *Pasteurella*-like bacillus with recovery following streptomycin therapy. *Ann Intern Med* 1947;26:780.
240. Tucker D, Slotnick I, King E, et al: Endocarditis caused by a *Pasteurella*-like organism. *N Engl J Med* 1962;267:913.
241. Perdue G, Dorney E, Ferrier F: Embolomycotic aneurysm associated with bacterial endocarditis due to *Cardiobacterium hominis*. *Ann Surg* 1968;32:901.
242. Midgley J, Lapage S, Jenkins B, et al: *Cardiobacterium hominis* endocarditis. *J Med Microbiol* 1970;3:91.
243. Snyder A, Ellner P: *Cardiobacterium hominis* endocarditis. *NY State J Med* 1969;69:704.
244. Weiner M, Werthamer S: *Cardiobacterium hominis* endocarditis: Characterization of the unusual organisms and review of the literature. *Am J Clin Pathol* 1975;63:131.
245. Savage D, Kagan R, Young N, et al: *Cardiobacterium hominis* endocarditis: Description of two patients and characterization of the organism. *J Clin Microbiol* 1977;5:75.
246. Wormser G, Bottone E, Tudy J, et al: Case report: *Cardiobacterium hominis:* Review of prior infections and report of endocarditis on a fascia lata prosthetic heart valve. *Am J Med Sci* 1987;276:117.
247. Johnson M, Wasilauskas B: *Cardiobacterium hominis* endocarditis. *Am J Med Technol* 1979;45:28.
248. Piot P, Dasnoy J, Eyckmans L: Bacterial endocarditis due to *Cardiobacterium hominis*. *Acta Clin Belg* 1978;33:308.
249. Pankey G, Horton J: *Cardiobacterium hominis* endocarditis: A case report. *J Miss State Med Assoc* 1978;19:107.
250. Wormser G, Bottone E: *Cardiobacterium hominis:* Review of microbiologic and clinical features. *Rev Infect Dis* 1983;5:680.
251. Panwalker A, Akalin H, Zimelis V, et al; *Actinobacillus actinomycetemcomitans* endocarditis in a patient with a prosthetic aortic valve. *Infection* 1977;5:104.
252. Stauffer J, Goldman M: Bacterial endocarditis due to *Actinobacillus actinomycetemcomitans* in a patient with a prosthetic aortic valve. *Calif Med* 1972;117:59.
253. Vogelzang R: Bacterial endocarditis due to *Actinobacillus actinomycetemcomitans* endocarditis in a patient with a prosthetic aortic valve. *Infection* 1977;5:104.
254. Serra P, Tonato M: Subacute bacterial endocarditis due to *Actinobacillus actinomycetemcomitans*. *Am J Med* 1969;47:809.
255. Macklon A, Ingham H, Selkon J, et al: Endocarditis due to *Actinobacillus actinomycetemcomitans*. *Br Med J* 1975;1:609.
256. Underhill E: Endocarditis due to *Actinobacillus actinomycetemcomitans*. *Can J Med Technol* 1968;30:125.
257. Goss J, Gutin R, Dizkhaus D: Bacterial endocarditis due to *Actinobacillus actinomycetemcomitans*. *Am J Med* 1967;43:636.
258. Mitchell R, Gillespie W: Bacterial endocarditis due to *Actinobacillus J Clin Pathol* 1964;17:511.
259. Thomas J: *Actinobacillus actinomycetemcomitans* endocarditis in a patient with bicuspid aortic valve coarctation of the aorta. *South Med J* 1967;60:783.
260. Overholt B: *Actinobacillus actinomycetemcomitans* endocarditis. *Arch Intern Med* 1966;177:99.
261. Affias S, West A, Stewart J, et al: *Actinobacillus actinomycetemcomitans* endocarditis. *Can Med Assoc J* 1978;118:1256.

262. Lalonde G, Hand R: Infective endocarditis due to *Actinobacillus actinomycetemcomitans* in a patient with a porcine prosthetic mitral valve. *Can Med Assoc J* 1980;122:316.

263. Reider J, Wehat J: Endocarditis caused by *Actinobacillus actinomycetemcomitans*. *South Med J* 1979;71:1219.

264. Geraci J, Wilson W, Washington J III: Infective endocarditis caused by *Actinobacillus actinomycetemcomitans*. *Mayo Clin Proc* 1980;55:415.

265. Bansky G, Russi E: *Actinobacillus actinomycetemcomitans* endocarditis. *Schweiz Med Wochensch* 1981;111:1136.

266. Kristinssen K, Thorgiersson G, Holbrook W: *Actinobacillus actinomycetemcomitans* and endocarditis. *J Infect Dis* 1988;157:599.

267. Sobel J, Carrizola J, Ziobrowski T, et al: Case report: Polymicrobial endocarditis involving *Eikenella corrodens*. *Am J Med Sci* 1981;282:41.

268. Geraci J, Herman J, Washington J: *Eikenella corrodens* endocarditis: Report of a cure in two cases. *Mayo Clin Proc* 1979;49:950.

269. Deber M, Graham B, Hunter E, et al: Endocarditis and infection of intravascular devices due to *Eikenella corrodens*. *Am J Med Sci* 1986;292:209.

270. Jenny D, Letendre P, Iveson G: Endocarditis due to *Kingella* species. *Rev Infect Dis* 1988;10:1065.

271. Swann R, Holmes B: Infective endocarditis caused by *Kingella denitrificans*. *J Clin Pathol* 1984;37:1384.

272. Ratner H: *Flavobacterium meningosepticum*. *Infect Control* 1984;5237.

273. Rulmondi A, Moosdeen F, Williams J: Antibiotic resistance pattern of *Flavobacterium meningosepticum*. *Eur J Clin Microbiol* 1986;5:461.

274. LeFrock J, Klainer A, Zuckerman K: *Edwardsiella tarda* bacteremia. *South Med J* 1976;69:188.

275. McCullough D, Menzies R, Corhere B: Endocarditis due to *Citrobacter diversus* developing resistance to cephalothin. *NZ Med J* 1977;85:182.

276. Perez R: Endocarditis with *Moraxella*-like M-A after cardiac catheterization. *J Clin Microbiol* 1986;24:501.

277. Silberfarb P, Lawe J: Endocarditis due to *Moraxella liquefaciens*. *Arch Intern Med* 1968;122:512.

278. Christensen C, Emmanouilides G: Bacterial endocarditis due to "*Moraxella* New Species I." *N Engl J Med* 1967;277:803.

279. Miridjanian A, Berrett D: Infective endocarditis caused by *Moraxella kingae*. *West J Med* 1978;129:344.

280. Bechard D, LeFrock J, Tillotson J: Endocarditis caused by *Moraxella nonliquefaciens*. *South Med J* 1979;72:1485.

281. Davis W II, Kane J, Garagusi V: Human *Aeromonas* infections: A review of the literature and a case report of endocarditis. *Medicine* 1978;57:267.

282. Janda J, Duffey P: Mesophilic aeromonas in human disease: Current taxonomy laboratory identification and infectious disease spectrum. *Rev Infect Dis* 1908;10:980.

283. Motyl M, McKinley G, Janda J: In vitro susceptibilities of *Aeromonas hydrophila*, *Aeromonas logria*, and *Aeromonas cartae* to 22 antimicrobial agents. *Antimicrob Agents Chemother* 1985;28:151.

284. Dale A, Geraci J: Mixed cardiac valvular infections: Report of case and review of literature. *Staff Meet Mayo Clin* 1961;36:288.

285. Masri A, Crieco M: *Bacteroides* endocarditis. *Am J Med Sci* 1972;263:357.

286. Tumulty H: Subacute bacterial endocarditis: *Bacteroides*. *Am J Med* 1948;4:37.

287. Scully R, McNeely B: Case records of the Massachusetts General Hospital: Weekly clinicopathological exercises. *N Engl J Med* 1974;291:242.

288. DeHay R, Bell J, Beebe J: *Bacteroides* bacterial endocarditis: Cure by massive doses of penicillin. *HA Med J* 1950;9:235.

289. Fisher A, McKusick V: *Bacteroides* infections; Clinical, bacteriological and therapeutic features of fourteen cases. *Am J Med Sci* 1953;225:253.

290. Nastro F, Sarma R: Infective endocarditis due to anaerobic and microaerophilic bacteria. *West J Med* 1902;137:18.

291. Jackson R, Dopp A: *Bacteroides fragilis* endocarditis. *South Med J* 1988;81:781.
292. Nastro L, Finegold S: endocarditis due to anaerobic gram-negative bacilli. *Am J Med* 1973;54:482.
293. Fredericka D: Endocarditis and brain abscess due to *Bacteroides oralis*. *J Infect Dis* 1982;145:918.
294. Seggie J: *Fusobacterium* endocarditis treated with metronidazole. *Br Med J* 1978;1: 960.
295. Felner J, Dowell V: Anaerobic bacterial endocarditis. *N Engl J Med* 1970;283:1188.
296. Barber M, Waterworth P: Antibacterial activity of the penicillins. *Br Med J* 1961; 1:1159.
297. Tze-Ying T, Wen-T'ao C, Fu W, et al: *Bacillus alkaligenes* infections: A clinical analysis of 33 cases. *Chin Med J* 1963;82:423.
298. Cole A, Marchall C: Infective endocarditis due to *Bacillus fecalis alcaligenes*. *Br Med J* 1952;2:867.
299. Auckenthaler R, Nicker-Hangehrow N, Pechere J: In vitro activity of new quinolones against *Aeromonas* species and *Pleisomonas shigelloides*. *Antimicrob Agents Chemother* 1986;17(Suppl B):29.
300. Hichlow K, Verghese A, Alvarez S: Dysgonic fermenter septicemia. *Rev Infect Dis* 1987;9:884.
301. Medfield S, Young E: Native valve endocarditis caused by dysgonic fermenter and bacilli. *Am J Med Sci* 1988;296:69.
302. Arlet G, Sanson-Lepore M-J, Casen I, et al: In vitro susceptibility of GU capnocytophagic stress, including a b-lactamase product of new b-lactam antibiotics and six quinolones. *Antimicrob Agents Chemother* 1989;31:1238.
303. Brancaccio M, Legendre G: *Megasphaera eisdenii* endocarditis. *J Clin Microbiol* 1979;10:72.
304. Wall T, Peyton R, Corey G: Gonococcal endocarditis: A new look at an old disease. *Medicine* 1989;68:375.
305. Dzindzio B, Myer L, Osterhold R, et al: Isolated gonococcal pulmonary valve endocarditis: Diagnosis by echocardiography. *Circulation* 1979;59:1319.
306. Voigt G, Bender H, Buckels L, et al: Gonococcal endocarditis with severe aortic regurgitation: Early valve replacement. *Johns Hopkins Med J* 1970;126:305.
307. Tahowitz H, Alder J, Chirito E: Gonococcal endocarditis. *NY State J Med* 1972;72: 2782.
308. John J, Nichols J, Eisenhower E, et al: Gonococcal endocarditis. *Sex Trans Dis* 1977; 4:84.
309. Gilson B, Trout M, Alleman H: Gonococcal endocarditis. *US Armed Forces Med J* 1960; 11:1375.
310. Davis D, Romansky M: Successful treatment of gonococcal endocarditis with erythromycin. *Am J Med* 1956;21:474.
311. Holmes K, Counts G, Beaty H: Disseminated gonococcal infection. *Ann Intern Med* 1971;74:979.
312. Hilless A, Molloy P: Urgent aortic valve replacement in disseminated gonococcemia associated with sinus of Valsalva aneurysm and fistula formation. *Aust NZ J Surg* 1976;46:246.
313. Dorset V, Spicknall C, Terry L: Penicillin therapy of gonococcic endocarditis. *Am Heart J* 1949;38:610.
314. Myers W: Penicillin therapy of gonococcal endocarditis of the pulmonary valve. *JAMA* 1947;133:1205.
315. Vogler W, Dorney E, Bridges H: Bacterial endocarditis. *Am J Med* 1962;32:910.
316. Sugar A, Utsinger P, Santoro J: Gonococcal endocarditis in a patient with mitral valve prolapse. Study of host immunology and organism characteristics. *Am J Med Sci* 1982;283:165.
317. Ebright J, Komorowski R: Gonococcal endocarditis associated with immune complex glomerulonephritis. *Am J Med* 1980;68:793.

318. Bonhoff M, Morello J, Lerner S: Auxotypes, penicillin susceptibility and serogroups of *Neissena gonorrhoeae* from disseminated and uncomplicated infections. *J Infect Dis* 1986;154:225.

319. Sternberg R, Smith J: Meningococcal endocarditis in an Ionescu-Shiley aortic valve prosthesis: Successful treatment with intravenous penicillin. *South Med J* 1989; 82:1314.

320. Doem G, Miller M, Winn R: *Branhamella (Neisseria)* catarrhisis systemic disease in humans. *Arch Intern Med* 1981;141:1690.

321. Dowling J, Lee W, Sacco R, et al: Endocarditis caused by *Neisseria mucosa* in Marfan's syndrome. *Ann Intern Med* 1974;81:641.

322. Brodie E, Adler J, Daly A: Bacterial endocarditis due to an unusual species of encapsulated *Neisseria: Neisseria mucosa* endocarditis. *Am J Dis Child* 1971;122:433.

323. Ghoneim A, Tandon A: Prosthetic valve endocarditis due to *Neisseria sicca:* A case report. *Indian Heart J* 1979;31:246.

324. Ghoneim A, Tandor A: Prosthetic valve endocarditis due to *Neisseria sicca:* A case report. *Indian Heart J* 1979;31:246.

325. Goldstein J: Endocarditis due to *Neisseria pharyngis* organism. *Am J Med Sci* 1934;187:672.

326. Graef I, de la Chapelle C, France M: *Pharyngis siccus* endocarditis. *Am J Clin Pathol* 1932;8:347.

327. Schultz O: Acute vegetative endocarditis with multiple secondary foci of involvement. *JAMA* 1918;71:1739.

328. Shiling M: Bacteriology of endocarditis with report of two unusual cases. *Ann Intern Med* 1939;13:476.

329. Weed M, Clapper M, Myers G: Endocarditis caused by the *Micrococcus pharyngis sicca:* Recovery after treatment with heparin and sulfa-pyridine. *Am Heart J* 1941;25: 547.

330. Zimmerman L: *Candida* and *Aspergillis* endocarditis. *Arch Pathol* 1950;50:591.

331. Seelig M, Goldverg P, Kozinn P, et al: Fungal endocarditis: Patients at risk and their treatment. *Postgrad Med J* 1979;55:632.

332. Henderson J, Nickerson J: Bacterial endocarditis with *Candida albicans* superinfection. *Can Med Assoc J* 1964;90:452.

333. Heineman H, Yunis E, Siemienski J, et al: Chlamydospores and dimorphism in *Candida albicans* endocarditis: Observations in fatal superinfection during treatment of *Staphylococcus* endocarditis. *Arch Intern Med* 1961;108:570.

334. Rubenstein E, Noriega E, Simberkoft M, et al: Fungal endocarditis: Analysis of 24 cases and review of the literature. *Medicine* 1975;54:331.

335. Andriole V, Dravetz H, Roberts W, et al: *Candida* endocarditis: Clinical and pathological studies. *Am J Med* 1962;32:251.

336. Kroetz F, Leonard J, Everett C: *Candida albicans* endocarditis successfully treated with amphotericin B. *N Engl J Med* 1962;26:592.

337. Robboy S, Kaiser J: Pathogenesis of fungal infection on heart valve prostheses. *Hum Pathol* 1975;6:711.

338. Climie A, Rachmaninoff N: Fungal (*Candida*) endocarditis following open-heart surgery. *J Thorac Cardiovasc Surg* 1965;50:431.

339. Fraser R, Rodman F, MacGregor J: *Candida* endocarditis in the right atrium following successful treatment of subacute bacterial endocarditis of the mitral valve. *Acta Cardiol* 1966;21:491.

340. Conway N, Kothari M, Lockey E, et al: *Candida* endocarditis after heart surgery. *Thorax* 1968;23:353.

341. Newman W, Cordell A: *Aspergillus* endocarditis after open-heart surgery. *J Thorac Cardiovasc Surg* 1964;48:652.

342. Luke J, Bolande R, Gross S: Generalized aspergillosis and *Aspergillus* endocarditis in infancy. *Pediatrics* 1963;31:115.

343. Caplan H, Firsch E, Houghton J, et al: *Aspergillus fumigatus* endocarditis: Report of a case diagnosed during life. *Ann Intern Med* 1968;68:378.

344. Mahvi T, Webb H, Dixon C, et al: Systemic aspergillosis caused by *Aspergillus niger* after open heart surgery. *JAMA* 1968;203:520.

345. Mershon J, Samuelson D, Layman T: Left ventricular fibrous bady aneurysm caused by *Aspergillus* endocarditis. *Am J Cardiol* 1968;22:281.

346. Kanawaty D, Stalker M, Munt P: Nonsurgical treatment of histoplasma endocarditis involving a bioprosthetic valve. *Chest* 1991;99:253.

347. Haust M, Wlodek G, Parker J: *Histoplasma* endocarditis. *Am J Med* 1962;32:460.

348. Segal C, Wheeler C, Tompsett R: *Histoplasma* endocarditis cured with amphotericin. *N Engl J Med* 1969;280:206.

349. Hartley R, Remsberg J, Sinaly N: *Histoplasma* endocarditis: Case report and review of the literature; *Arch Intern Med* 1967;119:527.

350. Gerber H, Schoonmaker F, Vazquez M: Chronic meningitis associated with *Histoplasma* endocarditis. *N Engl J Med* 1966;275:74.

351. Merchant R, Louria D, Geisler P, et al: Fungal endocarditis: Review of literature and report of three cases. *Ann Intern Med* 1958;48:242.

352. Colmers R, Irniger W, Steinberg D: *Cryptococcus neoformans* endocarditis cured by amphotericin B. *JAMA* 1967;199:762.

353. Shelburne P, Carey R: *Rhodotorula* fungemia complicating staphylococcal endocarditis. *JAMA* 1962;180:38.

354. Lees A, Rao S, Garrett J, et al: Endocarditis due to *Torulopsis glabrata*. *Lancet* 1971;1: 943.

355. Stein P, Folkens A, Hruska K: *Saccharomyces* fungemia. *Chest* 1970;58:173.

356. Silver M, Ruffnell P, Bigelow W: Endocarditis caused by *Paecilomyces varioti* affecting an aortic valve allograft. *J Thorac Cardiovasc Surg* 1971;61:278.

357. Scully R, Galdabini J, McNeely B: Case records of the Massachusetts General Hospital. *N Engl J Med* 1979;301:34.

358. Parker J: The potentially lethal problem of cardiac candidosis. *Am J Clin Pathol* 1980;73:356.

359. Joseph P, Himmelstein D, Mahowald J, et al: Atrial myxoma infected with *Candida:* First survival. *Chest* 1980;78:340.

360. Drexler L, Rytel M, Keelan M, et al: *Aspergillus terreus* infective endocarditis on a porcine heterograft valve. *J Thorac Cardiovasc Surg* 1980;79:269.

361. Mikulski S, Love L, Bergquist E, et al: *Aspergillus* vegetative endocarditis and complete heart block in a patient with acute leukemia. *Chest* 1979;76:473.

362. Walsh T, Hutchins G: *Aspergillus* mural endocarditis. *Am J Clin Pathol* 1979;71: 640.

363. Barst R, Prince A, Neu H: *Aspergillus* endocarditis in children: Case report and review of the literature. *Pediatrics* 1981;68:73.

364. Kaplan R, Duncalf D, Cizmar S: *Aspergillus* pancarditis and cardiac arrest during anesthesia. *Anesth Analg* 1981;60:440.

365. Blair T, Waugh R, Pollack M, et al: *Histoplasma capsulatum* endocarditis. *Am Heart J* 1980;99:783.

366. Goodwin R, Shapiro J, Thurman G, et al: Disseminated histoplasmosis. *Medicine* 1981;60:231.

367. Alexander W, Mowry R, Cobbs G, et al: Prosthetic valve endocarditis caused by *Histoplasma capsulatum*. *JAMA* 1979;242:1399.

368. Marier R, Zakhireh B, Downs J, et al: Case report: *Trichosporon cutaneum* endocarditis. *Scand J Infect Dis* 1978;10:255.

369. Arnold A, Gribbin B, DeLeval M, et al: *Trichosporon capitatum* causing recurrent fungal endocarditis. *Thorax* 1981;36:478.

370. DelRossi A, Morse D, Spagna P, et al: Successful management of *Penicillium* endocarditis. *J Thorac Cardiovasc Surg* 1980;80:945.

371. Holliday H, Keipper V, Kaiser A: *Torulopsis glabrata* endocarditis. *JAMA* 1980;140: 2088.

372. Rumisek J, Albus R, Clarke J: Late *Mycobacterium chelonei* from prosthetic valve endocarditis: Activation of implanted contaminants. *Ann Thorac Surg* 1905;39(3):277.

373. Laskowski L, Marr J, Spernoga J, et al: Fastidious mycobacteria grown from porcine prosthetic heart valve cultures. *N Engl J Med* 1977;297:101.

374. Tyras D, Kaiser G, Barnes H, et al: Atypical mycobacteria and the xenograft valve. *J Thorac Cardiovasc Surg* 1978;75:331.

375. Arroyo J, McDoff G: *Mycobacterium chelonei* infection: Successful treatment based on a radiometric susceptibility test. *Antimicrob Agents Chemother* 1977;11:763.

376. Lohr D, Goeken J, Dotty D, et al: *Mycobacterium gordonae* infection of a prosthetic aortic valve. *JAMA* 1978;239:1528.

377. Narasimhan S, Austin T: Prosthetic valve endocarditis due to *Mycobacterium fortuitum*. *Can Med Assoc J* 1978;119:154.

378. Cope A, Heber M, Wilkins E: Valvular tuberculosis endocarditis: A case report and review of the literature. *J Infect* 1990;21:293.

379. Baker R: Endocardial tuberculosis. *Arch Pathol* 1935;19:621.

380. Davie T: Tuberculous verrucosa endocarditis. *J Pathol Bacteriol* 1936;43:313.

381. Anyanwy C, Nassau E, Yacoub M: Miliary tuberculosis following homograft valve replacement. *Thorax* 1976;31:101.

382. Marmion B, Stoker M, McCoy J, et al: Q fever in Britain. *Lancet* 1953;1:503.

383. Robson A, Shimmin C: Chronic Q fever—I. Clinical aspects of a patient with endocarditis. *Br Med J* 1959;2:980.

384. Marmion B, Higgins F, Bridges J, et al: A case of subacute rickettsial endocarditis: With a survey of cardiac patients for this infection. *Br Med J* 1960;2:1264.

385. Krisinson A, Bentall H: Medical and surgical treatment of Q fever endocarditis. *Lancet* 1967;2:693.

386. Ferguson I, Craik J, Grist N: Clinical virological and pathological findings in a fatal case of Q fever endocarditis. *J Clin Pathol* 1962;15:235.

387. Grist N: Q fever endocarditis. *Am Heart J* 1968;75:846.

388. Peter O, Flepp M, Bestetto G, et al: Q fever endocarditis: Diagostic approaches and monitoring of theraputic effects. *Clin Invest* 1992;70:932.

389. Grist N, Bazaz G, et al: Pathological, rickettsiological and immunofluorescence studies of a case of Q fever endocarditis. *J Pathol Bacteriol* 1966;91:317.

390. Oakley C, Hainson R: Q fever (*Coxiella*) endocarditis. *Proc R Soc Med* 1970;63:282.

391. Lamb R, Boyd J, Grist N: Q fever endocarditis. *Scott Med J* 1969;14:10.

392. Wilson H, Neilson G, Gallea E, et al: Q fever endocarditis in Queensland. *Circulation* 1976;53:680.

393. Applefield M, Billingsley L, Tucker H, et al: Q fever endocarditis: A case occurring in the United States. *Am Heart J* 1977;93:669.

394. Pedoe H: Apparent recurrence of Q fever endocarditis following homograft replacement of aortic valve. *Br Heart J* 1970;32:568.

395. Morgans C, Cartwright R: Case of Q fever endocarditis at site of aortic valve prosthesis. *Br Heart J* 1969;31:520.

396. Tobin M, Cahill N, Gearty G, et al: Q fever endocarditis. *Am J Med* 1982;72:396.

397. Varma M, Adgey A, Connolly J: Chronic Q fever endocarditis. *Br Heart J* 1980;43:695.

398. Waters E, Romansky M, Johnson A, et al: *Actinomyces bovis* endocarditis: An uncommon and complex problem, in Sylvester JC (ed): *Antimicrobial Agents and Chemotherapy, 1962.* Proceedings of the Second Interscience Conference on Antimicrobial Agents and Chemotherapy. American Society of Microbiology, 1963, p 517.

399. Vlachakis N, Gazes P, Hairston P: Nocardial endocarditis following mitral valve replacement. *Chest* 1975;63:276.

400. Falk R, Dimock F, Sharkey J: Prosthetic valve endocarditis resulting from *Nocardia asteroides*. *Br Heart J* 1979;41:125.

401. Dutton W, Inclan H: Cardiac actinomycosis. *Chest* 1968;54:65.

402. Ward C, Ward A: Acquired valvular heart diseases in patients who keep pet birds. *Lancet* 1974;2:734.

403. Regan R, Dathan R, Treharne D: Infective endocarditis with glomerulonephritis associated with cat *Chlamydia* (*C. psittaci*) infection. *Br Heart J* 1979;42:349.

404. Jariwalla A, Davies B, White J: Infective endocarditis complicating psittacosis: Response to rifampin. *Br Med J* 1980;19:155.

405. Jones R, Priest J, Kuo C: Subacute chlamydial endocarditis. *JAMA* 1982;247:655.

406. Van der Bel-Kahn J, Watanakunakorn C, Menefee M: *Chlamydia trachomatis* endocarditis. *Am Heart J* 1978;95:627.

407. Dumont D, Mathieu P, Alemani M, et al: Osler's endocarditis possibly caused by *Chlamydia pneumoniae* (TWAR strain). *Presse Med* (Paris) 1990;19:1054.

408. Guze LB (ed): *Microbial Protoplasts, Spheroplasts and L-Forms.* Baltimore, Williams & Wilkins, 1967.

409. Madoff S (ed): *Mycoplasma and the L-Forms of Bacteria* (symposium). New York, Gordon and Breach, 1971.

410. Feingold D: Biology and pathogenicity of microbial spheroplasts and L-forms. *N Engl J Med* 1969;281:1149.

411. Charache P: Atypical bacterial forms in human disease, in Guze LB (ed): *Protoplasts, Spheroplasts and L-Forms.* Baltimore, Williams & Wilkins, 1967, p 484.

412. Wittler R, Malizia W, Kramer P, et al: Isolation of a *Corynebacterium* and its transitional forms from a case of subacute bacterial endocarditis treated with antibiotics. *J Gen Microbiol* 1960;23:513.

413. Nativelle R, Deparis M: Forme evolutive des bacteries dans les hemocultures. *Presse Med* (Paris) 1960;68:571.

414. Mattman L, Mattman P: L-forms of *Streptococcus fecalis* in septicemia. *Arch Intern Med* 1965;115:315.

415. Rosner R: Isolation of *Candida* protoplasts from a case of *Candida* endocarditis. *J Bacteriol* 1966;91:1329.

416. Neu H, Goldreyer B: Isolation of protoplasts in a case of enterococcal endocarditis. *Am J Med* 1968;45:784.

417. Zierdt C, Wertlake P: Transitional forms of *Corynebacterium acnes* in disease. *J Bacteriol* 1969;97:799.

418. Piepkorn M, Reichenbach D: Infective endocarditis associated with cell-wall deficient bacteria. *Hum Pathol* 1978;9:163.

419. Persand V: Two unusual cases of mural endocarditis with review of the literature. *Am J Clin Pathol* 1972;53:832.

420. Burch G, DePasquale N, Sun S, et al: Experimental *Coxsackie* virus endocarditis. *JAMA* 1965;191:862.

421. Burch G, DePasquale N, Sun S, et al: Endocarditis in mice infected with *Coxsackie* virus B4. *Science* 1966;151:447.

422. Burch G, Tsui C: Evaluation of *Coxsackie* viral valvular and mural endocarditis in mice. *Br J Exp Pathol* 1971;52:360.

423. DePasquale N, Burch G, Sun S, et al: Experimental *Coxsackie* Virus B4 valvulitis in cynomolgus monkeys. *Am Heart J* 1966;71:678.

424. Francis C: Cardiac involvement in AIDS. *Curr Probl Cardiol* 1990;15:571.

425. Niedt G, Schinella R: Acquired immunodeficiency syndrome: Clinico-pathologic study of 5 autopsies. *Arch Pathol Lab Med* 1985;109:727.

426. Baddour Q, Meyer J, Henry B: Polymicrobial infective endocarditis in the 1980's. *Rev Infect Dis* 1991;13:913.

427. Hobbs R, Downing S, Andriole V: Four-valve polymicrobial endocarditis caused by *Pseudomonas aeruginosa* and *Serratia marcescens. Am J Med* 1982;72:164.

428. Pankey G: Acute bacterial endocarditis at the University of Minnesota Hospitals. 1939–1959. *Am Heart J* 1962;64:583.

429. Saravolatz L, Burch K, Quinn E, et al: Polymicrobial infective endocarditis. *Am Heart J* 1978;95:163.

430. Rossiter S, Stinson E, Ayer P, et al: Prosthetic valve endocarditis comparison of heterograft tissue valves and mechanical valves. *J Thorac Cardiovasc Surg* 1978;76:795.

431. Karchmer A, Archer G, Dismukes W: *Staphylococcus epidermidis:* Microbiologic and clinical observation as guides to therapy. *Ann Intern Med* 1983;98:447.

432. Norenberg R, Sethi G, Scott S, et al: Opportunistic endocarditis following open-heart surgery. *Ann Thorac Surg* 1975;19:592.

433. Gaynes R, Gardner P, Causey W: Prosthetic valve endocarditis caused by *Histoplasma capsulatum. Arch Intern Med* 1981;141:1533.

434. Bailey I, Richards J: Infective endocarditis in a Sydney teaching hospital—1962–1971. *Aust NZ Med J* 1975;5:413.

435. Van Scoy R: Culture-negative endocarditis. *Mayo Clin Proc* 1982;57:149.

436. Pesanti E, Smith I: Infective endocarditis with negative blood cultures: An analysis of 52 cases. *Am J Med* 1979;66:43.

437. Pazin G, Saul S, Thompson M: Blood culture positivity, suppression by outpatient antibiotic therapy in patients with bacterial endocarditis. *Arch Intern Med* 1982;142:263.

438. Hilton e, Lerner C, Lowry F, et al: "Culture-negative" prosthetic valve endocarditis. *Arch Intern Med* 1984;144:2083.

6

Pathology

Vegetations, the hallmark of infective endocarditis, are present most often on the valvular leaflets and less frequently on the ventricular endocardium (mural thrombi), the atrium (MacCallum's patch), and the pulmonary or other arteries.[1] When fresh, these lesions are pink, red, yellow, or green in color. They become gray during healing, are usually larger and more friable than those present in patients with rheumatic valvulitis, and have an increased tendency to break off and embolize. Their size varies with the organism responsible for the disease. Fungal endocarditis is characterized by the presence of large vegetations that may occlude medium-sized and large arteries (Fig. 6.1). The valvular lesions are much smaller in individuals with bacterial infections. When *S. aureus, H. parainfluenzae,* and gram-negative, aerobic organisms infect valvular prostheses, the size of the vegetations may approach that of patients with infective endocarditis caused by fungi. On occasion, these may be very large, occlude blood vessels and valvular orifices, decrease cardiac output, and induce congestive cardiac failure. Rarely, new or healed rheumatic vegetations may be present in close proximity to those produced by infection.

Infective endocarditis affects the left side of the heart more often than the right. The valves involved are, in order of frequency, the mitral (28–45%), aortic (5–36%), or both (0–35%).[2–4] The aortic valve is involved more often in patients with acute endocardial infection. Infection of the pulmonic (less than 1%) and tricuspid (0–6%) valves is uncommon. However, the incidence of endocarditis of the tricuspid valve has grown over the past 15–20 years. This appears to be related to an increase in the number of intravenous drug addicts. The tricuspid valve is infected in 33% of these patients with right-sided endocarditis but in only 13.3% of those with concurrent infection of the left side of the heart.[5]

More often in acute than in subacute infective endocarditis, vegetations on the mitral valve may extend to the chordae tendinae and from there to the apex of the papillary muscles.[6–8] Valvular rupture occurs primarily in those patients who have not received treatment for an extended period. The chordae tendinae may be involved when an aortic valvular vegetation

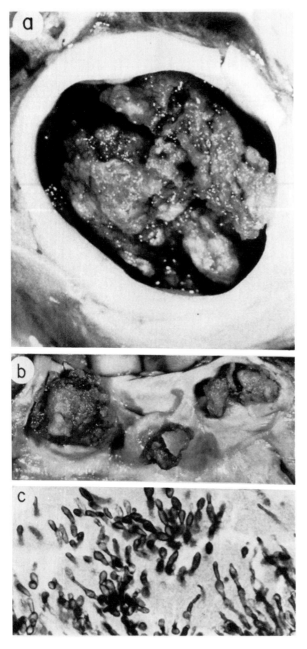

Fig. 6.1. *Candida parapsilosis* infecting the aortic valve. (A) Aortic valve viewed from above, with the vegetations blocking the valve orifice. (B) Opened valve with vegetations on each cusp. (C) Photomicrograph of the pseudomycelia of *C. parapsilosis* within the vegetation. (Methanamine silver stain). (Adapted from Ref. 11)

124

extends over the ventricular endocardium or when lesions on the ventricular surface of the anterior mitral cusp ulcerate. A "worm-eaten" appearance is a characteristic feature of a stenotic mitral valve infected in the course of subacute endocarditis. With healing, fibrous irregularities develop on the involved leaflets, giving them a coarse appearance resembling the skin of a shark.

Necrosis of an infected valve may lead to the development of aneurysms and/or perforation of the valvular cusps (Fig. 6.2). This occurs most often in

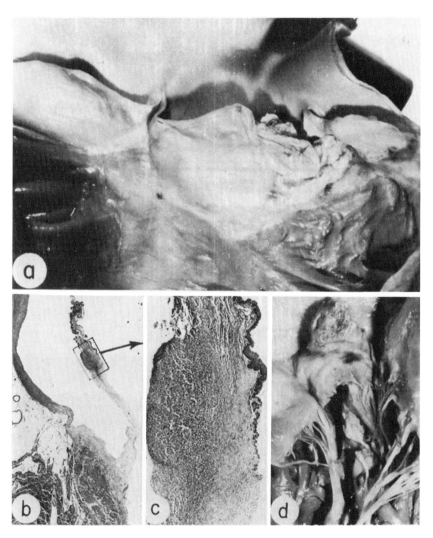

Fig. 6.2. *S. aureus* endocarditis involving the pulmonic (A–C) and mitral (D) valves. The vegetation on the pulmonic valve caused tearing of one leaflet. (B) Histological section through a portion of the infected pulmonic valve cusp. (C) Higher-power view of a portion of the same cusp. (Adapted from Ref. 2)

acute infective endocarditis, especially when it is caused by *S. aureus.* It may also appear during treatment of the subacute disease. Aneurysms that involve the sinus of Valsalva may be present at the base of the aorta; extend to the pericardial space between the aorta and pulmonary artery; and produce hemorrhagic, pyogenic, or fibrinous pericarditis. The infection may invade the upper or lower areas of the intraventricular septum (Fig. 6.3). Septal perforation occurs when endocarditis is acute; it is rare in subacute disease.[1]

The histological features of subacute infective endocarditis have been described by Libman and Friedberg.[1] They pointed out that the valvular vegetations contained platelet-fibrin collections in which bacterial colonies were present on and below the surface. This suggested that the thrombus

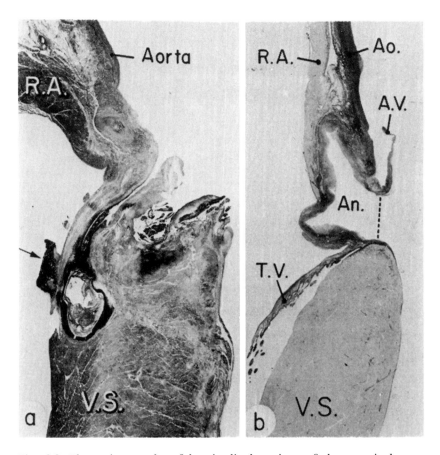

Fig. 6.3. Photomicrographs of longitudinal sections of the ventricular septum (V.S.) at two levels. (A) Section showing extension of the infective process through the entire thickness of the muscular V.S. A small vegetation (arrow) is apparent on the endocardium of the right side of the heart. R.A. = right atrium. (B) Section includes an aneurysm (An.) of the membranous portion of the V.S. The dashed line represents the normal site of the ventricular septum. T.V. = tricuspid valve leaflet; A.V. = aortic valve cusp; Ao. = aorta. (Adapted from Ref. 11)

was derived from destructive changes in the inflamed valve. The cellular reaction was composed primarily of mononuclear cells, lymphocytes, and histiocytes; very few polymorphonuclear cells were present. Giant cells containing phagocytized bacteria were common. The cusp below the vegetation was the site of a destructive process localized on the surface of one or both valves. At this stage, most of the organisms had disappeared and healing was prominent. In addition to inflammatory cells, the cusps contained numerous capillaries and fibroblasts. This "hypercapillarization" led to the formation of anastomosing cavernous channels that formed a distinctive "spongy lesion." Considerable fibroblastic replacement was present. When healing was prolonged, the vegetations were calcified. A variable degree of repair was present in some of the lesions; in others, the infection was still active. Fresh lesions were superimposed on healed ones when endocarditis recurred.

A number of pathological changes are present in the myocardium of patients with infective endocarditis. These usually consist of diffuse or localized collections of lymphocytes and mononuclear cells (the Bracht-Wächter bodies replace cardiac muscle and, unlike Aschoff bodies, are not present in the interstitium of the myocardium). Diffuse or localized collections of polymorphonuclear cells, with or without myocardial necrosis or miliary abscesses, are occasionally present. Gross suppuration is absent. Some muscle fibers have degenerated. Small scars in various stages of healing are often present. The endothelial cells of the capillaries and arterioles of the small branches of the coronary arteries are swollen and proliferating. Arteriolitis or necrosis of the media or adventitia, perivascular cellular infiltrates, and scars are present. In some instances, a large branch of a coronary artery may contain an embolus or is the site of a mycotic aneurysm.

The histopathology of infective endocarditis that involves the right side of the heart has been described by Buchbinder and Roberts[9] (Fig. 6.4). Among the lesions they noted were (1) myocardial abscesses that contained colonies of bacteria; (2) septic emboli (extra- or intramural) in one or more coronary arteries; (3) foci of necrosis in the ventricular wall or papillary muscles; (4) calcification of individual myocardial fibers; and (5) acute pneumonia with complicated pulmonary infarcts or abscesses.

The histological findings identified by Buchbinder and Roberts[9] in patients with infective endocarditis involving the left side of the heart who came to necropsy included myocardial fibrosis in the ventricle, papillary muscles, and ventricular free wall. Narrowing of the lumens of the coronary arteries to less than 25% of their normal diameter was present in 20% of the patients.

The microscopic anatomy of *acute* bacterial endocarditis is very different from that of *subacute* disease[10] (Figs. 6.5, 6.6). It is characterized by the rapid development of lesions containing no fibroblasts or other forms of organization that indicate an attempt to repair the process. The fibrin-platelet vegetations in untreated patients contain only polymorphonuclear leukocytes and large numbers of organisms in the necrotic areas of the

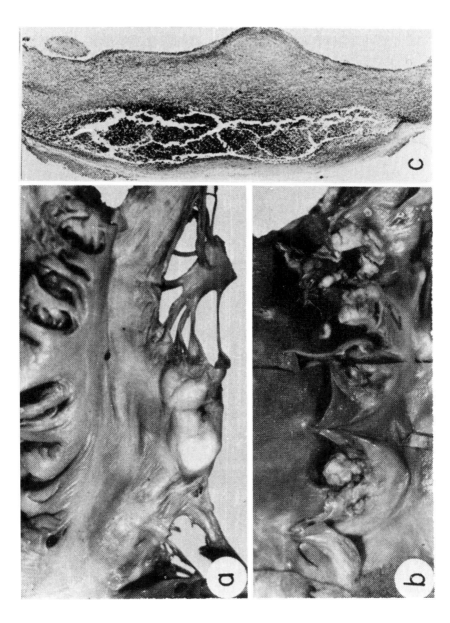

Fig. 6.4. Pneumococcal endocarditis involving the tricuspid (A) and aortic (B) valves. The vegetations on these valves are large and cause extensive destruction of the cusps. (C) Histologic section of a portion of the myxomatoid leaflet showing abscess formation. (Adapted from Ref. 2.)

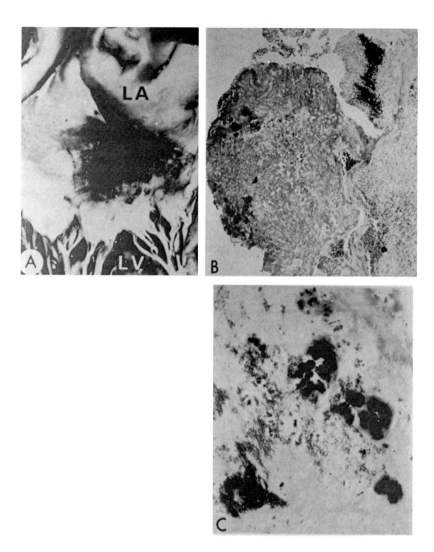

Fig. 6.5. Histology of infective endocarditis. *Staphylococcus aureus* endocarditis in a drug addict. (A) Opened left atrium revealing rheumatic mitral valvulitis and infective vegetations on the posterior mitral leaflets. (B, C) Histological sections of the vegetation. Note the darkly staining, gram-positive cocci near the periphery of the vegetation and the lack of vascular channels. (Adapted from Applefield M, Woodward T: Infective endocarditis: A clinical overview, in *Current Problems in Cardiology,* W Harvey et al (eds), Vol 2, No 1. Copyright © 1977. Year Book Medical Publishers, Inc, Chicago)

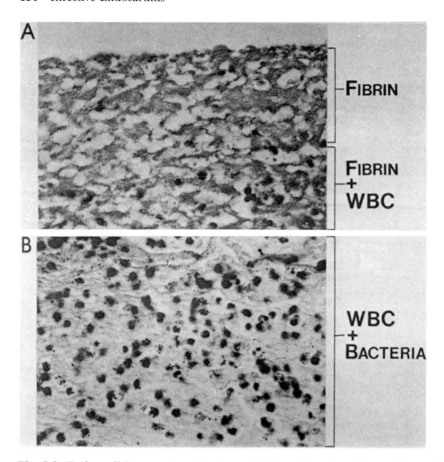

Fig. 6.6. Endocarditis vegetation showing a fibrin mesh on the valve surface and a dense interstitial infiltrate of inflammatory cells, polymorphonuclear leukocytes, and histiocytes (hematoxylin and eosin, ×300). (Adapted from Williams R, Kilpatrick K: Immunofluorescence studies of cardiac valve in infective endocarditis. *Arch Intern Med* 1985;145:297)

valve. These features satisfy the criteria for the diagnosis of acute or *ulcerative endocarditis* and explain the propensity of this disease to produce spontaneous rupture of valvular leaflets, papillary muscles, and chordae tendinae; the development of aneurysms; and the high incidence of suppurative and other intracardiac complications.

A study of 45 cases of acute infective endocarditis involving the left side of the heart, as well as a review of the literature by Buchbinder and Roberts,[9] have indicated that myocardial lesions were present in 88–100% of patients; 3–90% were necrotic and 4–64% were fibrotic. Evidence of infective endocarditis that involved previously normal valves was present in 42%. Fifty-three percent of patients had vegetations superimposed on anatomically normal valves. Autopsies indicated that cardiac failure caused by valvular dysfunction had been present in 59–74%. Necrosis of the papillary muscles without mitral regurgitation was present in 58% of the patients.

Pericarditis that appears in the course of infective endocarditis (8%) may be due to several causes. Most common is myocardial infarction following embolic occlusion of a coronary artery. Other reasons are (1) extension of a myocardial abscess; (2) spread from an infected aortic valve into the pericardium between the aortic root and the pulmonary artery; (3) bacteremia; (4) an increase in rheumatic fever; and (5) leakage of a mycotic aneurysm into the sinus of Valsalva.[6] Of 31 individuals with an infected aortic valve, 12 developed ring abscesses, evidence of severe destruction of the valvular cusps.

A study of the gross pathology of healed left-sided infective endocarditis in 59 patients has been reported by Roberts and Buchbinder.[11] The hearts of 42 patients were examined at autopsy. Fifty-one percent had lesions secondary to successfully treated endocarditis. Residua of valvular infection were more common in individuals with incompetent valves than in those with stenotic or mixed valvular disease. Fifty-one percent had perforation of the valvular cusps, probably related to the presence of a ring abscess. Rupture of chordae tendinae or aneurysms was less common. The organism most often involved was *S. viridans*. The mitral or aortic valve, or both, were either stenotic or incompetent. Sixteen patients had perforated valves; 13 developed regurgitation; and 3 had competent valves and ring abscesses. Stenotic valves were fibrosed and calcified. Focal or diffuse fibrosis usually was present in incompetent valves. Anatomical studies indicated that the infected valves on the left side of the heart were normal in 15% of the patients before they developed infective endocarditis. The involved valves were healed in 58%. All patients had bacteremia. Rheumatic cardiac disease was present in 41% of patients and congenital cardiac lesions in 29%. Other abnormalities, in order of frequency, were biscuspid valves, aortic regurgitation, ventricular septal defect, degenerative Marfan's syndrome, and unicuspid aortic valve.

The pathoanatomy of infective endocarditis that involved the right side of the heart in 12 patients has been described by Roberts and Buchbinder.[2] They noted that bacteria were present in the tricuspid or pulmonary valves. Other lesions included rupture of the chordae tendinae, necrosis of the papillary muscles, and suppurative or nonsuppurative myocarditis. The vegetations on the right side of the heart did not extend to the basal attachments of the leaflets or to the annuli in 9 of 12 patients. Mural lesions were present in three cases; two were situated on the right ventricular endocardium. The myocardium was involved in only 2 or 12 patients. Acute pneumonia was present in 10 and meningitis in 5 patients. Material resembling vegetations was present in the pulmonary artery in 7 of 10 individuals in whom infection of the lung was present. Renal abnormalities were present in nine patients; among these were glomerulonephritis, abscesses, and septic as well as healed infarcts.

The gross pathology of infective endocarditis involving prosthetic valves has been described by Arnett and Roberts[12] and Anderson et al.[13] (Fig. 6.7).

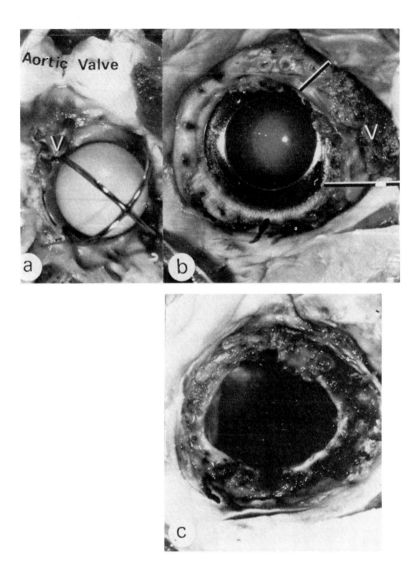

Fig. 6.7. Prosthetic mitral valve endocarditis caused by *S. epidermidis*. The infection appeared 10 years after replacement of both the mitral and tricuspid valves. At autopsy, only the mitral prosthesis was found to be infected. (A) Infected mitral valve prosthesis viewed from the left ventricle. Vegetative material (V) is present on the prosthetic annulus just below the aortic valve. (B) Prosthesis viewed from the left atrium, showing the vegetation (V) at the junction of the prosthetic and natural valve annuli. (C) Same view after removal of the prosthesis, showing even greater extension of the infection at the site of attachment of the prosthesis. (From Ref. 12)

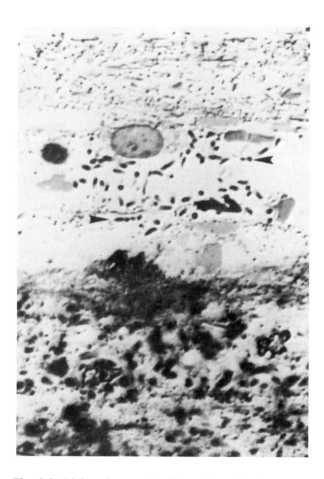

Fig. 6.8. Light micrograph of a section of a heterograft. A thick layer of fibrin overlies the surface of the heterograft, and a small cluster of bacteria is located between the fibrin and the valve collagen. Section of plastic-embedded tissue, 0.5 μm thick, stained with toluidine blue and viewed with Nomarski differential interference contrast optics (×1,600, reduced by 5%). (Adapted from Ferrans V, Boyle S, Billingham M, et al: Infecting glutaraldehyde-preserved porcine heterografts. *Am J Cardiol* 1979;43:1123)

Fifteen patients had infections of a rigid-frame aortic prosthesis; mitral involvement was present in seven. The infection appeared within 2 months after surgery in some individuals; in others, it was not apparent until after that period. *S. aureus* was identified most often. The infectious process was posterior to the area of attachment of the prosthesis to the valve ring and spread to the adjacent structures in 13 patients; 11 had aortic prostheses, most of which were detached. Defects in electrical conduction, left bundle branch block, or complete block were present in seven individuals. These were present most often when an aortic prosthesis was in place. This suggested that the conductive abnormalities were related to the presence of an abscess or to necrosis of the intraventricular septum.

Cardiac hypertrophy and/or dilatation of the left ventricle were present in 95% and 73%, of the patients, respectively.[13] Dysfunction of the prosthesis was a problem in 17% of patients and was associated with (1) ulceration of a valvular cusp; (2) a paravalvular leak; (3) entrapment of the poppet by a thrombus; (4) perforation of a ring abscess into the right ventricle; and (5) stenosis (most common). Infection of the aortic annulus was present in 57% of the patients. Other pathological findings included fibrinous or purulent pericarditis, aortic stenosis associated with exuberant vegetations, and embolic myocarditis (abscess and focal necrosis). Infective endocarditis involving the mitral annulus was present in 43% of the patients. Infection of a prosthetic valve did not spread to other valves. The A-V node and the bundle of His were obliterated by an abscess in one patient who developed complete heart block. The A-V node was extensively involved by an inflammatory process that spread from an abscess in the aortic ring in two individuals; the bundle of His was intact. Idiopathic atrophy and fibrosis of the proximal portion of the left bundle were present in two patients. Among other unusual findings were *peripheral, splenic* (59%), *renal* (50%), and *cerebral* (45%) emboli.

The pathological features of infected Hancock porcine prostheses have been described by Bortolloti et al.[14] They documented that the vegetations were friable, located primarily on the inflow surface of the involved valve, and ranged in size from small to so massive that they partially or completely obstructed the valvular openings. The infected cusps were frayed or perforated. Ring abscesses or calcification of the diseased valves were uncommon. Most of the bioprostheses exhibited morphological changes consistent with dysfunction. Histological examination disclosed mild to marked deposition of fibrin on the inflow surface of the involved valve. Disintegration of collagen led to the disappearance of collagen bundles, which were partially or completely replaced by homogeneous material. Macrophages and polymorphonuclear leukocytes were present in all patients; mild to marked subendothelial inflammation was identified in some. Clusters were often situated within the infected cusps. The inflammatory response was characterized by the presence of granulomas when a Hancock valve was invaded by a fungus.

Ferrans et al.[15] have described the features that distinguish the pathology of infected porcine valve heterografts from those involving other types of prostheses (Figs. 6.8, 6.9). They pointed out that "There are several characteristics of infection of rigid-framed prosthetic valves. The infection does not involve the prosthetic materials; instead it involves biologic products such as fibrin, organized thrombi and fibrous tissue that have covered the prosthetic valve; the infection is characteristically located at the site of attachment of the sewing ring to host tissue; valve ring abscesses are to be expected; and the infection does not destroy the prosthesis itself, although it may cause it to malfunction mechanically and to become detached from the valve ring.

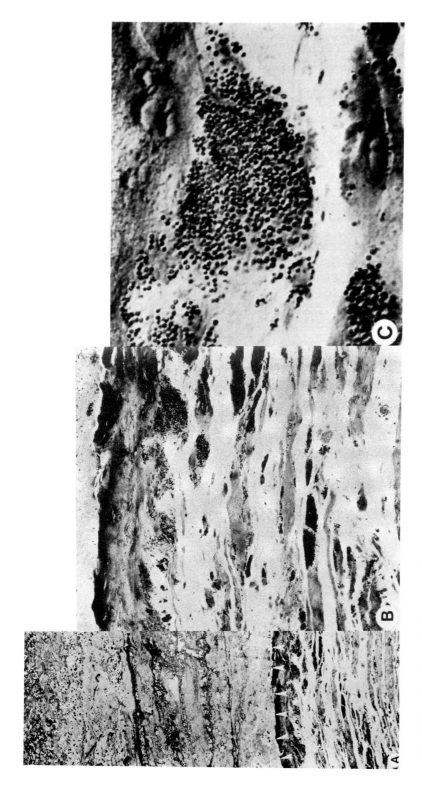

Fig. 6.9. View of a valve heterograft showing bacterial invasion of collagen bundles, which appear widely separated. Note the absence of inflammatory cells in this area of the heterograft (×400). (C) High-magnification micrograph (Normarski differential interference contrast optics) of a cluster of bacteria (same cluster as in upper right of B) with the typical morphological features of cocci (×1,600). (Adapted from Ferrans V, Boyle S, Billingham M, et al: Infecting glutaraldehyde-preserved porcine heterografts. *Am J Cardiol* 1979;43:1123)

Schoen and Levy described the differences between the pathoanatomical features of infection of mechanical and bioprosthetic valves.[16] They stated,

> "In contrast to these characteristics of infection of rigid-framed prosthetic valves, infection of porcine valve heterografts has the following features: it involves the prosthetic material itself as well as fibrin, organized thrombi and fibrous tissue from the host; it is localized in the cusps; it can destroy the prosthesis when it is uncommonly associated with ring abscesses. The destruction of bioprosthetic tissue is illustrated by our observation of invasion of the leaflet substance and severe breakdown of collagen in the heterografts from two of our patients. The pattern of localization of infection of porcine valve heterografts is similar to that recorded in other types of bioprostheses, including homografts, fascia lata valves and pericardial valves."

Bortolloti et al.[14] pointed out that the treatment of infected porcine valves with glutaraldehyde made the heterografts more resistant to infection. Stenosis of prosthetic valves with an infected vegetation is a common complication of infective endocarditis involving a porcine valve. Valvular ring abscesses and perivalvular leaks are uncommon. The incidence of valvular abscesses in patients with infected rigid-framed prosthetic valves may approach 100%; the death rate is very high. The entire circumference of the valvular bed is necrotic in about one-third of cases.

The extracardiac manifestations of endocarditis follow the deposition of a sterile or septic embolus at any site in the body. The pathogenesis of the peripheral manifestations of infective endocarditis in native valves is discussed in Chapter 8.

Marantic endocarditis occurs in patients with chronic disease, especially those who develop disorders other than infection. The distribution of embolic deposits is similar to that in infective endocarditis. The feature that distinguishes marantic from infective endocarditis primarily is the absence of a vigorous cellular response.[17] Microscopically, the valvular infection in patients with marantic endocardiosis contains platelets, fibrin, and a few mononuclear cells, but no organisms.[18]

References

1. Libman E, Friedberg CK: *Subacute Bacterial Endocarditis.* Oxford, Oxford University Press, 1941.
2. Roberts WC, Buchbinder NA: Right-sided valvular infective endocarditis. *Am J Med* 1971;53:7.
3. Come P: Infective endocarditis: Current perspective. *Compr Ther* 1982;8:57.
4. Pelletier LL, Petersdorf RG: Infective endocarditis: A review of 125 cases from the University of Washington Hospitals, 1963–1972. *Medicine (Baltimore)* 1977;56:287.
5. Watanakumakom C: Changing epidemiology and newer aspects of infective endocarditis. *Adv Intern Med* 1977;22:21.
6. Weinstein L, Schlesinger JJ: Pathoanatomic, pathophysiologic and clinical correlations in endocarditis. *N Engl J Med* 1974;291:832.
7. Robinson M, Ruedy J: Sequelae of bacterial endocarditis. *Am J Med* 1962;32:922.
8. Cohen L, Freedman L: Damage to the aortic valve as a cause of death in bacterial endocarditis. *Ann Intern Med* 1961;55:562.

9. Buchbinder NA, Roberts WC: Left-sided valvular active endocarditis. *Am J Med* 1972;53:20.

10. Arnett EC, Roberts WC: Acute infective endocarditis: A clinicopathologic analysis of 137 necropsy patients. *Curr Probl Cardio* 1976;1(No. 7):3.

11. Roberts WC, Buchbinder NA: Healed left-sided infective endocarditis: A clinicopathological study of 59 patients. *Am J Cardiol* 1976;40:876.

12. Arnett EN, Roberts WC: Prosthetic valve endocarditis: Clinicopathological analysis of 22 necropsy patients with comparison of observations in 74 necropsy patients with active infective endocarditis involving natural left-sided cardiac valves. *Am J Cardiol* 1976;38:281.

13. Anderson DJ, Buckley BH, Hutchins GM: A clinicopathologic study of prosthetic valve endocarditis in 22 patients: Morphologic basis for diagnosis and therapy. *Am Heart J* 1977;94:325.

14. Bortolloti V, Thiene G, Milano G, et al: Pathological study of infective endocarditis on Hancock porcine bioprostheses. *J Thorac Cardiovasc Surg* 1981;81:934.

15. Ferrans VJ, Boyce SW, Billingham ME, et al: Infection of glutaraldehyde-preserved porcine valve heterografts. *Am J Cardiol* 1979;43:1123.

16. Schoen F, Levy R: Bioprosthetic heart valve failure. Pathology and pathogenesis. *Cardiol Clin* 1984;2:717.

17. MacDonald RA, Robbins JL: The significance of nonbacterial thrombotic endocarditis: An autopsy and clinical study of 78 cases. *Ann Intern Med* 1957;46:255.

18. Bryar CJ: Nonbacterial thrombotic endocarditis with malignant tumors. *Am J Med* 1969;46:787.

7

Pathoanatomical, Pathophysiological, and Clinical Correlations

A clear understanding of any disease mandates a thorough knowledge of the specific pathophysiological and pathoanatomical processes involved in the onset and clinical course of a disease. It is interesting that in only some of the numerous disorders involving humans have the specific mechanisms been adequately defined. For example, the clinical syndromes and pathological features of atherosclerosis are well known, but the mechanisms involved in its pathogenesis are still debated. It is also not clear what actually occurs in patients overwhelmed by staphylococcus, nor are the anatomical and physiological bases for the symptoms and physical findings produced by the tubercle bacillus known with certainty.

Extensive laboratory and clinical studies have largely defined most of the mechanisms involved in the pathogenesis of infective endocarditis. The purpose of this presentation is to define the dynamics and ultimate effects of the pathoanatomical, pathophysiological, and immunological phenomena involved in the pathogenesis of acute and subacute infective endocarditis, as well as of noninfectious marantic endocarditis.

Pathogenesis of Infective Endocarditis

The pathoanatomical and pathophysiological processes involved in the development of subacute endocarditis are strikingly different from those responsible for the acute disease. Five mechanisms are involved in the initiation and localization of the subacute infection:[1] (1) a previously damaged cardiac valve; (2) a hemodynamic state in which a jet effect is produced by blood flowing from an area of high pressure to one of relatively low pressure, as in mitral insufficiency or the presence of a ventricular septal defect; (3) the presence of a sterile platelet-fibrin thrombus on a valvular leaflet; (4) transient or persistent bacteremia; and (5) a high titer of circulating, agglutinating antibodies specific for the invading organism.

Acute Infective Endocarditis

Acute infective endocarditis often does not share the factors underlying the genesis of the subacute disease. From 50% to 60% of acute cases involve previously normal valves. This underscores the fact that the development of a sterile platelet thrombus on a valve is not an absolute requirement for the development of the disease.[2] Organisms that produce fulminant valvular infection (*S. aureus, S. pneumoniae, S. meningitidis, S. pyogenes,* and *H. influenzae*) are highly invasive; only a small number are required to establish infection on an undamaged valve. It has been established that most of the pathogenicity of *S. aureus* may be accounted for by the fact that it stimulates the extrinsic clotting system when it infects a valve. The single most important factor in the initiation of acute endocarditis is an episode of bacteremia. It must be emphasized that acute infection may also occur in patients with underlying cardiac disease. In this situation, the sterile platelet-fibrin thrombi may already be present and serve as a site for the deposition of circulating microorganisms. The interaction between bacteria and platelets may provide another potential mechanism for the development of acute infective endocarditis. Platelets have been found to facilitate the adhesion of several microorganisms (*C. albicans* and *Ps. aeruginosa*).[3,4] The ability of bacteria to enhance the aggregation of platelets correlates positively with their capacity to infect cardiac endothelium. Platelets and bacteria are present in the peripheral bloodstream of patients with bacteremia[4] and act as building blocks for the growing valvular lesion.

The ability of organisms to adhere to the surfaces of cardiac valves plays a more important role than the interaction with platelets in the pathogenesis of acute infective endocarditis. Gould et al.[5] and Holmes and Ramirez-Ronda[6] examined the attachment of bacteria to normal dog and human valvular leaflets in vitro. The degree of adherence was highest for the enterococcus and *S. aureus*. Next, in order of decreasing activity, were viridans streptococci, *S. epidermidis, Ps. aeruginosa, E. coli,* and *K. pneumoniae*. These observations may explain the relative frequency with which some organisms, especially *S. aureus*, infect previously healthy cardiac valves. The low level of activity of *E. coli* and *K. pneumoniae* may account, in part, for the lower incidence of endocarditis despite the high frequency with which they produce bacteremia. Pelletier et al.[7] suggested that the tendency of *S. sanguis* to attach to endothelial surfaces may be related to its ability to produce dextran. Klotz[8] explored the methods by which *Candida* species attached to the vascular endothelium. The lining cells of blood vessels are relatively resistant to invasion by these organisms. However, *C. albicans* elaborates various enzymes (candidal acid proteases) that injure the membranes of these cells; this leads to enhanced adherence of fungi. In addition, the enzymatic attack exposes the extracellular matrix, which contains different proteins with which specific candidal receptors may form linkages (e.g., fibronectin, laminin, and types I and IV collagen).

Bacteremia

Transient or persistent bacteremia is crucial in the development of acute and subacute endocarditis. Microorganisms enter the circulation spontaneously from a focus of infection or following manipulation of the oral cavity, upper airway, genitourinary system, or intestinal tract, areas in which organisms are almost always present. The intensity of the bacteremia is related to the degree of trauma induced by a procedure and by the characteristics of the organism present at the site of intervention. An excellent review of this phenomenon has been presented by Everett and Hirschman.[9]

In the data presented by physcians, there are considerable differences regarding the frequency of transient bacteremia. This is probably due to a lack of uniformity with respect to obtaining blood for culture. Our experience and that of others has indicated that the quantity of blood obtained for culture must be at least 10 ml (less for young children).[10,11] The number of organisms in the circulation at any time is small and variable. Blood is usually drawn at 5, 10, 15, 20, and 30 min, or later in some cases. All the aliquots are added to appropriate media and incubated at 37°C for at least 4–6 days; longer periods of incubation are required for slowly growing organisms.

The reported incidence of transient bacteremia in patients who undergo dental extractions has ranged from 18% to 85%.[12] The organisms retrieved most often have been streptococci, usually viridans, and occasionally enterococci. Bacteria may be present in the bloodstream for more than 5–10 min when multiple teeth are extracted. The number of organisms in the circulation is usually small, ranging from a few to as many as 30 to 40 per millimeter. In addition, streptococci, diphtheroids, *S. epidermidis,* and anaerobic members of the oral microflora have been recovered. Dental manipulations other than extraction have led to the development of transient bacteremia. Among these have been chewing hard candy, scaling of gums and teeth, periodontal procedures, the use of unwaxed dental floss, and failure to floss for 1 to 2 days. Bacteremia has developed in 50% of patients using oral irrigation devices. This occurs in individuals with untreated periodontitis[13] and in those with mild gingivitis.[14] A study by Berger et al.[15] has indicated that individuals with normal gums who used a Water-Pik developed transient bacteremia. Brushing of healthy teeth and gums does not increase the risk of infection. Root et al.[16] have described a patient with periodontal disease who developed infection of a prosthetic valve by *H. aphrophilus.* The organism was recovered not only from the blood but also from dental plaque. This emphasizes the importance of effective therapy of dental infections in the prevention of infective endocarditis.

The incidence of bacteremia in patients with dental disease has been studied extensively by Winslow and Kobernick.[14] They divided their patients into three groups based on the severity of the gingival disease: (1) those with gingivitis; (2) those with mild disease of the gums; and (3) those with significant periodontitis. All patients underwent removal of calculus and curettage of the epithelium. Cultures of the blood obtained *prior to the procedure* grew organisms in two patients with severe gingivitis, in three with mild disease of the gums, and in none with simple gingivitis. Following the manipulation described above, bacteria were recovered from the circulation of larger numbers of individuals with periodontitis; organisms were present in small numbers in individuals with uncomplicated gingivitis. Statistical analysis of the data indicated that there is an increased risk of bacteremia when dental prophylactic procedures are carried out in the presence of periodontitis but not in individuals free of gingivitis. However, the authors made the comment that, in their opinion, "the bacteremia produced by prophylaxis and other dental procedures have no clinical importance in the great majority of instances." Other investigators have found that spontaneous bacteremia occurred in 9–11% of patients with gingival disease. This raised the question of whether interventional antibiotic prophylaxis is valid.[17]

There is some disagreement concerning the frequency of bacteremia in children who undergo dental manipulation. According to Hurwitz and associates,[18] cultures of blood obtained within 6 min after completion of routine oral prophylaxis were sterile. They suggested that the absence of significant periodontal disease may have been responsible for the failure of bacteria to invade the bloodstream. They also stated that it was possible to perform routine dental therapy in children without antimicrobial prophylaxis even when rheumatic or congenital cardiac disease had been present. However, De Leo et al.[19] failed to confirm these observations. They studied 39 children 7–12 years of age; 2 developed bacteremia before the procedure was initiated. Organisms were recovered from the blood of 11 (28%) children after the study was completed; only anaerobic species were present in seven patients. Peterson and Peacock[20] noted transient bacteremia in 35% of 101 children who had primary teeth removed, in 53% of those from whom diseased primary and permanent teeth were extracted, and in 61% of those in whom healthy teeth were removed. Restorative dental procedures were not associated with bacteremia. The organisms recovered from the blood were alpha streptococci (29%), diphtheroids (23%), *Peptostreptococcus* (10%), *Bacteroides* species (12%), coagulase-negative staphylococci (12%), *Veillonella* (4%), *Neisseria* species (9%), and *Vibiro* species (1%).

Transient intrusion of organisms into the bloodstream has not been limited to dental manipulation. Tonsilloadenoidectomy is often associated with bacteremia. A variety of organisms, most often streptococci, have been recovered from the blood of 27–38% of patients who have had dental surgery.[21–23] Transient bacteremia has followed rigid bronchoscopy and nasal and tracheal surgery.[24] Among the organisms recovered from the blood of patients who underwent these procedures have been *S. aureus*, streptococci, *Haemophilus* species, *S. pneumoniae*, and *S. epidermidis*. The results of a study of nasotracheal suctioning by LeFrock et al.[25] indicated that bacteremia persisted for 15 min in 17.6% of 68 patients. *E. coli*,

K. pneumoniae, B. melaninogenicus, Ps. aeruginosa, S. aureus, E. aerogenes, H. influenzae, and viridans streptococci were recovered from the blood. A comparison of nasotracheal and orotracheal suctioning with respect to the risk of transient bacteremia has been carried out by Barry and his colleagues.[26]

Gastrointestinal Tract

The incidence of transient bacteremia following fiberoptic endoscopy of the upper gastrointestinal tract has been studied by Shull and his colleagues.[27] They noted that 4 of 50 patients subjected to this procedure had organisms in their blood for 5–30 min after the instrument was removed. *Neisseria* species, streptococci, *Porpionbacterium acnes, A. calcoaceticus,* and/ or *S. epidermidis* were recovered. Only 1 of 100 patients examined by gastroscopy by Stray et al.[28] developed bacteremia. A study of 200 individuals subjected to this procedure by Baltch et al.[29] disclosed positive blood cultures in 8%; 12 different microbial species were identified.

Data indicating the frequency with which transient bacteremia is associated with sigmoidoscopy are conflicting. The reported incidence has ranged from 9% to 13%.[30,31] LeFrock and his colleagues,[32] using a minimum of 10 ml of blood for culture, recovered organisms from the circulation of 10% of 200 individuals who underwent sigmoidoscopy. Viridans streptococci were present in 18 individuals, and *E. coli* and *Bacteroides* species occurred in one patient each.

The administration of a barium enema may predispose patients to the risk of bacteremia. LeFrock et al.[33] noted that this occurred in 11% of their patients. However, Schimmel et al.[34] were unable to confirm this observation. It has been suggested that the mechanisms involved in the intrusion of organisms into the circulation during a barium enema are (1) trauma induced by pressure on the mucous membranes; (2) abrasion of the rectal wall by the enema tip; and (3) increased intraluminal pressure induced by the load of barium.[9]

Although transient bacteremia has been reported to occur in 2.5–5.3% of patients who undergo colonoscopy,[35] other studies have indicated that this may not be the case[36–38]. Hartong et al.[39] suggested that the higher incidence of invasion of bacteria into the circulation during barium studies compared to colonoscopy is related to the high pressure produced by the introduction of contrast material into the colon.

Biopsy of the liver may lead to the development of transient bacteremia in 3–13% of patients.[40,41] The presence of viral or alcoholic hepatitis and cirrhosis may increase the risk.[42]

The incidence of bacteremia associated with endoscopic injection sclerotherapy of esophageal varices has been studied by Camarra et al.[43] Eighteen patients were exposed to 40 sessions of this procedure. Cultures of the blood were collected 5 and 30 min and 24 hr after sclerotherapy was performed. The injector and endoscope were cultured before and after use. *E. cloacae* and a coagulase-negative staphylococcus were recovered from the circulation. *Ps. aeruginosa* was isolated from the injector after it was used. The authors concluded that "the incidence of transient bacteremia after sclerotherapy is no higher than after routine upper intestinal endoscopy." Microbial invasion of the bloodstream has been reported in individuals who have undergone appendectomy or cholecystectomy.[44]

Various manipulations of the urinary tract have led to the development of bacteremia.[9] This may occur even when the urine is sterile, but it is far more common when the urine contains a significant number of bacteria. The sources of the organisms, in addition to infected urine, are the normal microflora of the urethra, infection of the prostate, and contaminated instruments or irrigating fluids. The procedures, and the incidence of bacteremia with which they have been associated, are (1) internal urethrotomy (75%); (2) urethral dilatation or external urethrotomy (86%); (3) transurethral prostatecomy (12% overall but 10.8% when the urine is sterile); (4) 57.5% when bacteriuria is present; (5) the removal of indwelling catheters from patients with infected urine (26.3%); and (6) retropubic prostatectomy in individuals with sterile urine (7.4–12.8%) and in those with bacteriuria undergoing cystoscopy (82.4%).

Studies of the incidence of transient bacteremia during procedures that involve the female genital tract have produced variable results. The intrusion of organisms into the circulation during childbirth has been identified in about 5% of women.[45] However, some physicians have suggested that this does not occur in the course of uncomplicated childbirth. Genital strains of *Mycoplasma* have been recovered from the blood shortly after delivery.[46]

There is presently no agreement concerning the risk of invasion of the bloodstream in patients with intrauterine contraceptive devices. De Swiet et al.[47] have described a woman who developed infective endocarditis 6 weeks after insertion. However, the results of a study by Everett et al.[48] have indicated that the presence of this device is not associated with bacteremia.

Suction abortion may lead to transient bacteremia in about 85% of patients.[49] In some instances, microorganisms have been recovered from the blood after a bimanual pelvic examination. In some patients, bacteremia occurs intermittently; in others, it may be present for as long as 1 hr after an abortion has been completed. The organisms recovered from the circulation have included *Peptococcus, Peptostreptococcus, Lactobacillus, Veillonella*, and viridans streptococci. There is presently no evidence that biopsy of the cervix leads to the development of bacteremia.[50] Bacteremia is a rare event in patients subjected to cardiac catheterization or angiography performed under conditions of strict sterility.[51–53]

Infective endocarditis following closed-heart surgery occurs less often than it does after an open-heart procedure.[54,55] The risk of infection following insertion of a prosthetic valve is two to four times higher than it is in other open-heart procedures.[52] Intraoperative bacteremia has occurred in 20% of patients exposed to cardiopulmonary bypass units contaminated by microorganisms.[56–58] Twenty percent of patients exposed to this equipment have had an episode of bacteremia. The presence of intravascular catheters, infected wounds, and urinary and respiratory infections may lead to the development of bacteremia in the postoperative period.

Bacteremia is common in patients being treated for burns that involve more than 60% of the surface area of the body.[59] The incidence of the transient bacteremia is high during the massage of infected joints, tonsils, gums, prostate, and furuncles.[60] Bacteremia may be present in 2–8% of individuals who develop fever during hemodialysis. Bacteremia occurs in 2.5–4% of patients undergoing peritoneal dialysis.

A very interesting association of hepatic cirrhosis, especially that produced by alcohol and infectious hepatitis, has been reported by Snyder et al.[61] They noted that endocardial disease was present in 1.8% of 550 cirrhotic and 0.9% of 3,658 noncirrhotic individuals studied at autopsy. Rheumatic heart disease was absent in all patients; however, calcific aortic stenosis was common. Analysis of the incidence of endocarditis in 151 other patients admitted to the same hospital indicated that the disease was 3.5 times more common in those with alcoholic cirrhosis than in noncirrhotic individuals. Infective endocarditis was absent in patients with postnecrotic cirrhosis; it was present in one patient with hemochromatosis. Because peritonitis was twice as common in individuals with cirrhosis, this may have been the source of the bacteremia that led to the development of valvular infection. Gram-negative bacteria, enterococci, other streptococcal species, and *S. aureus* were involved.

Addiction to intravenous drugs has been an increasingly important factor in the pathogenesis of acute and subacute infective endocarditis.[62–70] A review of the literature by Reisbert[69] indicated that the incidence of valvular infection in these individuals was difficult to determine. Simberkoff[70] suggested that it was about 1.5 to 2 cases per 1,000 addicts. A study of 20,000 persons addicted to heroin living in a large city disclosed 50 cases of endocardial infection.[63] Patients addicted to heroin who developed valvular infection were usually young and became severely ill earlier than nonaddicted individuals. About 70% had respiratory symptoms and pulmonary infiltrates.[65,68] The tricuspid valve alone was involved in 28.5–72% of cases.[62] Endocarditis in narcotic addicts caused by *S. aureus* frequently involved the right side of the heart.[52,66] The source of the staphylococci responsible for the disease in these patients was the nasal mucosa, not needles, syringes, or drugs.[71]

The prolonged presence of polyethylene catheters or "long lines" in the peripheral venous system has increased the risk of infective endocarditis. This is due to colonization of the tip of the catheter and/or entry of organisms in the area on the skin through which the tube is passed. Infection of the tricuspid and pulmonic valves, as well as the right atrial and ventricular walls, occurs in patients with indwelling catheters in the pulmonary artery over an extended period.[72] *S. aureus* has been responsible for most of these infections. Hyperalimentation is associated with an increased risk of infection of cardiac valves;[73] yeasts and fungi are often the causative agents.

Burned patients are highly susceptible to the development of infective endocarditis. This occurred in 2% of 1,731 patients reported by Baskin et al.[74] They noted that 18 persons had involvement of the right side, 9 of the left side, and 8 of both sides of the heart. The disease was acute in 22 patients and subacute in 13. Murmurs were detectable in only two individuals. The organism most often involved was *S. aureus* (77%). A mixture of staphylococci and gram-negative bacteria has been recovered in 5% and *Providencia* and *Serratia* in 14% of patients. Suppurative thrombophlebitis was very common. Some patients had verrucous endocardiosis (marantic endocarditis) rather than infective endocarditis.

Although infections of transvenous cardiac pacemakers are common, endocarditis is relatively rare. In a review of years of experience with patients who had received pacemakers, Lemire et al.[75] failed to identify a single instance of infective endocarditis despite the fact that organisms were recovered from the generator pocket, electrodes, bloodstream, pericardium, and pleura.

A number of other infectious and noninfectious disorders and conditions that predispose patients to the development of infective endocarditis have been reported by Garvey and Neu.[76] Among these are neoplastic lesions, nonmalignant hematological disorders, collagen-vascular diseases, diabetes mellitus, chronic active viral hepatitis, renal failure, treatment with corticosteroids, antitumor chemotherapy and radiation therapy, perinephric abscess, obstruction or perforation of the bowel, and infections of sternal wounds following cardiac surgery. However, based on the results of a study of 7,840 patients with various cancers, Rosen and Armstrong[77] suggested that the incidence of infective endocarditis is equal to that of individuals free of neoplastic disease. Valvular infection that occurs in these patients is caused most often by staphylococci; next, in order of frequency, are streptococci, gram-negative bacilli, and *Candida*.

Other extracardiac foci of infection may be the primary sources of bacteremia that leads to the development of infective endocarditis. Among these are pimples and furuncles, especially when squeezed or subjected to inappropriate surgery. The organism usually responsible for valvular infection in these patients is *S. aureus*.

Pneumonia, especially that caused by *S. pneumoniae*, was a primary event in the pathogenesis of acute infective endocarditis prior to the availability of antimicrobial agents. Endocardial infection is presently an infrequent complication of respiratory disease. Among other extracardiac infections that predispose to endocarditis are acute hematogenous osteomyelitis, usually caused by *S. aureus*, acute pyelonephritis, meningococcemia, brucellosis, Q fever, rat bite fever, and a variety of immunosuppressive disorders, including the vasculitides when they are complicated by bacteremia and suprainfection by bacteria or fungi following exposure to antimicrobial agents.

Garvey and Neu[76] and Rosen and Armstrong[77] have pointed out that a significant number of individuals with active infection of structurally normal valves may develop endocarditis. Many of these patients had been immunosuppressed by major underlying disease or treatment with corticosteroids or radiation. They were also older, more likely to develop infection of the right side of the heart, and more susceptible to invasion of the valves by gram-negative bacilli and fungi than those who were immunologically competent. The presence of infective endocarditis had not been suspected during life in about one-third of the patients. The fatality rate in these patients was 57%; it was 28% in those with normal host defenses.

That infective endocarditis may be a subtle and often a lethal complication of hemodialysis has been pointed out by Cross and Steigbigel.[78] They suggested that the source of the invading organisms appeared to be contamination of access sites secondary to various manipulations, including dental procedures.[78] The incidence of infection was lower in individuals with arteriovenous fistulas than in those with arteriolvenous shunts. *S. aureus* was involved most often. *Ps. aeruginosa* was responsible for infection of access sites but produced endocarditis infrequently. Eradication of the valvular infection required treatment with antimicrobial agents in addition to removal of the shunt. The results reported by Cross and Steigbiegel have been duplicated by Leonard and his colleagues.[79,80] Eleven of their patients (2.7%) undergoing maintenance hemodialysis developed infective endocarditis. *S. aureus* was the cause in five cases, *L. monocytogenes* in two, and *Corynebacterium*, *N. israelii*, *S. epidermidis*, and *Enterococcus* in only one each. Valvular disease became apparent clinically about 28 months after the initiation of dialysis and was associated with microbial invasion of the vascular access site. In a review of 18 previously studied cases, Leonard et al.[79,80] noted that *S. aureus* was the most common pathogen.

That infective endocarditis is a serious diagnostic consideration in dialyzed individuals with prolonged bacteremia has been emphasized by Dobkin et al.[81] They suggested that the absence of the characteristic clinical manifestations of valvular disease or the isolation of gram-negative organisms from the bloodstream indicated that isolated invasion of the vascular access site was more likely. It is important to note that episodes of transient bacteremia may occur in 2% of apparently healthy individuals with intact mucous membranes.[82]

Since publication of the description of malignant endocarditis by Osler,[83] physicians have attempted to explain the constancy of the location of infected valvular vegetations. The concept that septic coronary artery emboli led to infection of the cardiac valves was first described by Luschka in 1852.[84–88] It was based on the misconception that normal human valvulor leaflets contained a large network of blood vessels fed by the coronary circulation (see Chapter 1). Unfortunately, many of the experiments that supported this theory were conducted in animals (oxen and cows); the valves of which are richly endowed with blood vessels. Injection studies demonstrated the vscularity of human valves involved hearts that had probably been injured by rheumatic fever.[89–92] When a clear distinction was made between rheumatic valvulitis and infective endocarditis during the second decade of this century, Luschka's hypothesis was finally discarded.

Lepeschkin[93] postulated that mechanical and hydraulic factors were important in the pathogenesis of infective endocarditis. Studies of 1,024 autopsied patients with this disease indicated that the mitral valve was involved in 86%, the aortic valve in 55%, the tricuspid valve in 19.6%, and the pulmonary valve in 1.1%. This suggested that the incidence of valvular infection was related to the pressure to which the valve was exposed and suggested that mechanical stress was a critical factor in the production of infective endocarditis.

It has been pointed out that quantitative and qualitative changes in the flow of blood influence the morphology and function of the endothelium of the circulatory system.[94–96] In areas in which laminar flow is present, the nuclei of the pyriform endothelial cells are aligned in parallel. This is not the case in areas in which blood flow is more turbulent; the nuclei and the cells themselves are not so lined up. The endothelial cells in the area of closure of valvular leaflets are polygonal in shape, with an increase in the amount of cytoplasmic filaments. Disruption of the laminar flow of blood may also lead to functional changes in the endothelium. Areas of increased turbulence augment the adhesion of leukocytes to the walls of blood vessels and to the surface of cardiac valves. In vitro studies have indicated an increase in the reactivity of platelets on the endothelial surface of cells exposed to low shear stress. Therefore, these normal-appearing endothelial cells may have a lower threshold for the development of a sterile platelet thrombus.

By injecting a bacterial aerosol into an air stream passing through an agar Venturi tube, Rodbard[97] proved that high pressure may force a contaminated fluid into a low-pressure sink. This explained the characteristic pattern of infection in which the maximal deposition of bacteria appeared in the low-pressure sink immediately beyond the constriction (Fig. 7-1). The application of the Venturi principle to the pathophysiology of infective endocarditis has been essential for understanding the distribution of lesions that develop on different valves, as well as those that appear on septal defects. The atrial side of the mitral valve and the adjacent segment of the atrium are the usual sites of infective endocarditis in patients with mitral insufficiency. A Venturi effect is produced when blood flows from the left ventricle (an area of high pressure) through an orifice (the nearly closed insufficient valve) into the atrium (a low-pressure sink). The regurgitant

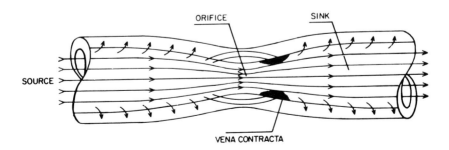

Fig. 7.1. Venturi model of a high-pressure source driving a bacterial aerosol into a low-pressure sink. (Adapted from Ref. 97)

bloodstream injures the endocardium of the left atrial wall and establishes an area of potential bacterial invasion (MacCallum's patch).

Infection of the aortic valve develops in a similar fashion. Some aortic insufficiency is critical. The high-pressure source is the aorta; the low-pressure source is the left ventricle. Vegetations develop on the ventricular surface of the aortic leaflets. Satellite lesions may be present on the chordae tendinae. These are produced by a regurgitant stream ejected at high speed through an incompetent valve (Fig. 7.2).

The development of a small hole in the ventricular septum induces a left-

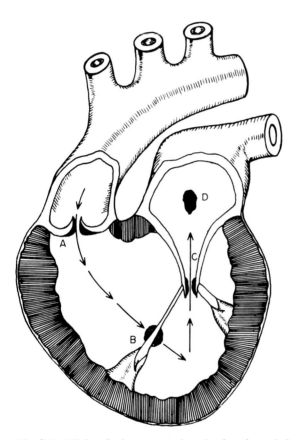

Fig. 7.2. High-velocity streams in mitral and aortic insufficiency and sites of endocarditic lesions. The arrow at the left indicates a high arterial pressure that generates regurgitant flow from the aorta to the ventricle. The vena contracta and endocarditic lesions appear at the ventricular surface of the aortic valve (A). The stream through the incompetent aortic valve may produce lesions on the chordae tendinae of the aortic leaf of the mitral valve (B). If the mitral valves cannot seal properly during ventricular systole, the regurgitant stream (arrow at right) will pass to the sink of the left atrium, and endocarditis will tend to become engrafted on the atrial surface of the mitral valve (C). The atrial endocardium in line with the regurgitant stream may produce a fibrous area, MacCallum's patch (D), which may become another site of endocarditic lesions. (Adapted from Ref. 97)

to-right shunt. The Venturi phenomenon is responsible for the development of lesions on the right side of the septum. These are usually in close proximity to a septal defect. Infective endocarditis may involve only the right ventricular wall at the point of impact of a high-pressure jet. Similar hemodynamic phenomena play a role in the pathogenesis of infection in individuals with tricuspid insufficiency, arteriovenous fistulas, coarctation of the aorta, or patent ductus arteriosus (Table 7.1). The jet and Venturi effects are attenuated in the presence of congestive cardiac failure and atrial fibrilation. This is probably the reason for the relative infrequency of subacute bacterial endocarditis in patients with these phenomena.[97] Large defects and those that connect chambers of equal volume minimize the

Table 7.1. Loci of Endocarditic Lesions

Condition	High Pressure Source	Orifice	Low-Pressure Sine	Location of Lesions (Add Adjacent Downstream Surfaces)	Satellite Lesions
Coarctation of aorta	Central aorta	Coarctation	Distal aorta	Down-stream wall	Lateral wall of aorta peripheral to stenotic lesion
Patent ductus arteriosus	Aorta	Ductus	Pulmonary artery	Pulmonary artery	Pulmonary valve
Arteriovenous fistula	Artery	Fistula	Vein	Communications and veins	
Ventricular septal defect	Left ventricle	Defect	Right ventricle	Right ventricular surface of defect	Pulmonary artery
Aortic insufficiency	Aorta	Closed aortic valves	Left ventricle	Ventricular surface of aortic valves	Mitral chordae
Mitral insufficiency	Left ventricle	Closed mitral valves	Left atrium	Atrial surface of mitral valves	Atrium
Pulmonary insufficiency	Pulmonary artery	Closed Pulmonary valves	Right ventricle	Ventricular surface of pulmonary valves	
Tricuspid insufficiency	Right ventricle	Closed tricuspid valves	Right atrium	Atrial surface of tricuspid valves	

Source: Adapted from Ref. 97.

differential in pressure and are usually not present in patients with endo-carditis. This may explain the paucity of this disease in individuals with isolated atrial septal defects, especially when they are small.

Sterile thrombotic lesions have been developed in animals by producing large arteriovenous fistulas, exposure to cold, simulated high altitudes, or passage of a sterile catheter through an artery or a vein and placement of its tip on the surface of a valve. Luxuriant platelet-fibrin thrombi develop on injured valves. The injection of potentially pathogenic organisms into the circulation leads to the development of infective endocarditis. Blood flow-ing over a cardiac valve the edges of which are rolled and irregular, chordae tendinae shortened due to rheumatic fever, or valvular leaflets deformed by the deposition of atherosclerotic plaques lose laminar flow. The resulting turbulence leads to the loss of platelets coated with fibrin. Over time, a small thrombus (vegetation) develops and increases the turbulence of blood over which it flows. This phenomenon is readily demonstrated in vitro by placing blood in two flasks, one of which contains small glass beads. When these are stirred vigorously, clotting occurs only in the flask that contains beads cov-ered by platelets and fibrin. Sterile platelet-fibrin thrombi have been devel-oped in animals in which large arteriovenous fistulas were produced,[98–100] exposure to cold,[101] treatment with hormones, simulated high altitude,[102] and passage of a catheter through the carotid artery, the tip of which lies just off the surface of the aortic valve.[103] Uninfected clumps of fibrin and platelets adherent to valvular tissue constitutes the syndrome known as *nonbacterial thrombotic endocarditis (NBTE).*

Gould et al.[5] have pointed out that organisms that adhere readily to canine cardiac valves are most often involved in the pathogenesis of infec-tive endocarditis in humans. The production of extracellular dextran by a variety of streptococci appears to be a significant factor in the ability of an organism to infect a damaged valvular leaflet. The importance of dextran has been reported by several investigators. Parker and Ball[104] pointed out that four streptococcal strains with the highest capacity to produce endocar-ditis elaborated significant quantities of dextran; the organisms were *S. mutans, S. bovis* I, *S. mitior,* and *S. sanguis* (Table 7.2). In vitro studies of the effect of dextran on the attachment of streptococci to NBTE were explored; the degree of adherence was related to the quantity of dextran generated. This was reversed by the addition of dextranase.[105] The gly-cocalyx was responsible for the partial resistance of streptococci to phagocytosis. It may also play a role in the relative resistance of these organisms to antimicrobial agents.[106]

Teichoic acids may enhance the adhesion of nondextran-producing gram-positive organisms to NBTE. These agents may be involved in the attachment to sterile thrombi of various microorganisms that do not pro-duce dextran.[107,108] The specific components of NBTE that come in contact with invading bacteria are unknown. Fibronectin, fibrinogen, and laminin are likely candidates for this role[109] (Table 7.3).

Some of the organisms commonly involved in the pathogenesis of infec-tive endocarditis (e.g., *S. sanguis* and staphylococci) aggregate platelets in

Table 7.2. Percentage of Cases of Bacteremia Caused by Various Strains of Streptococci That Represent Valvular Infection

Organism	Percentage
S. mutans*	93
S. bovis*	86
S. mitior*	77
S. sanguis*	75
S. faecalis	45
S. bovis II	37
S. milleri	28
S. agalactiae	18
S. pyogenes	3

*Producers of extracellular dextran.

Source: Modified from Pathogenesis and pathophysiology of infective endocarditis, in Sande M, Kaye D, Root R (eds): *Endocarditis.* Churchill Livingstone, New York, 1984, p 11

Table 7.3. Microorganism–NBTE Interaction in the Pathogenesis of Infective Endocarditis: Potentially Important Factors

Adhesion to NBTE
    Streptococcal dextran
    Lipoteichoic acid
    NBTE receptor (? fibronectin)
Host defense mechanisms
    Complement
    Humoral immunity
    Polymorphonuclear leukocytes
    Monocytes, macrophages
Growth of the vegetation
    Platelet aggregation
    Fibrin deposition
Bacterial division within the vegetation
Bacterial extracellular proteases

Source: Adapted from Scheld WM: pathogenesis and pathophysiology of infective endocarditis, in Sande M, Kaye D, Root R (eds): *Endocarditis.* New York, Churchill Livingstone, 1984, p 9.

protease-sensitive binding sites unrelated to dextran.[110] However, the importance of these cells in the development of valvular infections is not clear. Aspirin-induced thrombocytopenia and impairment of platelet function appear to have no effect on the development of the infected thrombus (vegetation) in experimental animals.[111,112]

There is some evidence that antibody directed to an organism in the bloodstream prevents infection of NBTE.[113–117] Agglutinating antibodies appear to play a critical role in the pathogenesis of subacute bacterial endocarditis.

Infected vegetations increase in size by the continuous deposition of platelet-fibrin. Monocytes may be important in this process. Phagocytosis of invading organisms leads to the release of thromboplastin and stimulates the constant deposition of fibrin.[118] Organisms that cause acute infective endocarditis (e.g., enterococci) may lead to the release of tissue thromboplastin from endothelial cells.[119]

Over time, the vegetation enlarges and the bacterial colonies are gradually buried below the accumulating layers of fibrin. Penetration of polymorphonuclear leukocytes into the vegetation is minimal. Very large numbers of organisms (10^9 to 10^{15} per gram of tissue) are the consequence of the unimpeded growth of the thrombus.[120] Fibrin has been noted to inhibit the function and chemotaxis of white cells in vitro.[121] Bacteria that live within the vegetations are less active metabolically. This dormant state may interfere significantly with the activity of antibiotics that rely on the presence of a rapid growth phase for optimum effect.[122]

There is an increase in the incidence of bacteremia, as manifested by the development of fever and chills. Anticoagulants do not prevent the initiation of disease, but instead promote the magnitude of the bacteremia and the incidence of the complications of the valvular infection.[123,124] Fibrinolytic agents (e.g., streptokinase) produce similar effects.[125]

It is important to point out that many of these effects may be related to the characteristics of the organism responsible for the disease. It has been noted that when NBTE is caused by proteolytic strains of *S. faecalis,* survival of the animals is shorter, the vegetations are more friable, bacteremia is more common, and the incidence of complications, including metastatic abscesses and septic emboli,[126] is increased.

That therapeutic levels of bactericidal agents in serum are required to prevent valvular infections has been questioned.[127] In vitro and in vivo studies have indicated that subinhibitory concentrations of an antimicrobial agent may be effective prophylactically by interfering with the attachment of organisms to NBTE. Exposure of *S. sanguis* to subinhibitory concentrations of penicillin releases lipoteichic acid from the cell wall. This alteration leads to a decrease in the ability of the streptococcus to adhere to the vegetation.[128,129] These observations are quite pertinent to a discussion of the antimicrobial prophylaxis of infective endocarditis.

Although transient bacteremia is common, it rarely results in the development of subacute endocarditis. This is the case even when a predisposing cardiac disorder is present. Despite multiple intrusions of organisms into the bloodstream, infection of a cardiac valve usually develops only after many years. The opposum and pig are the only animals that develop endocarditis spontaneously.[130] Several factors are responsible for the low incidence of infective endocarditis. The number of organisms present in the course of spontaneous bacteremia is usually small; it does not exceed 10–20 cfu per milliter of blood. A minimal number of organisms are required to initiate growth even when ideal media are employed. Failure to establish an infection is probably related to an inoculum too small to permit bacterial multiplication. This is so even when the organisms are trapped on a fibrin-platelet thrombus. Without the ability to replicate, the bacteria are washed away rapidly by the bloodstream and eventually cleared by the normal humoral and cellular defenses. A feature of the organism (e.g., the viridans streptococcus) that plays a significant role in the pathogenesis of subacute infective endocarditis is its low invasive capacity. The low level of pathogenicity and the small inoculum probably underlie the long delay between the initiation of the infectious process and the clinical manifestations of the subacute form of the disease. Recurrent bacteremia is required for the development of high titers of agglutinating antibody specific for the invading organism. Over time the titers of antibody become high enough to produce clumps of bacteria of sufficient size to initiate growth, on the surface and eventual invasion of NBTE. Evidence to support this series of events has been derived from experimental studies in which horses and rabbits[131] developed subacute endocarditis when they were immunized with pneumococci. Most important has been the observation that infected valvular vegetations did not develop until late in the course of immunization, when titers of agglutinating antibody were quite high.

More recent data have indicated that preformed antibody fails to promote NBTE but may prevent the development of infective endocarditis. This may be related to augmentation of the clearance of bacteremia by the reticuloendothelial system and/or interference with the attachment of circulating organisms to a fibrin thrombus.[113,114] Enhanced humoral immunity may exert no effect on the course of endocardial infection produced by gram-negative organisms.[132] It has been suggested that previously preformed antibody may play a role in the course of the subacute disease caused by *Ps. aeruginosa* in narcotic addicts.

The role of agglutinating antibody in facilitating infection in NBTE is based on both clinical observations in humans and the experimental studies described above. The manifestations of endocardial disease that are based on immunological processes support this concept. Several other mechanisms have been suggested to explain the adherence of microorganisms to abnormal cardiac endothelium. It is possible that a platelet-covered lesion provides a favorable surface for the attachment of organisms. It has been noted that platelets are capable of ingesting both latex particles and bacteria.[133] A variety of organisms, especially staphylococci and streptococci, aggregate platelets. Sequestration of large numbers of viable bacteria within these clumps of platelets may ensue.[134] The incidence of infective endocarditis produced by *E. coli* and other gram-negative bacteria is low.[135]

This is so despite the high frequency with which these organisms produce septicemia. One reason is that gram-negatives do not induce such aggregates of platelets. In addition, gram-negative organisms are serum sensitive and are lysed by complement before they are able to infect the NBTE.[136]

Agglutinating, complement-fixing, bactericidal antibodies and cryoglobulins have been identified by Cordiero et al.[137] in patients with subacute infective endocarditis. These authors also noted the presence of hypergammaglobulinemia characterized by an early increase in 19S and 7S globulins and a later rise in alpha-2 globulins. Some of these antibodies exhibited specific affinities for the renal glomerular basement membrane, vascular walls, and myocardial cells of healthy individuals. Their presence suggest that the immunological system plays an important role in the pathogenesis and clinical course of endocarditis. The immune system in these patients is altered in three major areas: (1) hypergammaglobulinemia caused by specific polyclonal B cells hyperactivity; (2) the presence of circulating antigen–antibody complexes; and (3) immune stimulation of an inflammatory response directed against the patient's tissues.[138]

Subacute infective endocarditis is characterized by persistent antigenic stimulation of the cellular and humoral immune systems. This is also the case in patients with malaria, syphilis, and leprosy. It is not surprising, therefore, that the levels of opsonizing, complement-fixing, agglutinating antibodies and cryoglobulins and immune complexes are elevated in patients with persistent valvular disease. The Raji cell assay detects the presence of complexes in almost all patients with endocardial infection. They contain IgG, IgA, and other components of the complement system. A prime example is rheumatoid factor, usually an IgM antibody directed against IgG.[139]

Rheumatoid factor is present in about 50% of patients with subacute infective endocarditis. The presence of this factor is established by studies involving sensitized sheep erythrocytes, aggregrated gammaglobulin, and anti-Rh antibody-coated erythrocytes; the reactive agent is 19S globulin. Rheumatoid factor is not specific for any organism. The highest titers are present when alpha-hemolytic streptococci are involved. High levels of rheumatoid factor have been detected in patients with active infection but who have sterile blood cultures. They are not present in those who have had multiple episodes of successfully treated infective endocarditis. Titers of circulating rheumatoid factor decrease rapidly with appropriate treatment. They reach zero about 2 months after the imitiation of therapy.[140,141] The more prolonged the clinical course of the disease, the higher the level in serum of this factor.

Carson et al.[142] have identified 19S and 7S anti-gammaglobulins in patients with infective endocarditis and rheumatoid arthritis. Both of these conditions are rich in kappa light chain–bearing antibodies in individuals with rheumatoid arthritis. Anti-gammaglobulins and 19S are enriched in kappa light chains in patients with subacute endocardial infection; 7S anti-gammaglobulins have normal kappa:lambda light chain ratios.

The properties of IgG and IgM rheumatoid factor, and their relation to circulating immune complexes in individuals with subacute endocarditis, have been described.[143] Significantly elevated concentrations of IgG and IgM rheumatoid factor are present in the sera of patients with subacute endocardial infection. These peak later in the course of the disease than do circulating immune complexes. Antimicrobial therapy decreases the level of rheumatoid factor but not as rapidly or completely as it does the levels of circulating immune complexes. Both IgG and IgM rheumatoid factors may be components of a polyvalent antibody response to elevated levels of circulating immune complexes.

Immunological abnormalities in individuals with infective endocarditis include antinuclear antibodies, depressed hemolytic complement, and C3 and C4. O'Connor et al.[144] studied 14 patients with infective endocarditis caused by *S. aureus*. Despite the severity of the disease, 10 individuals had decreases in complement and 10 had normal levels of C4 but low levels of C3. These data indicated that the alternate complement pathway had been activated. The level of factor B was low in three of six patients. Individuals with nonstaphylococcal endocardial disease had hypocomplementemia; the levels of C4, C3, and factor B were low, probably due to activation of C1 (classical pathway) with feedback to the alternate pathway. O'Connor et al. suggested that hypocomplementemia early in the course of infective endocarditis caused by *S. aureus* may be produced by a nonimmune reaction involving staphylococcal cell wall products (protein A), immunoglobulin, components of complement, and thrombocytes.

Elevated titers of rheumatoid factor have been reported in patients with acute infective endocarditis.[145] It has been noted that 13 or 55 parenteral drug users with valvular infections caused by *S. aureus* had circulating antibody at some time in the course of their disease. Only 2 of 30 noninfected patients had a positive reaction. The more severe the disease, as evidenced by the duration of fever after initiation of therapy, the more likely a positive latex fixation reaction would develop. Of 10 individuals studied over time, 7 had negative titers and 3 reduced titers of this antibody when they were discharged from the hospital.

Rheumatoid factor also appears to play a role in the pathogenesis of subacute infective endocarditis. IgM-IgG aggregates interfere with the phagocytosis of organisms by polymorphonuclear leukocytes. This modifies opsonic activity and interferes with the Fc portion of 7S gammaglobulins.[143,144] Rheumatoid factor and circulating immune complexes lead to an Arthus-like reaction by producing vascular damage. This initiates an inflammatory response in the tissues that activates the complement system, especially its chemotactic arm.[145] With successful therapy, the level of rheumatoid factor decreases and disappears in 50% of patients after 6 weeks of treatment. Failure to return to normal or an increase in the titer of rheumatoid factor indicates the presence of a mircobiological relapse.[146–151]

Bayer et al.[148] have used a Raji cell assay to distinguish endocarditic from nonendocarditic bacteremia. Of the 102 patients they studied, 50 had infective endocarditis. Ninety percent of those with endocardial disease, but only 50% of those with bacteremia alone, had circulating immune complexes.

The levels of these complexes were significantly higher in patients with endocardial disease than in those free of this disease. The authors stated that when infective endocarditis is suspected but the clinical and laboratory findings are not helpful, the levels of circulating immune complexes may be helpful in establishing a diagnosis.

Injury of tissue caused by circulating immune complexes has been responsible for many of the clinical manifestations of infective endocarditis. The presence of aggregates and end organ damage lead to the development of glomerulonephritis in patients with endocardial infection.[152–157] This is produced by the deposition of immune complexes ("lumpy-bumpy" pattern) on the glomerular basement membrane. Immunofluorescence studies have identified immunoglobulins and complement on the glomerular basement membrane; complement alone may be present. The exact site and size of the deposits in the glomerulus are determined by the mechanisms involved in their formation. Complexes that develop early in the course of the disease are smaller, form during antigen excess, and are present in the subepithelial area. Those that develop later are larger and are situated in the subendothelial mesangium. This type of glomerulonephritis is usually associated with the presence of rheumatoid factor. The morphologically different presentations on light microscopy (e.g., focal, diffuse, or membranous glomerulonephritis) probably share an underlying mechanism. These lesions may be partially healed by antimicrobial therapy.[143] Libman[156] described a bacteria-free stage of subacute infective endocarditis associated with severe renal failure. Prior to the availability of treatment, 25–35% of patients with this type of endocardial disease developed significant renal insufficiency; many cultures were sterile. The present incidence is 10%.[156]

Many of the peripheral manifestations of subacute bacterial endocarditis—purpuric lesions, Osler nodes, Roth spots, and subungual hemorrhages—may be due, in part, to a vasculitis caused by circulating immune complexes.[158–159] Deposition of these in the walls of blood vessels leads to the development of an Arthus reaction. Microscopy discloses a localized leukocytoclastic vasculitis with a mixture of polymorphonuclear leukocytes (monocytes and lymphocytes). One case report suggested that Roth spots consisted of clusters of lymphocytes surrounded by hemorrhage in the nerve layer of the retina.[159] Swelling and proliferation of endothelial cells is prominent. The pathogenesis of Osler nodes is different in patients with acute and subacute disease. Those that develop in patients with endocarditis caused by *S. aureus* and *C. albicans* are probably caused by septic emboli. The lesions appear to be associated with a sterile inflammatory reaction in individuals with infective endocarditis caused by viridans streptococci.

The mechanisms involved in the development of various musculoskeletal abnormalities are not clear.[160] Not all the peripheral manifestations of endocarditis are related to immunological phenomena. Janeway lesions are almost always produced by infected microemboli.[161]

Prior to the availability of antimicrobial agents, arterial embolization was responsible for many of the noncardiac complications of infective endocarditis. Formerly, 75–97% of patients experienced embolic episodes; these now occur in only 15–35%.[162–166] The most common areas for embolic deposition are the coronary arteries, kidneys, brain, and spleen. Although splenic embolization occurs in about 50% of patients, it is considered to be of little or no clinical importance. Albeit often not detected by electrocardiography, infective endocarditis has been identified at autopsy in about 50% of patients in whom embolization of one of the coronary arteries occurred. Renal emboli leading to infarction are common in patients who die (56%).

Cerebral emboli develop in more than a third of patients with infective endocarditis.[167–172] The middle cerebral artery is involved most often. Hemiplegia is the most common complication. Jochmann's comment, made in 1917,[170] that "in hemiplegia in young adults or children always think of subacute bacteria endocarditis" is relevant today. Arterial embolization may develop at any time in the course of the disease and as long as 1 year after it has been cured. Other neurological disorders caused by embolization include cerebral microabscesses, cranial nerve palsies, and cerebritis. Paraplegia may follow embolization of the spinal arteries. All the manifestations of peripheral neuropathy may follow an embolic event.[171]

Occlusion of large vessels by emboli deposited in patients with endocarditis is uncommon. In fact, this is more likely to be associated with fungal valvular disease, atrial myxoma, or marantic endocarditis. *S. aureus* and *Haemophilus* species may also produce large emboli. Macroembolization usually develops early in the course of infection but may appear, as in patients with cerebral emboli, 1 year or more after therapy has been begun.[162,173]

Although embolization develops in both acute and subacute infective endocarditis, the complications that follow the deposition of emboli differ. Infection is established peripherally when an embolus is deposited in patients with acute endocardial disease caused by *S. aureus*. Such metastatic infection is uncommon in subacute disease for the following reasons: (1) the limited ability of an organism to invade tissue locally; (2) a decrease in the number of bacteria in the inoculum; and (3) the presence of bactericidal antibody directed against the organisms present at a given site. Infarction of the myocardium, groin, and kidneys is fairly common in individuals with subacute disease; abscesses are uncommon.[1]

Mycotic aneurysms are more common in patients with subacute infection and develop more often when an organism with a low level of pathogenicity (e.g., *S. viridans*) is involved. The development of the lesions may be secondary to a number of mechanisms, including (1) embolic occlusion of the vasa vasorum; (2) deposition of immune complexes in the walls of a vessel; and (3) direct invasion of the walls of blood vessels.[1] Mycotic aneurysms are most common in the brain; abdominal aorta; superior mesenteric artery; splenic, coronary, and pulmonary arteries; the sinus of Valsalva; and a ligated ductus arteriosus.[174,175] When cerebral vessels are involved, the middle cerebral artery is impaired most often.[176] Mycotic aneurysms usually appear at the bifurcation of blood vessels and are generally silent prior to rupture. Cranial nerve palsies develop in 15% of patients.[172] Brain abscesses associated with embolic phenomena in individuals with acute endocarditis are usually multiple and small. Large lesions are rare and usually occur in the setting of cyanotic congenital heart disease.[177]

Marantic endocarditis is essentially NBTE. It is associated with a variety of diseases, especially terminal cancers, but may also be present in patients with congestive cardiac failure, pyelonephritis, or pneumonia.[178–182] Although the term *marantic* refers to wasting, the disease may involve healthy, young individuals or may be manifested by the presence of macroemboli. Sterile thrombi on the mitral and aortic valves are localized to the ventricular side of the latter and the atrial side of the former.

References

1. Weinstein L, Schlesinger J: Pathoanatomic, pathophysiologic and clinical correlations in endocarditis. *N Engl J Med* 1974;291:832.
2. Drake T, Rodgers G, Sande M: Tissue factor is a major stimulus for vegetation formation in enterococcal endocarditis in rabbits. *J Clin Invest* 1984;70:1750.
3. Clawson C: *Role of Platelets in the Pathogenesis of Endocarditis in Infective Endocarditis.* An American Heart Association symposium (Kaplan E, ed). Dallas, American Heart Association, 1977.
4. Scheld WM, Valone JA, Sande MA: Bacterial adherence in the pathogenesis of endocarditis: Interaction of bacterial dextran, platelets and fibrin. *J Clin Invest* 1978;61:1394.
5. Gould K, Ramirez-Ronda CH, Holmes RK, et al: Adherence of bacteria to heart valves in vitro. *J Clin Invest* 1975;56:1364.
6. Holmes RK, Ramirez-Ronda SH: *Adherence of Bacteria to the Endothelium of Heart Valves. Infective Endocarditis.* An American Heart Association Symposium. American Heart Association Monograph No. 52:12. Dallas, American Heart Association, 1977.
7. Pelletier LL Jr, Coyle M, Petersdorf R: Dextran production as a possible virulence factor in streptococcal endocarditis. *Proc Soc Exp Biol Med* 1978;158:415.
8. Klotz S: Fungal adherence to the vascular compartment: A critical step in the pathogenesis of disseminated candidiasis. *Clin Infect Dis* 1990;14:340.
9. Everett ED, Hirschman JV: Transient bacteremia and endocarditis: A review. *Medicine* 1977;56:61.
10. Aronson M, Bor D: Blood cultures. *Ann Intern Med* 1987;106:246.
11. Washington J II, Ilstrup D: Blood cultures: Issues and controversies. *Rev Infect Dis* 1986;8:792.
12. Goodman JS, Kolhouse JF, Koenig MG: Recurrent endocarditis due to *Streptococcus viridans* in an "edentulous" man. *South Med J* 1973;66:352.
13. Rushton MA: Subacute bacterial endocarditis following the extraction of teeth. *Guys Hosp Rep* 1930;80:39.
14. Winslow MB, Kobernick SD: Bacteremia after prophylaxis. *J Am Dent Assoc* 1960;61:69.
15. Berger SA, Weitzman S, Edberg SC, et al: Bacteremia after the use of an oral irrigation device: A controlled study in subjects with normal appearing gingiva: Comparison with use of toothbrush. *Ann Intern Med* 1974;50:510.
16. Root TE, Silva EA, Edwards LD, et al: *Hemophilus aprophilus* endocarditis with a probably primary dental infection. *Chest* 1981;80:109.
17. Loesche WJ: Indigenous human flora and bacteremia, in Kaplan EL, Taranta AV (eds): *Infective Endocarditis.* An American Heart Association Symposium. Dallas, American Heart Association, 1977, p 40.

18. Hurwitz G, Speck W, Keller G: Absence of bacteremia in children after prophylaxis. *Oral Surg* 1971;32:891.
19. Deleo A, Schoenknecht F, Anderson M, et al: The incidence of bacteremia following oral prophylaxis on pediatric patients. *Oral Surg* 1979;37:36.
20. Peterson LJ, Peacock R: The incidence of bacteremia in pediatric patients following tooth extraction. *Circulation* 1976;53:676.
21. Elliott SD: Bacteremia following tonsillectomy. *Lancet* 1939;2:589.
22. Fischer J, Gottdenker F: Transient bacteremia following tonsillectomy. Experimental bacteriological and clinical studies. *Laryngoscope* 1941;51:271.
23. Rhoads PS, Sibley JR, Billings CE: Bacteremia following tonsillectomy. *JAMA* 1955;157:877.
24. Burman SO: Bronchoscopy and bacteremia. *J Thorac Cardiovasc Surg* 1960;40:635.
25. LeFrock JL, Klainer AS, Wu WH, et al: Transient bacteremia associated with nasotracheal and orotracheal intubation. *Anesth Analg* 1973;52:873.
26. Barry FA Jr, Blankenbaker WL, Bail CG: A comparison of bacteremia occurring with nasotracheal and orotracheal intubation. *Anesth Analg* 1973;52:873.
27. Shull JH Jr, Greene BM, Allen SD, et al: Bacteremia with upper gastrointestinal endoscopy. *Ann Intern Med* 1975; 83:212.
28. Stray N, Midvedt T, Valnes K, et al: Endoscopy-related bacteremia. *Scand J Gastroenterol* 1978;13:345.
29. Baltch AL, Buhac I, Agrawal A, et al: Bacteremia after upper gastrointestinal endoscopy. *Arch Intern Med* 1977;137:594.
30. Buchman E, Berglund EM: Bacteremia following sigmoidoscopy. *Am Heart J* 1960; 60:863.
31. Unterman D, Milberg MB, Kranis M: Evaluation of blood cultures after sigmoidoscopy. *N Engl J Med* 1957;257:773.
32. LeFrock JL, Ellis CA, Turchik JB, et al: Transient bacteremia associated with sigmoidoscopy. *N Engl J Med* 1975;289:467.
33. LeFrock JL, Ellis CA, Klainer AS, et al: Transient bacteremia associated with barium enema. *Arch Intern Med* 1975;135:835.
34. Schimmel DH, Hanelin LG, Coehn S, et al: Bacteremia and the barium enema. *Am J Roentgenol* 1977;128:207.
35. Dickman MD, Farrell R, Higgs RH, et al: Colonoscopy associated bacteremia. *Surg Gynecol Obstet* 1976;142:173.
36. Norfleet RG, Mulholland DD, Mitchell PD, et al: Does bacteremia follow endoscopy? *Gastroenterology* 1976;70:20.
37. Hartong WA, Barnes WG, Calkins WG: The absence of bacteremia during colonoscopy. *Am J Gastroenterol* 1977;67:240.
38. Raforth AJ, Sorenson RM, Bond JH: Bacteremia following colonoscopy. *Gastrointest Endosc* 1975;22:32.
39. Hartong WA, Barnes WG, Calkins WG: The absence of bacteremia during colonoscopy. *Am J Gastroenterol* 1977;67:240.
40. LeFrock JL, Ellis CA, Turchik JB, et al: Transient bacteremia associated with percutaneous liver biopsy. *J Infect Dis* 1975;131S104.
41. McCloskey RV, Gold M, Weser E: Bacteremia after liver biopsy. *Arch Intern Med* 1973;132:213.
42. Loludice T, Buhac I, Balint J: Septicemia as a complication of percutaneous liver biopsy. *Gastroenterology* 1977;72:949.
43. Camara DS, Gruber M, Barde CJ, et al: Transient bacteremia following endoscopic infection. Sclerotherapy of esophageal varices. *Arch Intern Med* 1983;143:1350.
44. Seifert E: Uber Bakterien befunde im Blut nach Operationem. *Arch Klin Chir* 1925;138:565.
45. Redlead PD, Fadell EJ: Bacteremia during parturition. *JAMA* 1959;169:1284.
46. McCormack WM, Rosner B, Lee YH, et al: Isolation of genital mycoplasmas from blood obtained shortly after vaginal delivery. *Lancet* 1975;1:596.

47. DeSwiet M, Ramsay ID, Rees GM: Bacterial endocarditis after insertion of intrauterine contraceptive device. *Br Med J* 1975;3:76.

48. Everett ED, Reller LB, Droegemueller W, et al: Absence of bacteremia after insertion or removal of intrauterine devices. *Obstet Gynecol* 1976;47:207.

49. Ritvo R, Monroe P, Andriole VT: Transient bacteremia due to suction abortion. Implications for SBE prophylaxis. *Yale J Biol Med* 1977;50:471.

50. Regetz MJ, Starr SE, Dowell VR Jr, et al: Absence of bacteremia after diagnostic biopsy of the cervix. Chemoprophylactic implications. *Chest* 1974;65:223.

51. Kreidbert MG, Chernoff HL: Ineffectiveness of penicillin prophylaxis in cardiac catheterization. *J Pediatr* 1965;66:286.

52. Sande MA, Levision ME, Lukas DS, et al: Bacteremia associated with cardiac catheterization. *N Engl J Med* 1969;281:1104.

53. Shawker TH, Kluge RM, Ayella RJ: Bacteremia associated with angiography. *JAMA* 1974;299:1090.

54. Lerner PI, Weinstein L: Infective endocarditis in the antibiotic era. *N Engl J Med* 1966;274:199.

55. Yeh TJ, Anabtani IN, Cornett VE, et al: Bacterial endocarditis following open-heart surgery. *Ann Thorac Surg* 1967;3:29.

56. Killen DA, Collins HA, Koenig GA, et al: Prosthetic cardiac valves and bacterial endocarditis. *Ann Thorac Surg* 1970;9:238.

57. Blakemore WS, McGarrity GS, Thurer RJ, et al: Infection by airborne bacteria with cardiopulmonary bypass. *Surgery* 1971;70:830.

58. Ankeney JL, Parker RF: Staphylococcal endocarditis following open-heart surgery related to positive intraoperative blood cultures, in Brewer LA III (ed): *Prosthetic Heart Valves.* Springfield, IL, Charles C. Thomas, 1969, p 179.

59. Beard CH, Ribeiro CD, Jones DM: The bacteremia associated with burns and surgery. *Br J Surg* 1975;62:638.

60. Richards JH: Bacteremia following irritation of foci of infection. *JAMA* 1932;99:1496.

61. Snyder N, Atterbury CE, Correia JP, et al: Increased concurrence of cirrhosis and bacterial endocarditis. *Gastroenterology* 1977;73:1107.

62. Olsson RA, Romansky MJ: Staphylococcal tricuspid endocarditis in heroin addicts. *Ann Intern Med* 1962;57:755.

63. Banks T, Fletcher R, Nayab A: Infective endocarditis in heroin addicts. *Am J Med* 1966;284:199.

64. Dryer NP, Fields BN: Heroin-associated infective endocarditis: A report of 28 cases. *Ann Intern Med* 1973;78:699.

65. Stimmel B, Donoso E, Dack S: Comparison of infective endocarditis in addicts and non-drug users. *Am J Cardiol* 1973;32:924.

66. Tuazon CU, Cardells TA, Sheagren JN: Staphylococcal endocarditis in drug users; clinical and microbiologic aspects. *Arch Intern Med* 1975;135:1555.

67. Mills J, Drew D: *Serratia marcescens* endocarditis: A regional illness associated with intravenous drug abuse. *Ann Intern Med* 1976;84:29.

68. El-Khatib MR, Wilson FM, Lerner AM: Characteristics of bacterial endocarditis in heroin addicts in Detroit. *Am J Med Sci* 1976;271.

69. Reisber BE: Infective endocarditis in the narcotic addict. *Prog Cardiovasc Dis* 1979;22:193.

70. Simberkoff MS: Narcotic associated infective endocarditis, in Kaplan EL, Taranta AV (eds): *Infective Endocarditis.* Dallas, American Heart Association, 1977, p 46.

71. Tuazon CU, Sheagren JN: Staphylococcal endocarditis in parenteral drug abusers; source of the organism. *Ann Intern Med* 1975;82:788.

72. Sasaki TM, Panke TW, Dorethy JF, et al: The relationship of central venous and pulmonary artery catheter position to acute right-sided endocarditis in severe thermal injury. *J Trauma* 1979;19:740.

73. Gatti JE, Reichek N, Mulleu JL: Endocarditis complicating home hyper-alimentation. *Arch Surg* 1981;116:933.

74. Baskin RW, Rosenthal A, Bruitt BA Jr: Acute bacterial endocarditis: A silent source of sepsis in the burn patient. *Ann Surg* 1976;184:618.

75. Lemire G, Morin J, Dobell A: Pacemaker infections: A 12 year review. *Can J Surg* 1975;18:181.
76. Garvey GJ, Neu HC: Infective endocarditis, an evolving disease. A review of endocarditis at the Columbia-Presbyterian Medical Center, 1968–1973. *Medicine* 1978;57:105.
77. Rosen P, Armstrong D: Infective endocarditis in patients treated for malignant neoplastic disease. *Am J Clin Pathol* 1973;60:241.
78. Cross AS, Steigbigel NH: Infective endocarditis and access site infections in patients on hemodialysis. *Medicine* 1976;55:453.
79. Leonard A, Raij L, Shapiro FL: Bacterial endocarditis in regularly dialyzed patients. *Kidney Int* 1973;4:407.
80. Leonard A, Raij L, Comty CM, et al: Experience with endocarditis in a large kidney disease program. *Trans Am Soc Artif Intern Organs* 1973;19:278.
81. Dobkin JF, Miller MH, Steigbigel NH: Septicemia in patients on chronic hemodialysis. *Ann Intern Med* 1978;88:28.
82. Lowry F, Steigbigel H: Infective endocarditis: Prevention of bacterial endocarditis. *Am Heart J* 1977;96:689.
83. Osler W: Malignant endocarditis. *Lancet* 1885;1:415,459,505.
84. Luschka H: Das endocardium und die endocarditis. *Arch Pathol Anat Physiol* 1852;4:171.
85. Coombs C: The histology of rheumatic endocarditis. *Lancet* 1909;1:1377.
86. Rosenow EC: Experimental infectious endocarditis. *J Infect Dis* 1912;11:210.
87. Bayne-Jones S: The blood vessels of the heart valves. *Am J Anat* 1917;21:449.
88. Kerr WJ, Mettier SR: The circulation of the heart valves: Notes on the embolic basis for endocarditis. *Am Heart J* 1925;1:96.
89. Wearn JT, Moritz AR: The incidence and significance of blood vessels in normal and abnormal heart valves. *Am Heart J* 1937;13:7.
90. Gross L: Significance of blood vessels in human heart valves. *Am Heart J* 1937;13:275.
91. Allen AC: Mechanism of localization of vegetations of bacterial endocarditis. *Arch Pathol* 1939;27:399.
92. Harper WF: The structure of the heart valves, with special reference to their blood supply and the genesis of endocarditis. *J Pathol Bacteriol* 1945;57:229.
93. Lepeschkin E: On the relation between the site of valvular involvement in endocarditis and the blood pressure resting on the valve. *Am J Med Sci* 1952;224:318.
94. Davies PF, Remuzzi A, Gordon EJ, et al: Turbulent fluid shear stress induces vascular endothelial turnover in vitro. *Proc Natl Acad Sci USA* 1986;83:2114.
95. Langille BL: Integrity of arterial endothelium following acute exposure to high shear stress. *Biorheology* 1984;21:333.
96. Dewey CF, Bussolari SR, Gimbrone MA, et al: The dynamic response of vascular endothelial cells to fluid shear stress. *J Biomech Eng* 1981;103:177.
97. Rodbard S: Blood velocity and endocarditis. *Circulation* 1963;27:18.
98. Lillehei CW, Bobb JRR, Visscher MB: The occurrence of endocarditis with valvular deformities in dogs with arteriovenous fistulas. *Ann Surg* 1950;132:577.
99. Lee SH, Fisher B, Fisher ER, et al: Arteriovenous fistula and bacterial endocarditis. *Surgery* 1962;52:463.
100. Oka M, Shirota A, Angrist A: Experimental endocarditis: Endocrine factors in valve lesions on AV shunt rats. *Arch Pathol* 1966;82:85.
101. Highman B, Altland Pd: Effect of exposure and acclimatization in cold on susceptibility of rats to bacterial endocarditis. *Proc Soc Exp Biol Med* 1962;110:663.
102. Highman B, Altland P: A new method for the production of experimental bacterial endocarditis. *Proc Soc Exp Biol Med* 1950;75:573.
103. Garrison P, Freedman L: Experimental endocarditis I: Staphylococcal endocarditis in rabbits resulting from placement of a polyethylene catheter in the right side of the heart. *Yale J Biol Med* 1970;42:395.
104. Parker MT, Ball LC: Streptococci and aerococci associated with systemic infection in man. *J Med Microbiol* 1976;9:275.
105. Ramirez-Ronda CH: Adherence of glucan-positive and glucan-negative streptococci strains to normal and damaged heart valves. *J Clin Invest* 1978;62:805.

106. Dall L, Barnes WG, Lane JW, et al: Enzymatic modification of glycocalyx in the treatment of experimental endocarditis due to viridans streptococci. *J Infect Dis* 1987;156:736.

107. Thompson J, Meddens M, Thorig L, et al: The role of bacterial adherence in the pathogenesis of infective endocarditis. *Infection* 1982;10:196.

108. Beachey EH, Ofek I: Epithelial binding of group A streptococci by lipoteichoic acid on fimbriae denuded of M protein. *J Exp Med* 1976;14:759.

109. Scheld WM, Keeley JM, Balian G, et al: Microbial adhesion to fibronextin in the pathogenesis of infective endocarditis. *Clin Res* 1983;31:542A.

110. Herzberg MC, Brintzenhofe KL, Clawson CC: Aggregation of human platelets and adherence of *Streptococcus sanguis*. *Infect Immun* 1983;39:1457.

111. Durack DT, Beeson PB: Pathogenesis of infective endocarditis, in Rahimtoola SH (ed): *Infective Endocarditis*. New York, Grune and Stratton, 1977, p 1.

112. Levison ME, Carrizosa J, Tanphaichitra D, et al: Effect of aspirin on thrombogenesis and on production of experimental aortic valvular *Streptococcus viridans* endocarditis in rabbits. *Blood* 1977;49:645.

113. Adler SW II, Selinger DS, Reed WP: Effect of immunization on the genesis of pneumococcal endocarditis in rabbits. *Infect Immun* 1981;34:55.

114. Scheld WM, Thomas JH, Sande MA: Influence of preformed antibody on experimental *Streptococcus sanguis* endocarditis. *Infect Immun* 1979;25:781.

115. Durack DT, Gilliland BC, Petersdorf RG: Effect of immunization on susceptibility to experimental *Streptococcus mutans* and *Streptococcus sanguis* endocarditis. *Infect Immun* 1978;22:52.

116. Sande MA, Scheld WM: Bacterial adherence in endocarditis: Interaction of bacterial dextran, platelets, fibrin, and antibody. *Scand J Infect Dis* 1980;(Suppl 24):100.

117. Scheld WM, Calderone RA, Brodeur JP, et al: Influence of preformed antibody on the pathogenesis of experimental *Candida albicans* endocarditis. *Infect Immun* 1983;40:950.

118. Van Ginkel CJW, Thorig L, Thompson J, et al: Enhancement of generation of monocyte tissue thromboplastin by bacterial phagocytosis: Possible pathway for fibrin formation on infected vegetations in bacterial endocarditis. *Infect Immun* 1979;25:388.

119. Drake TA, Rodgers GM, Sande MA: Tissue factor is a major stimulus for vegetation formation in enterococcal endocarditis in rabbits. *J Clin Invest* 1084;70:1750.

120. Durack DT, Beeson PB: Experimental bacterial endocarditis. II. Survival of bacteria in endocardial vegetations. *Br J Exp Pathol* 1972;53:50.

121. Thorig L, Thompson J, Eulderink F: Effect of warfarin on the induction and course of experimental *Staphylococcus epidermidis* endocarditis. *Infect Immun* 1977;17:504.

122. Durack DT, Beeson PB: Experimental endocarditis. I. Colonization of a sterile vegetation. *Br J Exp Pathol* 1982;53:44.

123. Thorig L, Thompson J, Eulderink F, et al: effects of monocytopenia and anticoagulation in experimental *Streptococcus sanguis* endocarditis. *Br J Exp Pathol* 1980;61:108.

124. Hook EW III, Sande MA: Role of the vegetation in experimental *Streptococcus viridans* endocarditis. *Infect Immun* 1974;19:1433.

125. Thompson J, Eulderink F, Lemkes H, Van et al: Effect of warfarin on the induction and course of experimental endocarditis. *Infect Immun* 1976;14:1284.

126. Durack DT, Petersdorf RG: Chemotherapy of experimental streptococcal endocarditis. I. Comparison of commonly recommended prophylactic regimens. *J Clin Invest* 1973;52:592.

127. Johnson CE, Dewar HA, Aherne WA: Fibrinolytic therapy in subacute bacterial endocarditis. An experimental study. *Cardiovasc Res* 1982;14:482.

128. Scheld WM, Zak O, Vosbeck K, et al: Bacterial adhesion in the pathogenesis of infective endocarditis. Effect of subinhibitory antibiotic concentrations on streptococcal adhesion in vitro and the development of endocarditis in rabbits. *J Clin Invest* 1981;68:1381.

129. Moreillon P, Francioli P, Overholser D, et al: Mechanisms of successful amoxicillin prophylaxis of experimental endocarditis due to *Streptococcus intermedius*. *J Infect Dis* 1986;154:801.

130. Sherwood BF, Rowlands DT, Vakilzadeh J, et al: Experimental bacterial endocarditis in the opossum (*Didelphis virginiana*). *Am J Pathol* 1971;64:513.

131. Sande MA: Experimental endocarditis, in Kaye D (ed):*Infective Endocarditis*. Baltimore, University Park Press, 1976, p 11.

132. Thorig L, Thompson J, Van Furth R: Effects of immunization and anticoagulation on the development of experimental *Escherichia coli* endocarditis. *Infect Immun* 1980; 28:325.

133. Movat H, Weiser G, Glynn M, et al: Platelet pharyngitis and aggregation. *J Cell Biol* 1965;27:531.

134. Clawson CC, White JG: Platelet interaction with bacteria. I. Reaction phases and effects of inhibition. *Am J Pathol* 1971;65:367.

135. Clawson CC, White JG: Platelet interaction with bacteria. Fate of the bacteria. *Am J Pathol* 1971;65:381.

136. Durack DT, Beeson PB: Protective role of complement in experimental *Escherichia coli* endocarditis. *Infect Immun* 1977;16:213.

137. Cordeiro A, Costa H, Laghena F: Immunologic phase of subacute bacterial endocarditis. A new concept and general considerations. Editorial. *Am J Cardiol* 1865; 16:477.

138. Phair J, Clarke J: Immunology of infective endocarditis. *Prog Cardiovasc Dis* 1979;22:137.

139. Sheagren JN, Tauzon CU, Griffin C, et al: Rheumatoid factor in acute bacterial endocarditis. *Arthritis Rheum* 1976;19:887.

140. Messner R, Laxdal T, Quie P, et al: Rheumatoid factors in subacute bacterial endocarditis. Bacterium, duration of disease or genetic predisposition? *Ann Intern Med* 1968;68:746.

141. Williams R Jr, Kunbel H: Rheumatoid factors and their disappearance following therapy in patients with subacute bacterial endocarditis. *Arthritis Rheum* 1962;5:126.

142. Carson D, Bayer A, Eisenberg R, et al: IgM rheumatoid factor in subacute bacterial endocarditis: Relationship to IgG rheumatoid factor and circulatory complexes. *Clin Exp Immunol* 1970;31:100.

143. Bacon P, Davidson C, Smith B: Antibodies to candida and autoantibodies in sub-acute bacterial endocarditis. *Q J Med* 1979;43:535.

144. O'Connor D, Weisman M, Fierer J: Activation of the alternate complement pathway in *Staphylococcus aureus* and its relationship to thrombocytopenia, coagulation abnormalities and acute glomerulonephritis. *Clin Exp Immunol* 1978;34:179.

145. Sheagren JN, Tuazon CV, Griffin C, et al: Rheumatoid factor in acute bacterial endocarditis. *Arthritis Rheum* 1976;19:887.

146. Williams R: Rheumatoid factors in subacute bacterial endocarditis and other infectious diseases. *Scand J Rheum* 1988;75(Suppl):300.

147. Bayer AS, Theofilopoulos AN, Eisenberg R, et al: Circulating immune complexes in infective endocarditis. *N Engl J Med* 1976;295:1500.

148. Bayer AS, Theofilopoulos AN, Tillman DB, et al: Use of circulating immune complex levels in the serodifferentiation of endocarditic and nonendocarditic septicemias. *Am J Med* 1979;66:58.

149. Tu WH, Shearn MA, Lee JC: Acute diffuse glomerulonephritis in acute staphylococcal endocarditis. *Ann Intern Med* 1969;71:335.

150. Gutman RA, Striker GE, Gilliland BC, et al: The immune complex glomerulonephritis of bacterial endocarditis. *Medicine* 1972;51:1.

151. Levy RL, Hong R: The immune nature of subacute bacterial endocarditis (SBE) nephritis. *Am J Med* 1973;64:645.

152. Keslin MG, Messner RP, Williams RC Jr: Glomerulonephritis with subacute bacterial endocarditis. *Arch Intern Med* 1973;132:578.

153. Neugarten J, Baldwin D: Glomerulonephritis in bacterial endocarditis. *Am J Med* 1989;77:297.

154. Germuth F, Rodriguez E, Lovelle C, et al: Passive immune complex glomerulonephritis in mice: Models for various lesions in human disease to low avidity complexes and diffuse proliferative glomerulonephritis in the sub-epithelial deposits. *Lab Invest* 1979;41:366.

155. Feinstein E, Eknoyan G, Lister B, et al: Renal complications of bacterial endocarditis. *Am J Nephrol* 1985;5:457.

156. Libman E: Characterization of various forms of endocarditis. *JAMA* 1923;80:813.

157. Lerner PI, Weinstein L: Infective endocarditis in the antibiotic era. *N Engl J Med* 1966;274:199.

158. Alpert JS, Krous HF, Dalen JE, et al: Pathogenesis of Osler's nodes. *Ann Intern Med* 1976;85:471.

159. Silverberg HH: Roth spots. *Mt Sinai J Med* 1977;37:77.

160. Churchill M, Geraci J, Hunder G: Musculoskeletal manifestations of bacterial endocarditis. *Ann Intern Med* 1977;87:754.

161. Kerr A Jr, Tan J: Biopsies of the Janeway lesion of infective endocarditis. *J Cutan Pathol* 1979;6:124.

162. Cates JE, Christie RV: Subacute bacterial endocarditis: A review of 442 patients treated in 14 centres appointed by the Penicillin Trials Committee of the Medical Research Council. *Q J Med* 1951;20:93.

163. Kerr A Jr: *Subacute Bacterial Endocarditis*. Springfield, Il, Charles C Thomas, 1955.

164. Jackson JF, Allison F Jr: Bacterial endocarditis. *South Med J* 1961;54:1331.

165. Wenger NK, Bauer S: Coronary embolism: Review of the literature and presentation of fifteen cases. *Am J Med* 1958;25:549.

166. Menzies CJG: Coronary embolism with infarction in bacterial endocarditis. *Br Heart J* 1961;23:464.

167. Ziment I: Nervous system complications in bacterial endocarditis. *Am J Med* 1969;47:493.

168. Harrison MJG, Hampton JR: Neurological presentation of bacterial endocarditis. *Br Med J* 1967;2:148.

169. Jones HR Jr, Siekert RG, Geraci JE: Neurologic manifestations of bacterial endocarditis. *Ann Intern Med* 1969;71:21.

170. Jochmann G: *Lehrbuch der Infektionskrankheiten, fur Artze und Studierende*. Berlin, Julius Springer, 1914, p 144.

171. Kernohan JW, Woltman HW, Barnes AR: Involvement of the nervous system associated with endocarditis: Neuropsychiatric and neuropathologic observations in forty-two cases of fatal outcome. *Arch Neurol Psychiatry* 1939;42:789.

172. DeJong RN: Central nervous system complications in subacute bacterial endocarditis. *J Nerv Ment Dis* 1937;85:397.

173. Case records of the Massachusetts General Hospital (Case 45021). *N Engl J Med* 1959;260:82.

174. Morgan WL, Bland EF: Bacterial endocarditis in the antibiotic era: With special reference to the later complications. *Circulation* 1959;19:753.

175. Kauffman SL, Lynfield J, Hennigar GR: Mycotic aneurysms of the intrapulmonary arteries. *Circulation* 1967;35:90.

176. Greenlee J, Mandell G: Neurological manifestations of infective endocarditis: A review. *Stroke* 1983;4:958.

177. Matson DD, Salam M: Brain abscess in congenital heart disease. *Pediatrics* 1961;27:772.

178. MacDonald RA, Robbins SL: The significance of nonbacterial thrombotic endocarditis: An autopsy and clinical study of 78 cases. *Ann Intern Med* 1957;46:255.

179. Amromin GD, Wang SK: Degenerative verrucal endocardiosis and myocardial infarction: Report of two cases associated with mucus-producing bronchogenic carcinoma. *Ann Intern Med* 1959;50:1519.

180. Barron KD, Siqueira E, Hirano A: Cerebral embolism caused by nonbacterial thrombotic endocarditis. *Neurology (Minneapolis)* 1960;10:391.

181. Allen AC, Sirota JH: The morphogenesis and significance of degenerative verrucal endocarditis (terminal endocarditis, endocarditis simplex, nonbacterial thrombotic endocarditis). *Am J Pathol* 1944;20:1025.

182. Bryan CS: Nonbacterial thrombotic endocarditis with malignant tumors. *Am J Med* 1969;46:787.

8

Clinical Manifestations of Native Valve Endocarditis

The incubation period of infective endocarditis has been defined by Starkebaum et al.[1] as the interval between a procedure that may lead to transient bacteremia and the appearance of disease. This was determined in 76 patients with streptococcal valvular disease. The period of incubation was 1 week in 60 individuals infected by organisms other than enterococci. Symptoms of endocarditis were apparent within 2 weeks of dental or other procedures in 85% of patients. The diagnosis of valvular infection was established in only 16% over this period. An incubation period longer than 1 month was rare. A second time span was defined in 37 of the 60 patients described above. This was the duration between the onset of bacteremia and the diagnosis of valvular infection. The average of this interval was 6 weeks.

Among the reasons for delay in establishing the diagnosis of endocarditis are (1) the presence of mild, early, nonspecific manifestations of subacute disease; (2) reluctance to seek medical attention because the symptoms are mild; (3) failure to consider the diagnosis of infective endocarditis until the illness has been present for weeks or even months; and (4) treatment with antimicrobial agents for undefined disease that temporarily leads to defervescence and clearing of bacteria from the circulation. Endocarditis in 55 individuals with nonenterococcal disease and in 4 of 16 infected by enterococci followed dental surgery; 11 cases were associated with procedures that involved the genitourinary tract. The results of this study led Starkebaum et al.[1] to suggest that if endocarditis is causally related to a transient bacteremia, the manifestations of infection usually appear within 2 weeks. Patients with underlying cardiac valvular disease must be closely observed over this period and alerted to the need to report any symptoms compatible with endocarditis to their physician. Infection in which symptoms present longer than 2 weeks after discontinuation of antimicrobial prophylaxis is likely to originate from a bacteremia unrelated to the procedure. This would not constitute a failure of chemoprophylaxis.

Four mechanisms are involved in the pathogenesis of infective endocarditis:[2-4] (1) infection of a cardiac valve; (2) embolization of a thrombus (vegetation) situated on the infected leaflet; (3) metastatic infection involving extracardiac sites; and (4) the development of circulating abnormal globulins and immune complexes in various areas of the body of some individuals. There are striking qualitative and quantitative differences in the roles these play in subacute and acute infective endocarditis.

The onset of subacute valvular infection is variable. The early clinical manifestations are usually so subtle and nonspecific that patients or their physicians fail to consider the possibility of a potentially lethal disease. Delays in diagnoses are exacerbated when cultures of the blood are not carried out and empiric antibiotic therapy is instituted in response to the fever. As is often the case, the organism responsible for the endocardial disease is sensitive to the administered drug. Fever is absent as long as therapy is continued. With rare exceptions, however, it returns a few days to a week or more after therapy has been stopped. In some instances, this leads to one or more episodes of retreatment with the same antibiotic and the recurrence of fever when the drug is withdrawn. The more often this cycle is repeated prior to identification of the infection and initiation of appropriate management, the higher the risk that repeated exacerbations of the disease may occur, leading to permanent valvular damage and hemodynamic dysfunction.

Signs or symptoms indicating infection of the heart or other organs are often absent. The most common are presistent low-grade fever, lassitude, anorexia, fatigue, loss of weight, sleepiness, and an influenza-like syndrome. Libman and Friedberg[5] have pointed out that the clinical features of infective endocarditis may mimic those associated with a number of infected extracardiac sites. Among these are (1) generalized myalgia and a syndrome resembling influenza; (2) hemoptysis and pleuritic pain; (3) fever and arthritis suggesting rheumatic fever; (4) a dulled sensorium with fever, headache, and symptoms consistent with typhoid fever; (5) rigors treated intermittently with salicylates; (6) fever and pain in the right upper quadrant of the abdomen suggesting infection of the biliary tract; (7) vomiting and postprandial distress resembling carcinoma of the stomach; and (8) symptoms and signs that mimic acute appendicitis.

Other manifestations of subacute infective endocarditis are associated with complications caused by a delay of weeks or months in the initiation of appropriate antimicrobial therapy. Some of these are embolic; others are caused by the progressive destruction of an infected valve and the impact of a variety of immunological phenomena. Among the syndromes that appear after embolization are (1) hemiplegia caused by occlusion of the middle cerebral artery; (2) acute meningitis characterized by sterile spinal fluid, an increased number of white blood cells, an elevated concentration of protein, and a normal level of glucose; (3) the sudden onset of pain in the right or left upper quadrant of the abdomen following infarction of the kidney or spleen; (4) painless hematuria induced by multiple small renal infarcts; (5) acute unilateral blindness following occlusion of a retinal artery; and (6) myocardial infarction produced by embolization of a coronary artery. The earliest manifestation of infective endocarditis that involves the right side of the heart, especially the tricuspid valve, is the development of embolic pulmonary infarcts, a syndrome that mimics pneumonia. The presence of multiple pulmonary infiltrates in febrile patients with a murmur suggests the presence of infective endocarditis that involves the right side of the heart.

The onset of infective endocarditis in patients with unchecked disease is marked by a sudden change in the character of a preexisting murmur (uncommon in subacute disease) and the appearance of progressive cardiac failure caused by valvular insufficiency following scarring or destruction of the valvular leaflets.

Many of the initial manifestations of subacute infective endocarditis are caused by a variety of immunological processes. Subacute disease may present with anorexia, anemia, and renal failure related to interstitial nephritis or proliferative glomerulonephritis.

Arthralgias and arthritis are produced by the deposition of immune complexes in the synovia of various joints. They may be the initial sign of the disease. The development of cardiac palpitations and a variety of arrhythmias may be related to an immunologically mediated myocarditis. An immune-mediated vasculitis is involved in the production of the Osler node and Roth spot.

Significant pain in the lumbosacral area is common in patients with infective endocarditis[6] and, in rare cases, is due to vertebral osteomyelitis. Treatment with antimicrobial agents leads to rapid resolution of the pain. A very rare sign, unilateral nonsuppurative parotitis, present at the onset of endocarditis, may be immunological in origin.

The onset of infective endocarditis in intravenous drug addicts usually does not suggest the presence of valvular disease initially. An exception is infection of the tricuspid valve. Repeated episodes of pulmonary infarction should alert the physician to the possibility that a valve in the right side of the heart is infected. Individuals with fungal disease that involves the mitral and aortic valves may develop embolic occlusion of a major artery; the legs are involved most often. The diagnosis is established by studies of the thrombus recovered during embolectomy.[7]

The onset of acute infective endocarditis differs markedly from that of the subacute disease. Patients become ill rapidly despite the lack of initial signs and symptoms that indicate the presence of valvular disease. Progressive destruction of the involved valve leads to the development of a number of complications within a week of disease onset. Congestive cardiac failure is common, especially when the aortic valve is infected. The valvular vegetations are often large, friable, and poorly organized and pose a high risk of embolization. The earliest manifestations of the acute disease include multiple petechiae, purpuric lesions of the skin, and rapidly developing signs of neurological dysfunction. Multiple pulmonary infarcts or abscesses of the lung may appear when the right side of the heart is involved.

Signs and Symptoms

Fever is not universal in infective endocarditis; many patients are afebrile when they reach the hospital[8] and remain free of fever throughout the course of the disease. Osler[9] commented that "it is well recognized now that fever is not an invariable accompaniment of endocarditis." From 3% to 15% of individuals have normal or subnormal temperatures.[1,5,10–12] Elderly patients with subacute infective endocarditis are likely to be afebrile because basal and maximal daily temperatures gradually decrease with age. We have studied a number of individuals who were thought to be afebrile. However, when their temperature was monitored closely, it became clear that they experienced spikes of fever lower than those in young individuals; their temperature averaged 98.6°F. Low-grade fever is present in patients with massive intracerebral or subarachnoid hemorrhage, cardiac failure, or uremia.

Rigors are uncommon in children with subacute infective endocarditis. Treatment with salicylates may lead to the development of chills as the blood level of the antipyretic drug decreases. Patients with acute infective endocarditis may experience high-grade fever (up to 104°F) that may be preceded by a cluster of rigors even in the absence of treatment with salicylates.

About 15% of patients with subacute infective endocarditis have no detectable murmur early in the course of the disease. It often develops in the course of treatment or after treatment has been discontinued. A murmur may not be detected for many years after the disease has been cured. One of us has studied a 36-year-old man who had been well throughout life and then developed persistent low-grade fever. Numerous physical examinations disclosed no murmurs. However, a stroke occurred secondary to embolic occlusion of the right middle cerebral artery. Multiple cultures of blood grew viridans streptococci. The patient was treated with an appropriate antimicrobial agent for 4 weeks and recovered. No murmurs were audible during his hospitalization. Examinations carried out yearly for 15 years failed to identify a murmur by auscultation and/or phonocardiography.

Murmurs are absent in about one-third of patients with acute infective endocarditis that involves the left side of the heart.[13] Pankey[14,15] indicated that 1 of 167 individuals with subacute disease and 7 of 54 with acute disease were free of murmurs throughout the course of their illness. He noted that the characteristics of the murmurs changed in 16.7% of those with the subacute infection.

Based on extensive experience with infective endocarditis over the past 50 years, it has become clear that the absence of a murmur is rare in patients with subacute disease. This is not the case in acute infection. Murmurs are absent in two-thirds of patients with endocardial infection that involves the right side of the heart. This is also true for mural endocarditis.

The presence of a basal systolic murmur generated by blood flow from the left ventricle into an enlarged, tortuous aorta or by atherosclerotic changes in the aortic valve poses some difficulty in establishing the diagnosis of infective endocarditis, especially the subacute type. Murmurs present for many years usually do not change in character when infective endocarditis develops. The presence of subtle signs of infection in elderly individuals with unexplained fever and a murmur suggests the presence of endocardial infection. Sterile cultures of the blood do not rule this out. No murmur should be considered innocent when infective endocarditis is a diagnostic possibility. The assumption that a flow or ejection murmur is physiological may lead to failure to consider the possibility of endocardial disease.

An increase in the intensity of the murmur in mitral insufficiency must not be disregarded in patients in whom the level of fever and anemia has not changed. An effort must be made to rule out tricuspid insufficiency in individuals with staphylococcal bacteremia.[16]

Anemia and pallor of the skin and mucous membranes are almost always present in patients with acute or subacute infective endocarditis. A patient described by Libman and Celler[17] had erythema of the nose and cheeks that resembled the facial lesion of systemic lupus erythematosus.

Classical Peripheral Lesions of Infective Endocarditis

The classical peripheral lesions of infective endocarditis were present in about 85% of patients prior to the availability of antimicrobial therapy; they are now identified in only 19–40%.[5,18–21] Petechial lesions with pale centers are clinically more important than those with yellow centers[5] and are often present in the conjunctivae of the upper and lower eyelids, the dorsa of the hands and feet, the anterior chest and abdominal wall, the oral and pharyngeal mucosa, and the soft palate. Dermal purpuric lesions not associated with thrombocytopenia are present occasionally. Other conditions in which petechial lesions may be present are (1) various hematological disorders; (2) Libman-Sacks disease; (3) scurvy; (4) renal failure; (5) viral infections; (6) atrial myxoma; (7) marantic endocarditis; and (8) uncomplicated staphylococcal, streptococcal, meningococcal, gonococcal, pneumococcal, or influenzal bacteremia. Fifty percent of patients who undergo cardiopulmonary bypass surgery develop conjunctival petechiae due to the microembolism of fat.[21]

Subungual hemorrhages are now uncommon in patients with infective endocarditis.[22–24] These lesions appear most often in older individuals, as well as in typists and carpenters whose hands are traumatized by their occupation. The outstanding features of a splinter hemorrhage are its linearity and the fact that it fails to reach the distal edge of a nail. The number of involved fingers ranges from 1 to 10; 2 or more hemorrhages may be present in the toe nails. Multiple splinter hemorrhages of the nails are most common in individuals with trichinosis. Only the bleeding areas that appear not to be produced by trauma are consistent with infective endocarditis.[23]

Osler nodes are small, raised, tender nodules that range in color from red to purple. They are present in the pulp spaces of the terminal phalanges of the fingers, backs of the toes, soles of the feet, and thenar and hypothenar eminences of the hands. They are rarely present on the sides of the fingers, forearms, ears, and trunk. The development of an Osler node is sometimes preceded by an unusual sensation of pain at the site of the lesion. This lesion may be present for only a few hours, usually persists for 4–5 days, and is tender. However, the involved area remains tender for only 2–3 days. Necrosis is rarely a problem. Although essentially restricted to sub-acute infective endocarditis, these lesions may appear in the course of the acute disease; they are usually related to infected emboli and not to immunological phenomena. Lesions that resemble Osler nodes have been identified in marantic endocarditis, systemic lupus erythematosus, disseminated gonococcal disease, and cannulation of the radial artery. Since this lesion was described by Osler, its incidence has decreased from 70% to 10%.[5,12,15,25]

Janeway lesions are irregular, erythematous, painless macules that range in size from 1 to 4 mm in diameter and are most often present on the thenar and hypothenar eminences of the hands and soles of the feet. Less often, they occur on the tips of the fingers and plantar surfaces of the toes. They may also appear as a diffuse, macular, erythematous rash over the trunk and extremities that blanches with pressure. Kerr and Tan[26] have identified microabscesses in biopsy specimens of Janeway lesions from patients with endocarditis produced by *S. aureus*.

Although clubbing of the fingers and/or toes was once present in almost all patients with subacute infective endocarditis, it now occurs in only 10–12%. Our experience indicates that it is presently quite rare. Clubbing of the fingers and toes develops in individuals with prolonged, untreated infection. It disappears during antimicrobial therapy and in the bacteria-free stage of the disease.[5]

In addition to conjunctival petechiae, other ocular abnormalities may be present in patients with infective endocarditis. Circular or flame-shaped hemorrhages may appear in the sclera and retina. The Roth spot, as first described, is located in the retina and appears as a "cotton wool" exudate that contains aggregates of cytoid bodies. Roth suggested that this lesion was related to "varicose" hypertrophy of the retina and was not embolic in origin.[27] However, he failed to recognize the relationship of the ocular manifestation to endocardial infection because he had observed a similar retinal lesion in patients with disorders other than endocarditis. The cotton wool exudate, a perivascular collection of lymphocytes in the nerve layer of the retina, may or may not be surrounded by edema and hemorrhage. First described by Litten,[28] this became known as *Litten's sign*. The boat-shaped hemorrhages in the retina, erroneously identified as Roth spots, were first described by Doherty and Trubek,[29] who attributed them to recurrent showers of petechiae. Others[30,31] noted that the retinal lesions were composed of a central white zone containing inflammatory cells and surrounded by an area of diapadized erythrocytes. Roth spots and boat-shaped hemorrhages are presently identified in less than 5% of patients.[19,20]

Round "white spots" may be present in the retina of individuals with subacute infective endocarditis; optic neuritis may develop in the course of the disease.

Splenomegaly, common in patients with infective endocarditis (30%) prior to the advent of antimicrobial therapy,[32–34] is now less frequent. It develops more often in acute than in subacute disease.[35] There is no difference in its incidence in patients with prosthetic or native valves. Embolic infarction is the most common splenic complication of infective endocarditis (currently 1% of cases). This presents with acute pain in the left upper quadrant of the abdomen and is associated with the appearance of a left pleural effusion. About half of those who succumb to the disease have had splenic infarcts. Aneurysm of the splenic artery may develop.[36] The incidence of multiple small splenic abscesses is about 6%.[36] These are present most often in patients with acute infective endocarditis. Splenomegaly may persist long after therapy has been completed. Other uncommon manifestations of infective endocarditis include pericardial friction rubs, congestive cardiac failure, various arrhythmias, hematuria unrelated to renal infarction, cough, hoarseness, arthritis, and pain and tenderness in the long bones and sternum, especially when severe anemia is present.[37]

About 44% of individuals with infective endocarditis develop musculoskeletal disorders. Among these are arthralgia, arthritis, and synovitis (Table 8.1). Acute synovitis may involve the metacarpophalangeal, sternoclavicular, and acromioclavicular joints (Table 8.2). Arthritis associated with infective endocarditis is usually asymmetrical, monoarticular, or oligoarticular. The most common symptoms are myalgia and arthralgia.[38,39] The fluid present in the joints is usually sterile. However, it may be grossly purulent when *S. aureus* is the causative agent. Endocardial infection may present initially with symptoms and signs that may be confused with those of rheumatoid arthritis, Reiter's syndrome, or Lyme disease. The articular manifestations improve rapidly after the initiation of antimicrobial therapy. The cause of pain in the axial skeleton, especially the lumbar area, is unknown; it may be due to vertebral osteomyelitis. The organisms most often involved in the infection of bones are streptococci and *S. aureus*.[40] The most likely causes of low back pain are embolization of the vertebral blood vessels, aseptic necrosis of an intervertebral disc, or deposition of immune complexes in a disc space. Most striking is the disappearance of lumbar pain 8 to 10 days after antimicrobial therapy is initiated.

The Bacteria-Free Stage

The bacteria-free stage of infective endocarditis, first described by Libman in 1913,[41] has been defined as a syndrome in which patients with infective endocarditis have multiple sterile cultures of the blood over an extended period of time and in whom diagnosis and treatment may be delayed for months. The clinical features of this syndrome include congestive cardiac failure, arthralgias, edema of the legs, and severe pain in the thighs. Fever is

Table 8.1. Musculoskeletal Manifestations in 84 Patients with Bacterial Endocarditis

| | Number of cases (Mean and Range, Months)* | | |
	Developed before Diagnosis	Developed after Diagnosis	Total
Arthralgias	30 (2½, <¼–11)	2 (<¼, ½)	32
Arthritis	22 (3¼, <¼–11)	4 (¼, <¼–½)	26
Low back pain	19 (1½, 1–4)		19
Diffuse myalgias	16 (2½, <¼–12)		16
Leg myalgias	11 (2¼, ¼–6)		11
Disc space infection	5 (4¼, 1½–8)		5
Nail clubbing	4 (?)		4
Hypertrophic osteoarthropathy	1 (11)		1
Achilles tendinitis	1 (2)		1
Vascular necrosis		1 (6)	1
Total			121[†]

*Interval in which manifestations preceded or followed the diagnosis.
[†]Multiple complaints or findings occurred in some patients.
Source: Adapted from Ref. 38.

Table 8.2. Location of Arthritis in 26 Patients with Bacterial Endocarditis

Joint	Cases
Ankle	7
Knee	6
Wrist	5
Sternoclavicular	4
Elbow	4
Metatarsophalangeal	4
Metacarpophalangeal	3
Shoulder	2
Hip	2
Acromioclavicular	1
Total	38*

*Multiple joints were involved in some patients.
Source: Adapted from Ref. 38.

absent in most instances but may develop when embolization occurs; the emboli are always sterile. Although all patients have damaged mitral and/or aortic valves, new murmurs do not develop and preexisting ones may disappear. The kidney is almost always involved, and microscopic hematuria is common even in the absence of renal infarction, the cause of death in about one-third of patients. Anemia is universal. Leukopenia and granulocytopenia may develop in the course of the disease. The spleen is always enlarged; this may become the dominant clinical feature. Petechial lesions and Osler nodes are uncommon; purpuric ones are frequent in the early stage of the disease. Marked tenderness of the sternum and striking brown pigmentation of the face and dorse of the hands are outstanding features. Total body pain is frequent in the active stage of the disease. Aneurysms may be present in the mitral valve, septum membranaceum, sinus of Valsalva, and femoral and iliac arteries. The criteria for the diagnosis of the bacteria-free stage of subacute infective endocarditis are (1) the absence of clinical evidence suggesting endocardial infection; (2) sterile cultures of blood; (3) the presence of organisms in the valvular vegetations; (4) renal insufficiency;(5) severe progressive anemia; (6) embolic phenomena;[9] striking splenomegaly; (7) brown facial pigmentation; and (8) absence of fever. Patients with this syndrome may survive for as long as 3 years but eventually succumb to renal or cardiac failure or both.

Complications

The life-threatening complications of acute infective endocarditis are presented in Table 8.3. One of the most severe complications is rapidly progressive cardiac failure that fails to respond to intensive medical therapy or improves only incompletely or temporarily. The risk of this occurring is especially great when highly invasive organisms such as *S. aureus, S. pyogenes, S. pneumoniae, H. influenzae, N. gonorrhoeae,* and *N. meningitidis* are involved. When these organisms infect a normal valve, the suppuration can readily spread to the myocardium and produce a perivalvular abscess. Arrhythmias and varying degrees of heart block become predominant features when the conducting system is injured.[16] Congestive cardiac failure follows the appearance of aortic regurgitation and is the leading cause of death in patients with infective endocarditis.[42] The process may progress so rapidly that the involved valve requires replacement within 1 week. Cardiac failure characteristically develops over a prolonged period in patients with subacute endocarditis.

A study of 145 cases of subacute and acute infective endocarditis by Mills et al.[42] indicated that 55% of the patients had congestive cardiac failure; 80% developed aortic insufficiency after the valve was infected by enterococci. Cardiac decompensation developed in about 50% of patients with acquired mitral regurgitation and in 20% of those with congenital cardiac disease or involvement of the tricuspid valve. Five percent of the patients who developed cardiac failure within 6 months after the onset of endocar-

Table 8.3. Life-Threatening Complications of Infective Endocarditis

Intracardiac Complications	Extracardiac Complications
Intractable cardiac failure	Embolization of coronary arteries
Myocardial (or septal) abscess	Stroke
Rupture of papillary muscles	Embolus to spinal cord
Annular abscess	Abscess of spleen
Destruction of valvular leaflets	Mycotic aneurysm in brain
Mycotic aneurysm of sinus of Valsalva	Recurrence of endocarditis Cerebral abscess(es)
Aortocardiac and other fistulas	Multiple embolic episodes
Suppurative pericarditis	
Obstruction of outlet of Starr-Edwards valve	
Separation of prosthetic valve from annulus	
Infection of intracardiac patches	

Source: Ref. 102.

ditis had premonitory symptoms in the first month of illness. The organisms responsible for the disease were, in order of frequency, enterococci, *S. pneumoniae, S. aureus,* and viridans streptococci.

Cardiac decompensation is present in 15–65% of patients with infective endocarditis. It may appear as early as 1 month after and almost always within 6 months after the onset of the disease; it may also occur up to 1 year after the endocardial disease is cured. Although myocarditis may be responsible for congestive cardiac failure, it is now clear that the most common cause of failure is insufficiency of the aortic valve. The impact of the jet stream on the mitral valve produced by backflow from the diseased aortic valve may produce cardiac failure in patients with severe aortic regurgitation. This may lead to erosion or perforation of a valvular cusp or rupture of the chordae tendinae of the mitral valve.[43] Concurrent acute disease of the mitral valve, increases the overload of the left ventricle produced by aortic regurgitation and marked by the failing of the left side of the heart. Hemodynamically important valvular stenosis may be induced by unusually large vegetations in patients with fungal endocarditis. These produce obstruction of blood flow from the left ventricle.[44,45] A similar phenomenon has been observed in two cases of acute staphylococcal infection involving the mitral valve.[46] Pulmonary hypertension and decreased cardiac output have usually been present. Although mitral stenosis is usually present in this situation, murmurs are not identified during the acute stage of the disease.

The analyses of the hemodynamic severity of aortic regurgitation in patients with infective endocarditis has been evaluated by Mann et al.[47] They noted that the mean pulse, left ventricular end-diastolic pressure, and stroke volume are significantly reduced in patients with insufficiency of the aortic valve compared to those with chronic regurgitation. Ventricular pressures exceed those in the left atrium late in diastole. This produces premature closure of the mitral valve as the result of an increase in left ventricular end-diastolic pressure. Early closure of the mitral valve leads to the development of an Austin-Flint murmur; this has been confirmed by electrocardiography. Patients with very early mitral closure have severely volume-overloaded ventricles and are candidates for early replacement of their infected valves.

Intracardiac Complications

A number of potentially life-threatening intracardiac complications may develop in acute infective endocarditis; this is rare in subacute disease. Some acute infections are associated with rapid, progressive congestive cardiac failure and a change in the character of a present or previously undetected murmur. Disruption of infected valves and their supporting structures may lead to fenestration or tearing of the valvular leaflets, detachment of one or more areas of a valve from the annulus, and rupture of the chordae tendinae or papillary muscles.

Of 150 patients with infective endocarditis studied by Tompsett and Lubash,[48] 10 had intracardiac complications associated with subacute or acute disease. These included (1) the absence of hemodynamically significant aortic insufficiency prior to onset of the disease; (2) the development of hemodynamically important aortic regurgitation during or soon after initiation of treatment; and (3) evidence at autopsy of perforation or destruction of a valvular cusp, an important complication of acute infective endocarditis. Microbiological cure had been achieved in all individuals with progressive cardiac failure. The complexity of the clinical situation in which valvular perforation develops may obscure the fact that this has occurred and that the risk of development of intractable heart failure is high.

Other intracardiac complications that develop in patients with acute infective endocarditis are (1) aortocardiac and other fistulas; (2) aneurysms of the sinus of Valsalva; and (3) intraventricular abscesses that may perforate and lead to the appearance of acute pericarditis.[49–53] DeCock and Rees[54] have described a 16-year-old patient with staphylococcal bacteremia who developed pericarditis, a nodal rhythm, and right bundle branch block. During insertion of a valvular prosthesis, an infected, perforated bicuspid aortic valve and a communication between the aortic root and right atrium were identified. The defects were closed and the aortic valve replaced, but the patient died. Autopsy disclosed a large abscess in the intraventricular septum that was connected to the aortic root and the right atrium above the tricuspid valve.

Patients with acute infective endocarditis that involves the aortic valve may develop abnormalities of conduction when the infection spreads to the intraventricular septum. In a study correlating anatomical and electrocardiographic abnormalities in 24 patients with acute aortic valvular infection,

Roberts and Somerville[55] identified prolonged P-R intervals, unrelated to treatment with digitalis, in 18 patients and atrioventricular dissociation in 4. Aneurysms of the septum were present in four of six individuals with prolonged P-R intervals and in three of four with normal conduction and left bundle branch block. Four of six patients with delayed conduction died suddenly. Sapsford et al.[56] have described three persons in whom an aneurysm of the fibrous skeleton situated between the aortic and mitral valves complicated an infection of the aorta.

Multiple myocardial abscesses have been identified in about 20% of fatal cases of acute infective endocarditis caused by *S. aureus* and enterococci.[57,58] A staphylococcal abscess may rupture into the pericardial sac and cause rapid death due to the cardiac tamponade secondary to a massive pyohemopericardium. Septal abscesses are common in individuals with acute staphylococcal endocardial infection. These organisms may destroy an infected area in the septum and produce a left-to-right shunt. A patient with acute staphylococcal infection of the aortic valve who developed an aortopulmonary septal defect has been described.[59]

Destruction of cardiac tissue sufficient to allow shunting of blood is an uncommon complication of acute infective endocarditis. This occurs most often when an aneurysm of the aortic sinus ruptures into the septal wall of the right atrium or the posterior wall of the right outflow tract. In some instances, peripheral arteriovenous shunting may occur.[60–62] Septal abscesses that spread from an infected mitral valve are usually located at the lower end of the intraventricular septum.[61,62] The presence of these lesions is suspected when electrocardiography indicates a gradual increase in the P-R and Q-T intervals and left bundle branch block; the right bundle is involved less often. Early recognition of these changes is critical because surgical removal of the abscess is indicated (Table 8.4).

Abscesses in the upper septum in patients with acute infective endocarditis pose a serious threat and must be removed. The electrocardiographic abnormalities in this area are not as specific as they are in the lower septum. The presence of an abscess in the upper septum may not be identified until it is beyond effective surgical treatment. Serial electrocardiography may identify a variety of arrhythmias, including third-degree or complete heart block and/or episodes of ventricular tachycardia. Early surgical removal of an abscess is mandatory and usually requires placement of a pacemaker.

Abscesses that involve the valvular ring have been described by Arnett and Roberts[63] in 27 fatal cases of acute infective endocarditis. They notice that these lesions were located in the aortic annulus more often than in the mitral annulus or atrioventricular ring. The development of an abscess in the valvular ring was not related to the age or sex of the patient, the status of the valve prior to the onset of infection, the organism involved, or the type of antimicrobial therapy employed. The criteria required to establish the diagnosis of annular abscess are (1) infection of the aortic valve; (2) the recent development of valvular regurgitation; (3) the presence of pericarditis; (4) a high level of atrioventricular block; and (5) a short duration of

Table 8.4. Types of Conduction Abnormalities in
20 Patients with Unstable Atrioventricular Block*

Type	Frequency (%)
First-degree AV block	9 (45)
Isolated	5
+ Left BBB	3
+ LAHB	1
Second-degree AV block	3 (15)
Isolated	2
+ Right BBB (incomplete)	1
Third-degree AV block	4 (20)
Isolated	2
+ Left BBB	1
+ Right BBB	1
Left BBB (isolated)	1 (5)
Right BBB (isolated)	2 (10)
LPHB	1 (5)

*Patients with varying degrees of AV block are classified according to the highest degree of block documented in their medical record, even if this was a transient episode.

AV = atrioventricular; BBB = bundle branch block; LAHB = left anterior hemiblock; LPHB = left posterior hemiblock.

Source: Adapted from DiNubile et al.[64]

symptoms followed by the rapid development of severe disability and death.[64]

Pericarditis is uncommon in patients with subacute infective endocarditis.[65] When present, it results from the deposition of immune complexes in the pericardium. The pericarditis that complicates the acute type of endocardial infection is almost always pyogenic in origin. Organisms commonly enter the pericardium in the course of a bacteremia. Rupture of a myocardial abscess often produces pericarditis. Other causes of pericarditis are (1) erosion of a mycotic aneurysm in the sinus of Valsalva; (2) extension of infection from the aortic valve to the pericardial wedge situated between the roots of the aortic and pulmonary arteries; (3) uremia secondary to glomerulonephritis; and (4) a flare of rheumatic fever triggered by active endocarditis (Fig. 8.1).

Myocarditis that appears in the course of infective endocarditis may be caused by ischemic injury associated with (1) vasculitis that involves the coronary arteries; (2) embolic occlusion of one or more of these vessels; (3) injury produced by microbial toxins; (4) invasion by organisms; and (5) deposition of immune complexes in the walls of the coronary vessels.[66–68] The prominent histological features in the heart are the Bracht-Wachter bodies, collections of lymphocytes, and aggregates of polymorphonuclear leukocytes. Miliary abscesses, arteriolitis, medial necrosis, and adventitial and perivascular infiltrates are present in some patients.

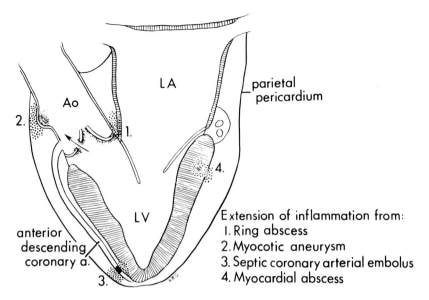

Fig. 8.1. Schematic portrayal of the pathogenesis of pericarditis in infective endocarditis. Ao, aorta; LV, left ventricle; LA, left atrium. (From Roberts, WC, Buchbinder, NA: Healed left-sided infective endocarditis. A clinicopathological study of 59 patients. *Am J Cardiol* 1976;40:876)

The development of a midsystolic "click," loudest over the tricuspid valve in two heroin addicts with infective endocarditis, has been reported by Bashour and Lindsay.[69] They suggested that dysfunction of the chordae tendinae was responsible for the adventitious sound.

Embolization

Arterial embolization is the second most common complication in patients with both subacute and acute infective endocarditis. This ranged from 70–97% in the preantibiotic era to 15–35% today. Over this period, major emboli have decreased in frequency from 40% to 25%. The incidence of multiple episodes of embolization has declined due, in part, to early diagnosis and effective therapy.[70,71] Clinical profiles have been developed to identify patients at risk of this complication. It occurs most often in patients 20–40 years of age and in those with disease involving the mitral and aortic native or prosthetic valves. Valvular infection caused by *Candida* species, *S. aureus, H. parainfluenzae, Aspergillus* species, group B streptococci, and nutritionally variant streptococci[72–74] is characterized by the presence of large, friable vegetations that give rise to large emboli.

Most of the extracardiac complications in patients with acute and subacute infective endocarditis are related to embolization. The organs most often involved are the spleen, kidneys, coronary arteries, meninges, and brain; less common are the skin, muscles of the eyes, joints, and bones. Postmortem studies have disclosed a much higher incidence of embolization of the kidneys and central nervous system than was identified during life.[75–77] Embolization occurs most often in the lower legs (45%) and less often in the carotid artery (23%) and upper arms (14%).[78]

Although the total incidence of embolization of various organs in patients with infective endocarditis has been defined, the frequency with which this occurs in a given patient is not predictable. In some individuals only a single episode may occur; in others, multiple emboli are deposited throughout the active stage of the disease or even after cure has been accomplished. Because the vegetations in subacute endocarditis are usually small and firm, it has been suggested that embolization may be uncommon, except in acute disease in which the presence of large, friable valvular thrombi predisposes patients to embolization. However, this is not the case. There appears to be little difference in the incidence of embolization in the two types of infective endocarditis. The risk appears to be related to the nature of the organism responsible for the infection rather than to the clinical nature of the disease.

Although often not recognized clinically, embolic infarction of the kidney was identified at necropsy in about 50% of patients in the past; it is now less common.[79] Renal embolization of the kidney may lead to the development of embolic glomerular lesions in 52% of patients with subacute endocarditis and in 7% of those with acute endocarditis.[80,81]

Myocardial infarction, often small and occasionally multiple, has been identified at autopsy in 40–60% of patients with embolization of the coronary arteries. Because electrocardiographic abnormalities are not common during life, the possibility of infarction has often not been considered. The loss of myocardium often leads to the development of congestive cardiac failure, especially when the tissue surrounding the aortic valve has been injured.[82–85]

Embolization of major cerebral vessels occurs in about one-third of patients with infective endocarditis. The middle cerebral artery and its branches are involved most often.[86] About 3% of all cerebral emboli develop late in the course of subacute or acute disease[87] or occur years after it has been cured. Occlusion due to embole of the blood vessels of the spinal cord is rare. It may present with pain in a girdle distribution or with parplegia.[88] Embolic involvement of the blood vessels that supply the peripheral nerves leads to the appearance of localized tenderness, peripheral neuropathy, various sensory disturbances, and pain.[89–92]

Embolization of the retinal arteries may lead to the appearance of ipsilateral blindness. Other complications include retinal infarction with formation of a hole in the visual field and retinopathy.[93,94] Prepapillary emboic abscesses are very rare.[95] Examination of the eyes of patients with ocular abscesses discloses pus over the optic disc, star figure exudates in the macula, retinal hemorrhages with white centers, and Roth spots (Fig. 8.2).

Infarction of the gallbladder and liver, produced by emboli has been identified in a patient with acute staphylococcal endocarditis.[96] Angiography disclosed emboli in the liver and in a major branch of the cystic artery. The gallbladder was completely necrotic. Histological study disclosed coagulation necrosis of the hepatic cells and relative preservation of the adjacent portal areas.

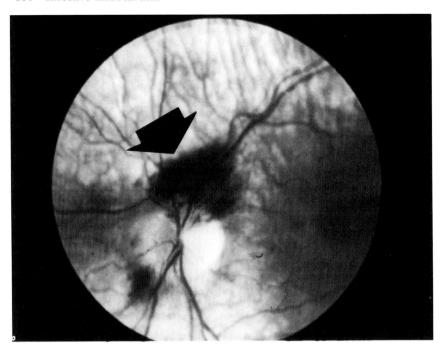

Fig. 8.2. The arrow indicates a Roth spot in the fundus of a 26-year-old man with subacute infective endocarditis.

Embolic occlusion of large arteries is very uncommon. The most likely causes are fungal infection or the presence of an atrial myxoma. It is important to note that patients infected by staphylococci, nutritionally variant streptococci, or *H. influenzae* may produce large, friable vegetations. Rarely, subacute endocardial disease caused by viridans streptococci may be complicated by embolization of a large artery. Embolization may occur weeks to months after a valvular infection has been cured. Three to 6 months of therapy may be required for the complete endothelialization of valvular vegetations. Although cardiac catheterization during active infective endocarditis has been considered hazardous, there is no evidence that catheterization-induced emboli poses any real risk.[97]

Metastatic Infections

The complications of embolization that occur in acute infective endocarditis are, with few exceptions, different from those present in the subacute disease. Abscesses almost always develop in areas where emboli are deposited in patients infected by *S. aureus*. Fatal disease caused by this organism is associated with the presence of multiple abscesses in almost every organ, especially the kidneys and heart. Staphylococcal infection of the brain may produce single or multiple lesions (Fig. 8.3). Features that suggest the presence of metastatic abscesses are (1) defervescence after initiation of therapy; (2) recurrent episodes of fever during or shortly after treatment is discontinued; (3) failure to respond initially to therapy with an appropriate antibiotic; and (4) the presence of bacteremia during treatment.

Metastatic infection following embolization is rare in patients with subacute infective endocarditis. The embolus usually produces a sterile infarct because it contains such a small number of organisms. The bacteria, especially *S. viridans*, are usually not very invasive. Most patients have high levels of specific bactericidal antibody for the pathogens of subacute disease. Abscesses and other infections rarely develop at the site of such an embolus. Aseptic meningitis or diffuse encephalitis may be the initial manifestation of subacute infective endocarditis.

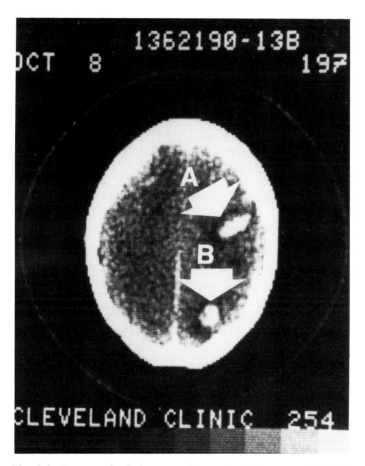

Fig. 8.3. Two cerebral abscesses demonstrated on a cerebral CT scan of a patient with *S. aureus* endocarditis.

Mycotic Aneurysms

Life-threatening mycotic aneurysms are present in about 2.5% of patients with infective endocarditis. Some of these are rarely identified premortem because they remain asymptomatic throughout the course of the disease.[98] Infected aneurysms that usually appear in the active phase of endocarditis may not be identified for months to years after the valvular infection has been cured. Mycotic aneurysms are most often produced by organisms with a low invasive capacity, such as viridans streptococci. Paradoxically, mycotic aneurysms are less common in individuals infected by the more aggressive organisms, such as *S. aureus* and *Aspergillus* species.[99] Several pathological processes are involved in the development of a mycotic aneurysm.[100] Among these are (1) injury of the arterial wall caused by the deposition of immune complexes; (2) sterile infarction following the deposition of microemboli in the vasa vasorum; (3) microbial invasion of the vascular wall in the course of bacteremia; and (4) an abscess in the wall of an infarcted artery in which rupture is common. The brain; the sinus of Valsalva; a ligated ductus arteriosus; the abdominal aorta and its branches; and the superior mesenteric, splenic, coronary, and pulmonary arteries are the most common sites of aneurysms. About 20–30% are present in the arteries of the limbs, especially the legs; 10–20% involve the mesenteric artery; and 4% affect the splenic arteries. The descending aorta is now involved in 6% compared to 23% prior to the availability of antimicrobial agents.[21,25,101,102]

Infected aneurysms are usually silent, making their presence known only after a slow leak or hemorrhage occurs. Those in the brain rarely produce headache or cranial nerve palsies. Although any artery may be involved, those in which aneurysms pose a danger to life are the cerebral vessels; abdominal aorta; superior mesenteric, splenic, and coronary arteries; and a ligated ductus arteriosus.[103]

Neurological Complications

It has been known for many years that neurological complications may develop in patients with infective endocarditis.[104,105] These may be the initial presentation is 42–58% of patients with acute or subacute disease.[106,107] Sex, age, and the nature of the underlying cardiac disease play no role in the development of the neurological manifestations of endocardial infection. The fatality rate ranges from 22% to 92% when neurological dysfunction is present.[108–113] By contrast, it is 6–24% in those free of neurological disorders.

Among the neurological complications in patients with infective endocarditis are (1) vascular phenomena associated with embolization; (2) rupture of an intracerebral mycotic aneurysm; and (3) meningitis or meningoencephalitis. *S. aureus* is responsible for 55–70% of the neurological complications and 75% of cerebral hemorrhages.[106,108] This organism is most often the cause of septic meningitis.[114] Gram-negative bacteria are increasingly involved in a number of neurological syndromes.

The mitral valve appears to be the source of emboli in more than 50% of patients with infective endocarditis.[106] The incidence of significant embolic events is higher in individuals with large, friable vegetations, especially in those infected by *H. parainfluenzae*.[115,117] Anticoagulation appears to promote embolization. A study by Pruitt et al.[106] indicated that 23% of hemorrhagic events occurred in about 3% of patients treated with anticoagulants; about 50% developed a cerebral hematoma.[107] In individuals with infective endocarditis there appears to be no relation between either cerebral hemorrhage and thrombocytopenia or between cardiac arrhythmias and cerebral emboli. Patients with staphylococcal infection of the mitral valve receiving anticoagulants must be monitored closely for the appearance of severe complications that involve the central nervous system.

The neurological manifestations of infective endocarditis have been classified by Ziment[105] on the basis of their etiology. He defined them as follows: (1) *toxic manifestations*—headache, decreased concentration, insomnia, drowsiness, vertigo, and irritability; (2) *psychiatric disorders*—neurosis, psychosis, confusion, disorientation, emotional instability, delirium, auditory and visual disturbances, apathy, and altered personality; (3) *stroke*—aphonia, hemi-, di-, para-, or quadriplegia, stupor, and coma; (4) *meningoencephalitis*—acute brain syndrome; (5) *involvement of the cranial nerves*—visual disturbances and cranial nerve sensory impairment; (6) Dyskinesia—tremor, ataxia, parkinsonism, seizures, chorea, hemifacial dyskinesia, iccups, and myoclonus; and (7) *spinal cord* or *small nerves*—girdle pain, weakness, paraplegia, paresis, sensory disturbances, myalgia, and peripheral neuropathy.

Embolic abscesses develop in 1% of subacute and 25% of acute infective endocarditis. Encephalomalacia and endarteritis appear to be related to vasculitis of the cerebral arteries. Petechial and purpuric lesions are present mainly in the white matter close to the lateral ventricles and in the gray matter along the aqueduct and corpus callosum. Meningitis and cerebral edema may develop. Embolic retinal artery occlusion and retinal or conjunctival hemorrhages may be present. Papilledema, iridocyclitis, panophthalmitis, nystagmus, and conjugate deviation of the third cranial nerve have been identified.

Embolic cerebral infarction appears to be the most common complication of infective endocarditis that involves the central nervous system. The affected area may be macroscopic or microscopic in size. About 11% of patients have multiple microembolic-punctate lesions. At least 50% of those with cerebral emboli experience embolization of other organs. When highly invasive organisms (e.g., *S. aureus*, enterococci, and *E. coli*) produce the disease, cerebral infarction usually develops within 2 weeks. When less agressive organisms are involved, infarction of the brain occurs as early as 2–4 weeks or as late as 1–3 months after the onset of endocarditis.

Mycotic aneurysms of the cerebral vessels develop in 2–10% of patients with infective endocarditis. Molinari et al.[115] suggested that aneurysmal dilatation is produced by material carried to the adventitial layers of the vasa vasorum, where an embolus triggers an inflammatory reaction which weakens the adventitia and muscular layers of the artery. It has been suggested that in some instances the primary injury of the vascular wall is produced by the deposition of immune complexes.

Eighty percent of 85 individuals with cerebral mycotic aneurysms studied by Bohmfalk et al.[118] died after rupture of the lesion. Multiple aneurysms were present in 17.7%; a second one developed after the first was identified. Angiographic studies indicated that single or multiple lesions were peripheral to the first bifurcation of a major intracranial artery (Fig. 8.4). Sixty-five percent of the aneurysms ruptured spontaneously; they disappeared in 10 patients. It has been suggested that the true incidence of cerebral mycotic aneurysms is unknown. The reported incidence of 6.2–29% of multiple lesions may be low.

Cerebral abscesses have been present in about 4% of patients with acute infective endocarditis;[106] none were detected during life (Fig. 8.3). The lesions have been less than 1 cm^3 in size in eight cases. Multiple microabscesses of the brain and other organs have been identified. With one exception, the endocardial disease was caused by *S. aureus*, enterococci, or *Serratia*. A large cerebral abscess was present in one patient. It was considered to be secondary to an episode of otitis media probably unrelated to the endocarditis. One of us has studied a patient with acute staphylococcal endocardial disease who had had two large and multiple small abscesses in the brain; staphylococci were recovered only from the heart.

Cerebrospinal fluid was found by Pruitt et al.[106] to be abnormal in about 72% of patients with infective endocarditis; all had neurological dysfunction. Polymorphonuclear leukocytes were predominant when the endocardial disease was caused by *S. aureus,* gram-negative bacteria, or *S. pneumoniae.* When the infective endocarditis is caused by relatively avirulent organisms, such as viridans streptococci, the abnormalities of the spinal fluid were usually characteristic of aseptic meningitis. Blood was present in the cerebrospinal fluid in about 15% of the patients.[106]

Renal Complications

Involvement of the kidney is relatively common in patients with acute or subacute infective endocarditis (Table 8.5). Five major types of renal disease have been identified.[119–121] Two are caused by embolization. The others are associated with immunological phenomena. Large, uninfected infarcts of the kidney, accompanied by gross or microscopic hematuria, were common in subacute disease 35–40 years ago but are presently infrequent.[119] However, multiple small areas of infarction are now often identified at autopsy. Focal embolic glomerulonephritis is presently the second most common renal disorder in patients with subacute infective endocarditis; it is present in 50% of untreated and 15% of treated patients. Pathologically, it

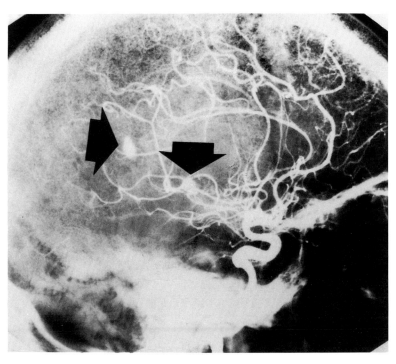

Fig. 8.4. Two cerebral artery mycotic aneurysms documented by arteriography.

Table 8.5. Renal Complications of Endocarditis

Renal infarction	Most common lesion: present in ²/₃ of of untreated cases. Occurs in 10 to 15% of right-sided endocarditis.
Focal glomerulonephritis	Second most common lesion. Occurs in 50% of untreated cases and 15% of treated ones. May be associated with renal failure and nephrotic syndrome.
Diffuse glomerulonephritis	30 to 60% of untreated cases and 10% of treated cases.
"Flea-bitten" kidney	Multiple emboli and hemorrhages.
Renal abscess(es)	Usually with highly invasive organisms, e.g., *Staph aureus*.
Cortical necrosis	In patients with disseminated intravascular coagulation
Renal lesions related to antimicrobial therapy	Interstitial nephritis, toxic nephropathy, acute tubular necrosis. Renal failure may occur in the course of subacute endocarditis.

Source: Ref. 103.

is a localized process characterized by proliferation of endothelial and mesangial cells, infiltration by neutrophils, and localized bleeding. Fibrinoid necrosis with crescent formation may develop in the kidney. Multiple renal microabscesses secondary to infection of the infarcted sites are common in acute endocardial disease caused by *S. aureus*. Immunological phenomena may produce clinically important renal complications. Interstitial nephritis and acute or chronic proliferative glomerulonephritis have been identified by Bell[80] in 64% of patients with subacute infective endocarditis and in 28% of those with acute disease.[122] Valvular disease caused by *S. epidermidis* may be complicated by the development of membranoproliferative glomerulonephritis.[122] Acute renal failure may be associated with untoward reactions to antimicrobial agents.[123]

Infection of the Right Side of the Heart

The right side of the heart is infected in about 5% of patients with infective endocarditis.[124–126] In most instances, the tricuspid valve is the site of disease. *S. aureus* (55%), yeasts, and fungi are involved. Two-thirds of patients with involvement of the right side of the heart have been classified as having acute disease.[127] Pulmonary complications are common. Murmurs, splenomegaly, multiple cutaneous abscesses, and renal abscesses are present in about one-third of patients with acute right-sided endocarditis. Blood cultures are almost invariably positive. *S. aureus, S. pneumoniae, N. gonorrhoeae*, streptococci (*viridans, faecalis*, and *pyogenes*), and gram-negative organisms most commonly infect the right side of the heart. Although normal hearts may be involved in some cases, congenital defects, narcotic abuse, septic abortion, and infections of the skin, respiratory tract, or genitourinary tract have been the usual predisposing factors. A murmur may be absent in 80% of individuals with infection of the tricuspid valve. The disease is frequently unsuspected during life. Sixty-five percent of patients with renal disease have glomerular and tubular hemorrhages, focal embolic glomerulonephritis, renal abscesses, and pyelonephritis.

Emboli are deposited almost exclusively in the lungs early in the course of infective endocarditis when congenital abnormalities, including a predominant left-to-right shunt, defects in the intraventricular septum, and patent ductus arteriosus, are present.[128] This may lead to hemoptysis, pleurisy, or pneumonia. Embolization of the systemic circulation usually occurs late in the course of the infection. When congenital heart disease or valvular insufficiency is present, the infected thrombus is always located downstream of the orifice through which an elevated pressure gradient pushes the blood at high velocity.[129] When an intraventricular septal defect is present, infection is most likely to occur when the opening is small because a large pressure gradient is generated. In this situation, the vegetations are situated around the opening in the right septal wall and ventricular endocardium at the point of impact of the jet stream. The pulmonary artery, immediately beyond its junction with the ductus arteriosus, is the usual site of infection. An atrial septal defect is rarely infected.

The lungs are the primary site of emboli deposited on the right side of the heart. When the organism responsible for the valvulitis is avirulent, such as *S. viridans*, pulmonary infarcts are sterile. However, when a highly invasive organism such as *S. aureus* is involved, the infarcts are almost always infected and may lead to the development of abscesses. Among other complications of infected pulmonary emboli are pneumonia, thrombosis, and septic arteritis of the branches of the pulmonary artery. Repeated episodes of pulmonary infarction may be complicated by the development of recurrent pneumonia, hepatomegaly, jaundice, and progressive renal failure. When these are present in an afebrile patient, the possibility of infective endocarditis involving the right side of the heart must be given serious consideration. Murmurs are usually absent. Cultures of the blood are very often sterile when a poorly invasive organism is involved.

Relapse and Recurrence of Infective Endocarditis

Early relapse in infective endocarditis has been defined as recurrence of the clinical manifestations of the disease plus bacteremia during treatment or within 3 months after it has been completed. It must be emphasized, however, that the longer the interval between disease onset and relapse, the more likely cultures of the blood will be sterile. The organisms responsible for the initial infection and relapse may be identical or different. A number of factors play a role in the development of early relapses. Among these are (1) an inappropriate antimicrobial agent; (2) improper dosing regimen; (3) inadequate duration of therapy; (4) infection by a tolerant organism; (5) suprainfection, usually caused by a bacterium, fungus, or yeast; (6) intrusion of an organism into the bloodstream from colonized intravenous catheters or suppurative thrombophlebitis; (7) development of drug resistance in the organism initially involved; and (8) appearance of cell wall–deficient organisms (microbial persisters), especially when drugs that inhibit synthesis of the bacterial cell wall are administered. A syndrome that appears to be an early relapse but is actually related to an intra- or extracardiac complication may appear occasionally in patients with infective endocarditis caused by *S. aureus*. The persistence of an abscess in one or more organs is usually associated with a return of fever, with or without bacteremia. This represents failure of treatment of an extracardiac complication of the valvulitis, not of the primary valvular disease.

Late relapse is defined as the return of all manifestations of infective endocarditis 3–6 months after treatment has been discontinued. The organism responsible for the relapse may be the one initially involved or it may be different. This may be the case when an infected vegetation is present in a ventricular aneurysm. Late relapses are often caused by fungi, the growth of which has been stimulated by prolonged treatment with antibiotics. Failure to sterilize the interior of luxuriant vegetations and the tendency of fungal disease to spread to areas in the heart adjacent to an infected valve are common. Relapses of fungal endocarditis occur frequently in individuals with prosthetic valves.

Recurrent endocardial infection has been defined as the return of the signs and symptoms of the disease and positive cultures of the blood after 6 months of treatment with an effective antimicrobial agent. Recurrences have been documented many years after an initial episode of infective endocarditis. Recurrences that appear 6 or more months after effective therapy has been discontinued represent new infections caused either by the organism initially involved or more often by a different bacterium or fungus.

The incidence of recurrent endocarditis ranges from 1% to 10%.[130] The mechanism involved in its pathogenesis has been proposed by Cordeiro and Pimental.[131] They noted that organisms were often present in healed valvular lesions more than 10 months after patients had been "cured." They compared this situation to instances of persistent endocardial infection recorded by Morgan and Bland in 8.5% of their patients.[132] Recurrence occurred in 9.5% of patients with subacute endocarditis;[15] 2.5% experienced a third episode. Relapse of the infection occurred in 31% of the patients studied by Welton et al.[133] Intravenous drug addicts are especially prone to develop recurrent infective endocarditis. The incidence of the disease in these individuals was 41% compared to 17% in nonaddicts.

Recurrences of infective endocarditis may be multiple. A remarkable case has been described by Mokotoff et al.[134] The patient was addicted to the parenteral use of narcotics and had had seven episodes of infective endocarditis over 9.5 years. The organisms involved were *S. aureus* (five episodes) and enterococci (one episode). No bacteria were recovered from the seventh attack. The authors pointed out that recurrent infections were probably related to inadequate treatment of each episode. Baddour[135] speculated that the incidence of repeated infections may be as high as 75% in some populations. He identified a group of individuals in whom three or more factors (e.g., an underlying cardiac disorder, periodontal disease, or the chronic use of drugs) posed a danger of recurrence. It was clear that a variety of surgical procedures, such as insertion of prosthetic valves and various grafts in patients with congenital cardiac defects, were risk factors for recurrent infection. Congestive cardiac failure and simultaneous bacterial invasion of the mitral and aortic valves are more common in the early stages of recurrent disease than during the initial episode of infective endocarditis.

References

1. Starkebaum M, Durack D, Beeson P: The "incubation period" of subacute bacterial endocarditis. *Yale J Biol Med* 1977;50:49.
2. Lerner P, Weinstein L: Infective endocarditis in the antibiotic era. *N Engl J Med* 1966;247:199.

3. Weinstein L, Schlesinger JJ: Pathoanatomic, pathophysiologic and clinical correlations in endocarditis. N Engl J Med 1974;291:832.
4. Weinstein L, Rubin RH: Infective endocarditis—1973. *Prog Cardiovasc Dis* 1974;16:239.
5. Libman E, Friedberg CK: *Subacute Bacterial Endocarditis*. Oxford, Oxford University Press, 1948.
6. Geraci J, Harkonen J, Olin P, et al: Severe backache as a presenting sign of bacterial endocarditis. *Acta Med Scand* 1981;210:329.
7. Vo N, Ruvall J, Becker D: Mycotic emboli of the peripheral vessels. Analysis of forty-four cases. *Surgery* 1981;90:541.
8. Nager F: Changing clinical spectrum of infective endocarditis, in Horstkotte D, Bodnar D (eds): *Infective Endocarditis*. London, ICR Publishers, p 25.
9. Osler W: Malignant endocarditis. *Lancet* 1885;1:415.
10. Vogler WR, Dorney ER, Bridges HA: Bacterial endocarditis: A review of 148 cases. *Am J Med* 1962;32:910.
11. Cooper ES, Cooper JW, Schnabel TG Jr: Pitfalls in the diagnosis of bacterial endocarditis. *Arch Intern Med* 1966;118:55.
12. Newman W, Torres JM, Guck JK: Bacterial endocarditis: Analysis of 52 cases. *Am J Med* 1954;16:535.
13. Weinstein L: Infective endocarditis: Past, present, and future. *J R Coll Phys Lond* 1972; 6:161.
14. Pankey GA: Subacute bacterial endocarditis at University of Minnesota Hospitals, 1939–1959. *Ann Intern Med* 1961;55:550.
15. Pankey GA: Acute bacterial endocarditis at University of Minnesota hospitals. *Am Heart J* 1962;64:583.
16. Hermans PE: The clinical manifestations of infective endocarditis. *Mayo Clin Proc* 1982;57:15.
17. Libman E, Celler HL: The etiology of subacute infective endocarditis. *Am J Med Sci* 1910;140:516.
18. Uwaydah MM, Weinberg AN: Bacterial endocarditis—a changing pattern. *N Engl J Med* 1965;273:1231.
19. Garvey G, Neu H: Infective endocarditis, an evolving disease: A review of endocarditis at the Columbia Presbyterian Medical Center 1968–1973. *Medicine* 1982;57:105.
20. Kerr A Jr: *Subacute Bacterial Endocarditis* (Pullen RL ed). No. 24, American Lecture Series Monograph of the Bannerstone Division of American Lectures in Internal Medicine. Springfield, IL, Charles C Thomas, 1955, p 343.
21. Willerson JT, Moellering RC Jr, Buckley MJ, et al: Conjunctival petechiae after open-heart surgery. *N Engl J Med* 1971;284:539.
22. Gross NJ, Tall R: Clinical significance of splinter hemorrhages. *Br Med J* 1963;2:1496.
23. Kilpatrick ZM, Greenberg PA, Sanford JP: Splinter hemorrhages—their clinical significance. *Arch Intern Med* 1965;115:730.
24. Dowling RH: Subungual splinter hemorrhages. *Postgrad Med J* 1964;40:595.
25. Freedman C: Consequences of intravascular infection in infective endocarditis and other intravascular infections, in Greenough W III, Merrigan J (eds): *Current Topics in Infectious Diseases*. New York, Plenum, 1982, p 25.
26. Kerr A Jr, Tan JS: Biopsies of the Janeway lesion of infective endocarditis. *J Cutan Pathol* 1979;6:124.
27. Roth M: Ueber Netzhautaffectionem bie Wundfiebern. *Deutsch Z Chic* 1872;1:471.
28. Litten M: Ueber akute maligne endocarditis und die dabei vorkommender retinalveranderungen. *Charit Ann* 1878;3:137.
29. Doherty WB, Trubeck M: Significant hemorrhagic retinal lesions in bacterial endocarditis (Roth's spots). *JAMA* 1931;97:308.
30. Mendel DL, Daibil M: A case of subacute bacterial endocarditis with brain abscess. *Can Med Assoc J* 1937;37:53.
31. Victor M, Banker BQ: Brain abscess. *Med Clin North Am* 1963;47:1355.
32. Von Reyn C, Levy B, Arbeit R: Infective endocarditis: An analysis based on strict case definitions. *Ann Intern Med* 1981;94:505.

33. Terpenning M, Baggy B, Kauffman C: Infective endocarditis: Clinical features in young and elderly patients. *Am J Med* 1987;83:626.
34. Cherubin C, Neu H: Infective endocarditis at the Presbyterian Hospital in New York City from 1958–1967. *Am J Med* 1971;51:83.
35. Leport C, Vilde J, Bricaire F: Fifty cases of late prosthetic valve endocarditis: Improvement in prognosis over a 15 year period. *Br Heart J* 1982;58:66.
36. Colin A. Godeau F: Les aneurysms des endocardites bacterienne. *Sem Hop Paris* 1960;36:2502.
37. Weinstein L: Infected prosthetic valves: A diagnostic and therapeutic dilemma. *N Engl J Med* 1972;286:1100.
38. Churchill M, Geraci J, Hunder G: Musculoskeletal manifestations of bacterial endocarditis. *Ann Intern Med* 1977;87:755.
39. Thomas P, Allal J, Bontoux D: Rheumatological manifestations of bacterial *endocarditis*. *Ann Rheum Dis* 1989;93:716.
40. Phillipe P, Lopitaux R, Heligenstein D: Association de spondylodiscite a streptocooques D'endocardir: Deux nouvelles observations. *Sem Hop Paris* 1983;59:327.
41. Libman E: The clincial features of cases of subacute bacterial endocarditis that have spontaneously become bacteria-free. *Am J Med Sci* 1913;146:625.
42. Mills J, Utley J, Abbott J: Heart failure in infective endocarditis: Predisposing factors, course and treatment. *Chest* 1974;66:151.
43. Gonzales-Lavin L, Lise M, Ross D: The importance of the "jet lesion" in bacterial endocarditis involving the left heart: Surgical considerations. *J Thorac Cardiovasc Surg* 1970;59:185.
44. Roberts WC, Ewy GA, Glancy DL, et al: Valvular stenosis produced by active infective endocarditis. *Circulation* 1967;36:449.
45. Sacks PV, Lakier JB, Barlow JB: Severe aortic stenosis produced by bacterial endocarditis. *Br Med J* 1969;3:97.
46. Matula G, Karpman LS, Frank S, et al: Mitral obstruction from staphylococcal endocarditis, corrected surgically. 1975;233:58.
47. Mann T, McLaurin L, Grossman W, et al: Assessing the hemodynamic severity of acute regurgitation due to infective endocarditis. *N Engl J Med* 1975;293:108.
48. Thompsett R, Lubash GD: Aortic perforation in bacterial endocarditis. *Circulation* 1961;23:662.
49. Bjork VO, Olin C: Ventricular septal defect and aortic insufficiency in the same patient caused by bacterial endocarditis. *Scand J Thorac Cardiovasc Surg* 1968;2:92.
50. Ebringer A, Goldstein G, Sloman G: Fistula between aorta and atrium due to bacterial endocarditis. *Br Heart J* 1969;31:133.
51. Rose RL Jr, Higgins LS, Helgason AH: Bacterial endocarditis, pericarditis and cardiac tamponade. *Am J Cardiol* 1967;19:447.
52. Chesler E, Korns ME, Porter GE, et al: False aneurysm of the left ventricle secondary to bacterial endocarditis with perforation of the mitral aortic interventricular fibrosa. *Circulation* 1968;37:518.
53. Layman TE, January LE: Mycotic left ventricular aneurysm involving the atrioventricular body. *Am J Cardiol* 1967;20:423.
54. DeCock KM, Rees JR: Staphylococal aortic valve endocarditis with aortic root to right atrial fistula. *Postgrad Med J* 1978;54:413.
55. Roberts NK, Somerville J: Pathological significance of electrocardiographic changes in aortic valve endocarditis. *Br Heart J* 1969;31:395.
56. Sapsford RN, Fitchett DH, Tarin D, et al: Aneurysm of left ventricle secondary to bacterial endocarditis. *J Thorac Cardiovasc Surg* 1979;78:79.
57. Gopalakrishna KV, Kwan K, Shah A: Metastatic myocardial abscess due to group F streptococci. *Am J Med Sci* 1977;274:329.
58. Kim HS, Weilbacher DG, Lie JT, et al: Myocardial abscesses. *Am J Clin Pathol* 1978;70:18.
59. Vieweg WYR, Oury JH, Tretheway DG, et al: Aortopulmonary septal defect due to staphylococcal endocarditis. *Chest* 1974;65:101.
60. Kerr A Jr: Bacterial endocarditis—revisited. *Mod Concepts Cardiovasc Dis* 1964;33:831.

61. Sanson J, Slodki S, Gruhn JG: Myocardial abscesses. *Am Heart J* 1963;66:301.
62. Ryon DS, Pastor BH, Myerson RM: Abscess of the myocardium. *Am J Med Sci* 1966;251:698.
63. Arnett EN, Roberts WC: Valve ring abscess in active infective endocarditis; frequency, location and clues to clinical diagnosis from the study of 95 necropsy patients. *Circulation* 1976;54:140.
64. Di Nubile MJ, Calderwood SB, Steinhaus DM, et al: Cardiac conduction abnormalities complicating native valve active infective endocarditis. *Am J Cardiol* 1986;58:1215.
65. Weinstein L: Life-threatening infective endocarditis. *Arch Intern Med* 1986;46:953.
66. Perry EL, Fleming RG, Edwards JE: Myocardial lesions in subacute bacterial endocarditis. *Ann Intern Med* 1952;36:126.
s67. Blankenhorn MA, Gall EA: Myocarditis and myocardiosis: Clinicopathological appraisal. *Circulation* 1956;13:217.
68. Saphir O, Katz LN, Gore I: The myocardium in subacute bacterial endocarditis. *Circulation* 1950;1:1155.
69. Bashour R, Lindsay J Jr: Midsystolic clicks originating from tricuspid valve structures: A sequela to heroin-induced endocarditis. *Chest* 1975;67:620.
70. Cates JE, Christie RV: Subacute bacterial endocarditis. A review of 442 patients treated in 14 centres appointed by the Penicillin Trials Committee of the Medical Research Council. *Q J Med* 1951;20:93.
71. Vogler WR, Dorney ER: Bacterial endocarditis in congenital heart diseae. *Am Heart J* 1962;64:198.
72. Geraci J, Wilkowske C, Wilson W, et al: *Haemophilus* endocarditis: Report of 14 patients. *Mayo Clin Proc* 1977;52:209.
73. Cohen P, Maguire J, Weinstein L: Infective endocarditis caused by gram-negative bacteria: A review of the literature 1945–1977. *Prog Cardiovasc Dis* 1980;22:205.
74. Merchant R, Louria D, Geisler P: Fungal endocarditis: Review of the literature and report of three cases. *Ann Intern Med* 1958;48:292.
75. Kerr A: Bacterial endocarditis—revisited. *Mod Concepts Cardiovasc Dis* 1964;33:831.
76. Jones HR, Seikert RG, Geraci JE: Neurologic manifestation of bacterial endocarditis. *Ann Intern Med* 1969;71:21.
77. McDevitt EL: Treatment of cerebral embolism. *Mod Treat* 1965;2:52.
78. Elliott JP, Smith RF: Peripheral embolization, in Magilligan DJ, Quinn EL (eds): *Endocarditis: Medical and Surgical Management.* New York, Marcel Dekker, 1986, p 165.
79. Glassock RJ, Cohen AG: Secondary glomerular disease, in Brenner BM, Rector FC (eds): *The Kidney.* Philadelphia, Saunders, 1981, p 1536.
80. Bell ET: Glomerular lesions associated with endocarditis. *Am J Pathol* 1932;8:639.
81. Heptinstall RH: Focal glomerulonephritis, in *Pathology of the Kidney.* Boston, Little, Brown, 1974, p 438.
82. Jackson JF, Allison F Jr: Bacterial endocarditis. *South Med J* 1961;54:1331.
83. Pfeifer JF, Lipton MJ, Oury JH, et al: Acute coronary embolism complicating bacterial endocarditis: Operative treatment. *Am J Cardiol* 1976;37:920.
84. Menzies CJG: Coronary embolism with infarction in bacterial endocarditis. *Br Heart J* 1961;23:464.
85. Brunson JG: Coronary embolism in bacterial endocarditis. *Am J Pathol* 1953;29:689.
86. Horder TJ: Infective endocarditis: With an analysis of 150 cases and with special reference to the chronic form of the disease. *Q J Med* 1909;2:289.
87. McDevitt E: Treatment of cerebral embolism. *Mod Treat* 1965;2:52.
88. Harrington AW: Embolism of the spinal cord. *Glasgow Med J* 1925;103:28.
89. Harrison MJG, Hampton JR: Neurological presentation of bacterial endocarditis. *Br Med J* 1967;2:148.
90. Hernohan JW, Woltman HW, Barnes AR: Involvement of the nervous system associated with endocarditis: Neuropsychiatric and neuropathological observations in forty-two cases of fatal outcome. *Arch Neurol Psych* 1938;42:789.
91. Krinsky CM, Merritt HH: Neurologic manifestations of subacute bacterial endocarditis. *N Engl J Med* 1938;218:563.

92. Dejong RN: Central nervous system complications in subacute bacterial endocarditis. *J Nerv Ment Dis* 1937;75:397.
93. Schocket S, Braver D: Cilioretinal artery occlusion in a patient with suspected subacute bacterial endocarditis. *South Med J* 1970;63:1.
94. Jones HR Jr, Siekert RG: Embolic mononeuropathy and bacterial endocarditis. *Arch Neurol* 1968;19:535.
95. Manor RS, Mendel I, Savir H: Prepapillary metastatic abscess in a case of subacute bacterial endocarditis. *Ophthalmologica* 1975;170:22.
96. Henrich WL, Huehnergarth J, Rosch J, et al: Gallbladder and liver infarction occurring as a complication of acute bacterial endocarditis. *Gastroenterology* 1975;68:1602.
97. Welton DE, Young JB, Raizner AE, et al: Value and safety of cardiac catheterization during active infective endocarditis. *Am J Cardiol* 1979;44:1306.
98. Roach MR, Drake CG: Ruptured cerebral aneurysms caused by microorganisms. *N Engl J Med* 1963;273:240.
99. Choyke PL, Edmonds PR, Markowitz RI, et al: Mycotic pulmonary artery aneurysm: Complications of aspergillus endocarditis. *Am J Roentgenol* 1982;138:1172.
100. Kauffman SL, Lynfield J, Hennigar GR: Mycotic aneurysms of the intrapulmonary arteries. *Circulation* 1967;35:90.
101. Lau J, Mattox KL, de Bakey ME: Mycotic aneurysm of the inferior mesenteric artery. *Am J Surg* 1979;138:443.
102. Trevisani MF, Ricci MA, Michaels RM, et al: Multiple mesenteric aneurysms complicating subacute bacterial endocarditis. *Arch Surg* 1987;122:823.
103. Weinstein L: Infective endocarditis, in Braunwald E (ed): *Heart Disease: a Textbook of Cardiovascular Medicine,* ed 3. Philadelphia, Saunders, 1988, p 1108.
104. Le Cam B, Guivarch G, Boles JM, et al: Neurologic complications in a group of 86 cases of bacterial endocarditis. *Eur Heart J* 1984;5:97.
105. Ziment I: Nervous system complications in bacterial endocarditis. *Am J Med* 1969;47:593.
106. Pruitt AA, Rubin RH, Karchmer AW, et al: Neurologic complications of bacterial endocarditis. *Medicine* 1978;57:329.
107. Wolff M, Witchitz S, Regnier B, et al: Neurologic complications of *S. aureus* endocarditis. In *Program and Abstracts of the Twenty-Seventh Interscience Conference on Antimicrobial Agents and Chemotherapy. New York, 1987.*
108. Ben Ismail M, Hannachi N, Abid F, et al: Prosthetic valve endocarditis. *Br Heart J* 1987;58:72.
109. Leport C, Vilde JL, Bricaire F, et al: Fifty cases of late prosthetic valve endocarditis: Improvement in prognosis over a 15 year period. *Br Heart J* 1987;58:66.
110. Salgado AV, Furlan AJ, Keys TF: Neurologic Complications of native and prosthetic valve endocarditis; a longitudinal study. In Program and Abstracts of the Twenty-Seventh Interscience Conference on Antimicrobial Agents and Chemotherapy. New York, 1987.
111. Terpenning MS, Buggy BP, Kauffman C: Infective endocarditis: Clinical features in young and elderly patients. *Am J Med* 1987;83:626.
112. Von Reyn CF, Levy BS, Arbeit RD, et al: Infective endocarditis: An analysis based on strict case definitions. *Ann Intern Med* 1981; 94 (Part 1):505.
113. Venezio FR, Westerfielder GO, Cook FV, et al: Infective endocarditis in a community hospital. *Arch Intern Med* 1982;142:789.
114. Hart RJ, Kgan-Hallet K, Joerns SE: Mechanisms of intracranial haemorrhage in infective endocarditis. *Stroke* 1987;18:1048.
115. Molinari GF, Smith L, Goldstein MN, et al: Pathogenesis of cerebral mycotic aneurysms. *Neurology* 1974;23:325.
116. Geraci JE, Wilkowske CJ, Wilson WR, et al: *Haemophilus* endocarditis. *Mayo Clin Proc* 1977;52:209.
117. Merchant RK, Louria DB, Geisler PH, et al: Fungal endocarditis: Review of the literature and report of three cases. *Ann Intern Med* 1958;48:242.

118. Bohmfalk GL, Story JL, Wissinger JP, et al: Bacterial intracranial aneurysm. *J Neurosurg* 1978;48:369.
119. Baehe G: Renal complications of endocarditis. *Trans Am Assoc Phys* 1931;46:87.
120. Villarreal H, Somoloff J: The occurrence of renal insufficiency in subacute bacterial endocarditis. *Ann Intern Med* 1977;87:754.
121. Feinstein E, Eknoyan G, Lister B: Renal complications of bacterial endocarditis. *Am J Nephrol* 1985;5:457.
122. Weinstein L: "Modern" infective endocarditis. *JAMA* 1975;223:260.
123. Moore R, Smith C, Lipsky J, et al: Risk factors for nephrotoxicity in patients treated with aminoglycosides. *Ann Intern Med* 1989;100:352.
124. Bashour FA, Winchell CP: Right-sided bacterial endocarditis. *Am J Med Sci* 1960;240:411.
125. Panidis I, Kotler M, Mintz G: Right heart endocarditis: Clinical and echocardiographic features. *Am Heart J* 1989;107:759.
126. Hubbell G, Cheitlin M, Rapaport E: Presentation, management, and follow-up evaluation of infective endocarditis in drug addicts. *Am Heart J* 1981;102:185.
127. Bain R, Edward J, Scheiffen C: Right-sided bacterial endocarditis and endarteritis: Clinical and pathologic study. *Am J Med* 1958;29:9.
128. Altschule MD: Subacute bacterial endocarditis of the right heart. *Med Sci* 1964;15:50.
129. Rodbard S: Blood velocity and endocarditis. *Circulation* 1963;27:18.
130. Garvey GJ, Neu HC: Infective endocarditis: An evolving disease. *Medicine* 1978;57:105.
131. Cordeiro A, Pimental C: Novas fisionomias da endocardite subaguda. *Ref Medica Angola* 1961;13:5.
132. Morgan WL, Bland EF: Bacterial endocarditis in antobiotic era. *Circulation* 1959;19:753.
133. Welton DE, Young JB, Gentry WO, et al: Recurrent infective endocarditis: Analysis of predisposing factors and clinical features. *Am J Med* 1979;66:932.
134 Mokotoff D, Young JB, Welton DE, et al: Recurrent infective endocarditis in a drug addict. Multiple separate episodes in nine years. *Chest* 1979;76:592.
135. Baddour L: Twelve year review of recurrent native valve infective endocarditis: A disease of the modern antibiotic era. *Rev Infect Dis* 1988;10:1163.

9

Endocarditis in Intravenous Drug Abusers

The exact incidence of infective endocarditis in intravenous drug abusers (IVDA) has been difficult to determine. This is due, in part, to the haphazard use of the health care system by these patients.[1] Levine et al.[2] suggested that 60% of admissions of IVDA to hospitals are prompted by a variety of infections. From 5% to 8% of these patients have infective endocarditis. It has been estimated that this occurs in 1.5 to 2 per 1,000 IVDA per year. Despite the high incidence of endocardial infection in this population, only 72 instances of endocarditis in IVDA were reported prior to the 1970s.[3] Hussey and Katz[4] described the clinical features of infective endocarditis in eight individuals with IVDA; in seven, the tricuspid valve was infected by *S. aureus; Pseudomonas* was recovered from the aortic valve of one patient. The clinical syndrome of endocarditis in IVDA has increased greatly over the past 40 years.

The bacteria involved most often in infections in IVDA have remained fairly constant. This is probably related to the fact that organisms present in the bloodstream originate from the skin.[2,5] There may be significant differences in the microbiological profile in various urban areas. In the 1970s, *Ps. aeruginosa* was identified as the most common cause of IVDA-associated endocardial disease in Chicago and Detroit. Over the same period, clusters of endocarditis caused by *Serratia* were noted in San Francisco.[6–8]

S. aureus is responsible for more than 50% of infective endocarditis in IVDA.[2,9] This organism is often recovered from the mucocutaneous surfaces of drug addicts. Forty percent of *S. aureus* recovered from IVDA have been found to be resistant to methicillin. *S. epidermidis*, an uncommon cause of IVDA-associated endocardial disease, usually invades damaged natural or prosthetic valves. Streptococcal species, including enterococci, presently account for about 20% of the cases. Although *S. viridans* was involved in 40% of IVDA 20 years ago,[10] it now affects less than 5% of patients and does not infect normal valves. Group A streptococci have been reported to cause 10–25% of endocarditis in IVDA.[2,11,12] The incidence of enterococcal disease in these patients declined from 55% in 1976 to about 8% in 1986. As the recovery of enterococci from valvulitis in IVDA has declined,[13] other streptococci have been identified more often.[14] *S. pneumoniae* is now rarely implicated. Occasionally, other gram-positive bacteria, *Bacillus* species, or *Corynebacterium* have produced infection in IVDA.[15–22]

Gram-negative aerobic organisms, primarily *Ps. aeruginosa,* are involved in 10% of patients. This has been especially common in those treated with pentazocaine (Talwin) or tripelennamine.[23,24] The incidence of infective endocarditis caused by *Serratia* reached a peak in the San Francisco Bay Area in the 1970s; it no longer occurs except very sporadically.[8]

Most fungal infections are caused by candidal species other than *C. albicans.*[25,26] *C. parapsilosis* is most common.[27] Other species involved are *C. tropicalis, C. guilleromondi, C. krusei,* and *C. stellatoidea.*[28]

Among the bacterial species observed in infections in IVDA are *H. influenzae,*[29] *Neisseria* species,[30–32] *Ps. maltophilia,*[33] and *E. corrodens.*[34,35] The last example cited produces dermal abscesses in patients addicted to methylphenidate or methamphetamine.

About 5% of IVDA-related infective endocarditis is polymicrobial in origin.[36,37] More than two organisms are rarely involved; *S. aureus* is almost always present. Other species are members of the human oral flora. This is probably related to the habit of IVDA of licking the needle before inserting it into the vein.[38] Organisms rarely implicated in the pathogenesis of infective endocarditis (e.g., *H. parainfluenzae*) are often present in polymicrobial infections. It has been suggested that in one patient a streptococcus may have provided the V factor that facilitated the growth of a strain of *Haemophilus* in the valvular vegetation.[38]

Epidemiology

Infective endocarditis in IVDA mainly affects men (male: female ratio is 3:1).[39] Infection caused by some organisms (e.g., *S. pyogenes*) is not related to the sex of the patient. There may be intrinsic differences between men and women in host defenses and techniques of intravenous injection. The briefer use of drugs among women, accounts for the better maintenance of the normal microbial flora of the skin. Overgrowth of drug-resistant organisms (e.g., *S. aureus, Ps. aeruginosa*) occurs less often.[40] A decrease in the frequency of self-medication with antibiotics by women is very important in preserving their microflora.[41]

From 6% to 25% of IVDA with infective endocarditis have preexisting valvular disease.[42] The incidence of predisposing disorders in these patients is much lower on the right than on the left side of the heart (13% vs. 27%).[43–45] These values have declined in concert with the decrease in frequency of rheumatic fever. Valvular injury produced by a prior infection may be the most important predisposing factor for the development of endocarditis in IVDA. Overall, cardiac disease, both in the present and in the past, is a very minor determinant of whether an episode of bacteremia may produce valvular disease.

Pathogenesis

Several features of infective endocarditis in IVDA are not only clinically distinctive but also pose a challenge to a clear understanding of the pathogenesis of this disease. Narcotic-associated endocarditis predisposes patients to infection of the right side of the heart. The tricuspid valve alone has been involved in 70% of patients studied by Nievel.[46] Multiple valves were infected in 10% of patients. In 1977, Watanakunakorn[47] reported that the clinical manifestations of infective endocarditis in IVDA were as follows: (1) the tricuspid valve was involved, alone or together with other valves, in 52.2%; (2) the aortic valve alone was infected in 18.5%, the mitral valve alone in 10–18%, and the aortic and mitral valves in 12.5%. Later studies revealed a similar distribution.[48,49] *S. aureus* is the predominant organism. It accounts for 80% of tricuspid valvular disease among IVDA. Infection of the aortic and mitral valves occurs in previously damaged structures caused by the organisms responsible for valvular disease in nonaddicted patients (*S. viridans,* enterococci).[43] In addition, *Ps. aeruginosa* and *Serratia* have often been involved.

Initial clinical studies of infective endocarditis in IVDA have emphasized the frequent involvement of the right side of the heart and have pointed out that the disease of the tricuspid valve is much more benign than that of the mitral or aortic valve.[50–53] Early studies at autopsy indicated that infections of the left side of the heart were predominant in IVDA. A study of individuals dying during the first episode of infective endocarditis has revealed that the right side of the heart alone was infected in 30%; both the right and left sides were involved in 13% and the mitral or aortic valve in 41% (Table 9.1). A postmortem study reported by Buchbinder and Roberts, [54,55] indicated a decreased incidence of mitral and aortic valvular disease than had been recognized previously. Of the patients studied, 33% had right-sided disease and 13.3% had disease of the aorta or mitral valve. The authors also emphasized significant pathological differences between right- and left-sided endocardial infection in IVDA. Cultures of the lesions on the right side of the heart usually grew *S. aureus.*

Buchbinder and Roberts [54,55] have pointed out that the infectious process did not extend beyond the cusps of the valves. Abscesses of the valvular ring boring into the myocardium were unusual. Perforation of the leaflets did not occur. Invariably, the endocarditis involved a previously normal tricuspid valve. The pulmonic valve was rarely infected. Because there is usually no previous valvular disease, the presenting symptoms often do not point to the heart as the primary site of the disease but are related to metastatic infection.

S. aureus is less likely to be recovered from cultures of the blood of patients with infection on the left side of the heart. The organisms isolated are identical to those that cause infective endocarditis in patients who do not abuse drugs. Abscesses of the myocardium and valvular rings and purulent pericarditis are often present. Because this type of IVDA-associated endocardial infection occurs in patients with previous valvular disease, it is

Table 9.1. Location of Valvular Vegetations During the First Episode of Active Infective Endocarditis in Opiate Addicts (80 Necropsy Cases)

Valves with Vegetations*	No. Of Patients	Died During First Episode of Active Disease without Surgery
Single right-sided		
TV	23	14
PV	1	0
Single right-sided plus		
TV + MV	8	2
TV + AV	4	2
PV + MV	1	1
PV + AV	0	0
Single left-sided		
MV	15	10
AV	18	8
Double left-sided		
AV + MV	10	5
Total	80 (100%)	42 (53%)

*Mitral valve excised and replaced; tricuspid valve excised without replacement; aortic valve excised and replaced; tricuspid valve excised without replacement;[1] aortic valve replaced after active disease had disappeared in two of the three patients; site of recurrence was a bioprosthetic or prosthetic valve in the aortic valve position in two patients.

AV = aortic vlave; MV = mitral valve; PV = pulmonic valve; TV = tricuspid valve.

Source: Adapted from Ref. 2.

obvious early in the course of the disease that the patient has infective endocarditis.

In the absence of a platelet-fibrin thrombus, the mechanisms involved in the adhesion of circulating organisms to a normal cardiac valve are not clear. One possible explanation is injury to the valvular endothelium produced by multiple injections of the particulate matter present in illicit drugs. It appears that IVDA with long experience with injectable drugs have the highest incidence of right-sided endocardial infection. Continuous exposure of a cardiac valve to various adulterants is an important factor in the development of infective endocarditis. Supporting evidence has been provided by a study that detected talc embedded in the valves of IVDA.[56] In addition, it has been recognized that repeated injections of foreign protein may produce nonbacterial thrombotic endocarditis by a variety of immunological mechanisms. This then may serve as a nidus for the deposition of circulating organisms.[57]

Various forms of stress may lead to the deposition of a fibrin-platelet thrombus on the surface of valvular leaflets of rats.[58,59] The pathological changes may resolve when the initiating stress is removed. An important counterpart may be the continuous drive of the addict to acquire and use drugs. Cocaine, with its ability to induce sympathetic stimuli, may add to a highly enhanced state of stress.

The increasing incidence of infection produced by the human immunodeficiency virus (HIV) among IVDA is well known. The role of immunosuppression produced by infection with this agent in the pathogenesis of infective endocarditis is unclear.[60]

Patients who use intravenous drugs are infected by their own microflora. This has been pointed out by Tuazon and Sheagran[61] in individuals invaded by *S. aureus*. They noted that in 60–100% of cases, a single strain of *S. aureus* was recovered from the blood, skin, anterior nares, and oropharynx. When the organism was present in the pharynx, it was transferred to the skin and bloodstream. Similar mechanisms have been involved in the transmission of streptococci. The illicit drug, alone or with the equipment used to inject it, may be an important reservoir of pathogens.[61] Some strains of *Pseudomonas* may survive in tripelennamine.[62]

Clinical Manifestations

The signs and symptoms of IVDA are determined by the organism and the cardiac valve involved.[46] Infection of the right side of the heart often presents with pulmonary, pleuropulmonary, or nonspecific complaints.[46] The symptoms and signs are often no different from those of enmpyema and pneumonia. Metastatic spread may predominate early in the course of the disease when *S. aureus* infects the tricuspid valve.[63–65] Endocardial infections caused by *Pseudomonas* involve the mitral or aortic valve and are associated with a high incidence of neurological injury and persistent bacteremia even when appropriate antimicrobial agents have been administered.[66] Mycotic aneurysms and abscesses of the brain may be present.

Patients with infective endocarditis that involves the right side of the heart rarely develop congestive cardiac failure. Fever is universal. Nonfocal symptoms are present in 25–50% of patients.[67–69] The interval between the onset of symptoms and diagnosis is 14 days in individuals with both right- and left-sided endocardial infection.[46] The presenting features in 50% of IVDA with infection of the tricuspid valve are cough and pleurisy.[30–74] Fifty percent to 95% of these individuals experienced septic pulmonary emboli, and 12–13% develop empyema. Mycotic aneurysms of the pulmonary artery are rare.[75] The source of the emboli is usually the heart but may be thrombophlebitis of the pelvic veins.

About 5% of patients with infection of the tricuspid valve develop a murmur. This is often difficult to detect.[75] Murmurs associated with disease of the mitral and aortic valves are identified more easily.[69,73] About 20% of patients with bacteremia unrelated to cardiac infection may develop a murmur.

Endocarditis involving the left side of the heart in IVDA is often complicated by arterial embolization to the renal and cerebral arteries. The organisms responsible for this are *S. aureus* and a variety of streptococcal species.

The integumentary hallmarks of infective endocarditis are present much less often in IVDA than in nonaddicts.[69–71] Clubbing of the fingers is rare. Splinter hemorrhages are present in about 10%; these are not specific for endocarditis. Conjunctival petechiae are present in 50% of patients.[76]

Severe abdominal pain may be a problem in patients with abscesses, infarction of the spleen, ileus, or ischemic colitis.[77] The presence of a splenic abscess may lead to persistent bacteremia despite potentially effective therapy for the valvular disease.[72,73] A number of septic states often complicate the course of staphylococcal and beta-hemolytic streptococcal endocarditis.

Lesions of the central nervous system in IVDA are similar to those present in nonaddicts. Two distinct clinical features are present in IVDA: panophthalmitis in 10% of patients[78] and a high incidence of cerebral mycotic aneurysms that often rupture. Toxic encephalopathy develops in 30%. Although the concentrations of glucose and protein in the spinal fluid are within normal limits,[2,12] the organisms responsible for the infection are easily recovered from it. The parenteral use of drugs plays an increasingly important role in the pathogenesis of stroke in patients younger than 25 years.[79]

Septic arthritis develops in 10–20% of IVDA with infective endocarditis caused by *S. aureus*.[80] Arthralgia induced by the deposition of immune complexes in the synovium of the joints is common. Table 9.2 and Fig. 9.1 summarize the clinical features of endocarditis in IVDA.

Diagnosis

Drug addicts who present with fever or other manifestations of sepsis require at least three cultures of blood. Even in the absence of treatment, these cultures may fail to grow the responsible organism(s).[81,82] This can be the case when *S. aureus* is the causative agent.[72,73] In some instances, cultures of blood drawn several days after antimicrobial therapy has been discontinued may yield the causative agent. Persistent sterile cultures over several days mandates reconsideration of the diagnosis.[83] The longer the interval between obtaining blood samples, the greater the possibility that the organism responsible for the disease will be identified. Blood drawn at 5-min intervals from different sites of a blood vessel may yield the organism responsible for the disease. Inserting a needle into the site in which the illicit drug is injected is dangerous and should be avoided. Manipulation of an underlying mycotic aneurysm may lead to its rupture.

Noninfectious disorders may cause fever in IVDA. This condition, labeled *cotton fever,* is caused by pyrogens present in the drugs used by addicts. Fever, chills, and dyspnea develop shortly after injection of a drug and disappear within a few hours. Although this syndrome is usually thought to represent a noninfectious disorder, it may occur in patients with infective endocarditis that involves the right side of the heart.[83,84]

A detailed physical examination, cultures of the blood, and radiography

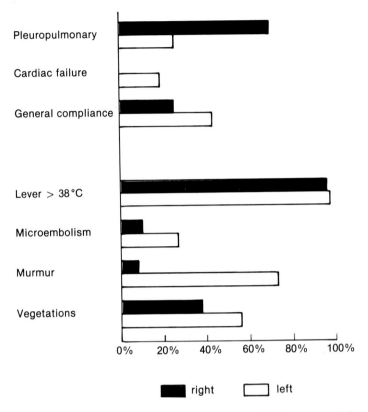

Fig. 9.1. Infective endocarditis with drug addiction: complaints and findings. (From Ref. 41)

of the chest are mandatory in the febrile addict. There appears to be little difference in the results of these studies in IVDA with or without bacteremia and/or endocarditis.[85] The use of illicit drugs and the development of infection by HIV pose a challenge to clinicians treating infected addicts. The many disorders that produce fever in HIV-positive patients adds to the diagnostic dilemma. The HIV status of an IVDA plays no role in determining the early clinical manifestations of infective endocarditis. The fatality rate is 40% in HIV-positive, symptomatic individuals (CDC group IV). In HIV-positive, asymptomatic patients, it is identical to that in HIV-negative patients: 10%.[86]

The high-tech modality most often used to establish the diagnosis of infective endocarditis is echocardiography. Clinicians are often unaware of the type of echocardiogram required or when sonography of the heart may be helpful. Echocardiography using the two-dimensional or M-mode technique is unreliable in about 50% of individuals with IVDA-associated endocarditis.[2] The tricuspid valve is difficult to image by these methods. False valvular vegetations have been described in patients with endocardial infec-

Table 9.2. Clinical Features of Patients by Endocarditis Classification

	Endocarditis (n = 11)	Other (n = 76)
History, n (%)		
Chills	9 (82)	52 (68)
Back pain	2 (18)	17 (22)
Pleuritic chest pain	4 (36)	36 (47)
Weight loss	1 (9)	31 (41)
Physical/laboratory findings, n (%)		
Heart murmur	2 (18)	25 (33)
Splenomegaly	0 (0)	5 (7)
Peripheral emboli	1 (9)	1 (1)
Lymphadenopathy	10 (91)	58 (76)
Pyuria (<5 leukocytes per high-power field)	3 (50)	2 (4)
Median physical/laboratory findings (Interquartile range)		
Temperature, °C	39.2 (38.6–40.0)	38.8 (38.3–39.4)
Serum NA$^+$, mmol/liter	132 (131–134)	136 (133–138)
Serum K$^+$, mmol/liter	3.6 (3.4–4.1)	4.1 (3.9–4.4)
Leukocyte count, × 10^9/liter	11 (10–17)	8 (6–13)
Erythrocyte sedimentation rate, mm/hr	48 (39–74)	60 (25–90)
Length of stay, days	30 (16–31)	6 (3–12)

Source: Adapted from Ref. 82.

tion of the left heart. Transesophageal echocardiography (TEE) eliminates many of the problems associated with other techniques. It identifies vegetations as small as 1.5 mm. The transthoracic approach defines lesions 3–5 mm in diameter and is highly effective (90%) in identifying valvular vegetations.[80–92] TEE is not the first approach to the diagnosis. Studies that support its sensitivity and specificity have been based on observations in patients in tertiary care hospitals. When used in a community hospital, its value has not been established.

TEE appears to be useful in two situations. The first is defined by cultures of the blood that are sterile after several days of incubation. This is often the case in infection caused by fastidious organisms, such as fungi or nutritionally deficient streptococci. An echocardiogram that identifies vegetations on a valve or an abscess of the aortic root mandates continued incubation and the use of special microbiological techniques that accelerate identification of the pathogen. The other condition in which TEE may be helpful in corroborating the presence of valvular infection is when cultures of blood are positive in the absence of radiological, laboratory, or clinical data supportive of the diagnosis of endocarditis.

Treatment

Patients who appear to be well, are afebrile, do not appear to be deteriorating, and have no clinical evidence of infective endocarditis on admission to a hospital, do not require immediate therapy unless they have a prosthetic valve in place. In fact, a significant minority of individuals (20%) defervesce within a few hours after hospitalization.[93,94] The subsequent clinical course of this subset of patients, as well as the results of laboratory studies, never support the presence of infective endocarditis.

Watchful waiting is helpful in dealing with the problem posed by sterile cultures of blood in individuals who have taken antibiotics obtained on the street or from physicians.

Obtaining cultures not only at the time of admission, but also at intervals that permit clearance of the antibiotic from the blood, significantly increases the opportunity to establish a diagnosis. If, during the period of observation, the patient deteriorates clinically or develops signs of infective endocarditis, or if cultures of blood become positive, antimicrobial therapy must be instituted immediately.

In most instances, treatment is initiated before the results of the medical evaluation are known. Physicians must pay close attention to the clinical and laboratory findings in order to choose a valid antimicrobial therapy (Table 9.3). Answers to the following three questions are important in reaching therapeutic decisions: (1) Do gram-negative aerobic bacteria, such as *Pseudomonas*, play a significant role in IVDA-associated endocarditis in the community? (2) Is methicillin resistant *S. aureus* (MRSA) a significant factor in relation to the residence of a patient? (3) Which side of the heart is involved? There is considerable evidence that the treatment of infections caused by *S. aureus* with oxacillin is adequate for the management of infective endocarditis of the right side of the heart. Vancomycin is the drug of choice when MRSA is present. Other drugs, including rifampin, trimethoprim-sulfamethoxazole, and the quinolones, are less effective.[95] Combinations of vancomycin plus rifampin or vancomycin plus gentamicin have

Table 9.3. Organisms That Should Be Included in Empiric Antibiotic Coverage of Infective Endocarditis in IVDA in Certain Clinical Situations

Clinical Setting	Organism
No previous history of cardiac pathology; absence of murmur; no evidence of septic pulmonary emboli or other signs of right-sided endocarditis	*S. aureus:* methicillin sensitive, methicillin resistant
Previous history of cardiac pathology, ± unimpressive murmur, or classic murmur of aortic or mitral valvular disease; with signs and symptoms of systemic embolization, especially of the central nervous system	*S. aureus:* streptococcal species, especially enterococci, *S. viridans,* and *Ps aeruginosa*

been employed for the treatment of endocarditis caused by MRSA. The first pair may produce an indifferent or antagonistic effect against many strains of MRSA[96,97] and the second occasionally leads to nephrotoxicity.[98]

Kozeniowski[99] reported that a combination of nafcillin and an aminoglycoside produced rapid defervescence, a decrement in the white blood cell count, and a decrease in the duration of bacteremia in patients infected by methicillin-sensitive *S. aureus* (MSSA). However, there was no effect on the fatality rate. Treatment for 2 weeks with a beta-lactam antibiotic plus gentamicin cured an uncomplicated infection of a tricuspid valve caused by MSSA.[100] Patients with infective endocarditis involving the right side of the heart respond better to medical therapy than do those with disease of the left side.

Except for outbreaks of infections caused by a number of other gram-negative organisms, *Pseudomonas* is the only bacterium involved in IVDA-associated endocarditis in which the clinical course is indolent.

Large dosages of aminoglycosides (e.g., 8 mg/kg/day of gentamicin) are required to achieve therapeutic levels in the serum of IVDA with infective endocarditis. Delay in initiating treatment until a definite diagnosis is made, does not appear to adversely affect the clinical outcome.[101,102] The clinical echocardiographic and microbiological findings in 10 individuals who succumbed to endocarditis are presented in Table 9.4

Fungal endocarditis in IVDA[42] is chiefly a surgical disease. Treatment with antimicrobial agents is indicated after the infected valves are excised.[103]

Surgical Therapy

The indications for the replacement of an infected valve in drug-addicted patients with infective endocarditis are similar to those for other types of valvular disease. However, there is disagreement concerning the role of surgery in individuals with vegetations larger than 1 cm and unremitting fever,[104-106] especially when the tricuspid valve is infected. It has been suggested that this condition may require valvular surgery to prevent embolization.[107-109] Some physicians have adopted a conservative approach, basing their therapeutic decisions not only on the echocardiographic findings but also on their close clinical observations. The presence of intractable sepsis, the onset of congestive cardiac failure, or the development of emboli indicates the need for valvulectomy.[107,108] It has been suggested that medical treatment is eventually effective in most patients with right-sided endocarditis. Persistent infection and the development of congestive cardiac failure are valid indications for surgery.[109,110]

Whether replacement of a tricuspid valve should be routine is questionable. The long-term fatality rate in surgically treated patients has been reported to be 60% after 13 months. Only 33% per cent treated medically for 20 months survived.[111] The major cause of failure of treatment in the former group was the development of paravalvular leaks in 50% of the

Table 9.4. Clinical, Echocardiographic, and Bacteriological Findings in 10 Patients Who Died*

Patient Number[†]	Age (years), Sex	Vegetation Size	Number of Days of Treatment	Organism	Affected Valve	Cause of Death	Other Findings
1	21, F	2.1	21	*S. aureus*	Tricuspid	Pulmonary embolus	Left-sided heart failure, renal failure
2	44, M	2.5	6	*S. aureus*	Tricuspid	Adult respiratory distress syndrome, sepsis	Left-sided heart failure
3	30, M	2.4	95	*S. aureus, Pseudomonas*	Tricuspid	Multiorgan failure, sepsis	
4	35, M	4.3	3	*S. aureus*	Tricuspid	Multiorgan failure sepsis	
5	42, F	3.6	12	*S. aureus*	Tricuspid	Adult respiratory distress syndrome, sepsis	Renal failure
6	33, F	2.9	25	*S. aureus*, methicillin resistant	Tricuspid	Multiorgan failure, sepsis	
7	26, M	1.6	4	*S. aureus*	Tricuspid	Pulmonary embolus	Left-sided heart failure
	49, F	1.1	50	*S. aureus*, methicillin resistant	Tricuspid, aortic	Cerebrovascular accident	Left-sided heart failure
9	35, M	2.4	10	*S. aureus*	Tricuspid, aortic, mitral	Aortic valve perforation, sepsis	
10	24, F	4.0	10	*S. aureus*	Tricuspid, porcine	Sepsis	Tricuspid valve excision, renal failure

*Number of days of treatment = duration of treatment with antibiotic therapy; renal failure = creatine range, 203 to 566 μmol/liter; sepsis = overwhelming systemic infection.
[†]Patients 1 to 7 include those with visible vegetations confined to native right-sided valves; patients 8 to 10 include those with either concomitant left-sided vegetations or prosthetic valve endocarditis.
Source: Adapted from Ref. 103.

patients. Almost two-thirds of them required repeated surgery. Most of the excess morbidity and mortality in these patients was probably related to the continued use of illicit drugs. Recurrent valvular infection occurs in 20–40% of IVDA with prostheses; by contrast, the incidence is only 4% in non-IVDA with prosthetic valves.[73] Excision of an infected tricuspid valve is curative and leads to a hemodynamically normal state in most cases. However, symptoms of tricuspid regurgitation may be quite bothersome for some individuals. A prosthetic valve may be implanted safely when the patient stops using illicit drugs.[112,113]

It is important to note that the presence of a splenic abscess must be ruled out prior to surgery. This condition may mimic infective endocarditis and is refractory to antimicrobial therapy.[114] Experience has indicated that a replacement valve may be inserted without risk in an infected bed as long as the patient is receiving appropriate perioperative antibiotics.[115–119]

References

1. Reisberg B: Infective endocarditis in the narcotic addict. *Prog Cardiovasc Dis* 1979;22:193.
2. Levine D, Crane L, Servos M: Bacteremia in narcotic addicts at the Detroit Medical Center. II. Infectious endocarditis: A prospective study. *Rev Infect Dis* 1986;8:374.
3. Ramsey RG, Gunnar RM, Tobin JR Jr: Endocarditis in the drug addict. *Am J Cardiol* 1970;25:608.
4. Hussey H, Katz S: Infections resulting from narcotic addiction. *Am J Med* 1980;9:186.
5. Tuazon CW, Sheagran JW: Increased rate of carriage of *Staphylococcus aureus* among narcotic addicts. *J Infect Dis* 1974;129:725.
6. Reyes MP, Palutke WA, Wylin RF: *Pseudomonas* endocarditis in the Detroit Medical Center 1969–1972. *Medicine* 1973;52:173.
7. Reyes MP, Brown WJ, Lerner AM: Treatment of patients with *Pseudomonas* endocarditis with high dose aminoglycoside and carbenicillin therapy. *Medicine* 1978;57:37.
8. Mills J, Drew D: *Serratia marcescens* endocarditis: A regional illness associated with intravenous drug abuse. *Ann Intern Med* 1976;84:29.
9. Julander I: Staphylococcal septicemia and endocarditis in 80 drug addicts. Aspects on epidemiology, clinical and laboratory findings and prognosis. *Scand J Infect Dis* 1983;41(Suppl):49.
10. Pelletier LL, Petersdorf RG: Infective endocarditis: A review of 125 cases from the University of Washington Hospitals 1963–72. *Medicine* 1977;56:287.
11. Barg NL, Kish MA, Kauffman CA, et al: Group A streptococcal bacteremia in intravenous drug abusers. *Am J Med* 1985;78:569.
12. Reiner NE, Gopalarkrishna KV, Lerner PI: Enterococcal endocarditis in heroin addicts. *JAMA* 1976;235:1861.
13. Crane L, Levine D, Zervos M, et al: Bacteremia in narcotic addicts at the Detroit Medical Center. I. Microbiology, risk factors and empiric therapy. *Rev Infect Dis* 1986;8:364.
14. Gallagher PG, Watanakunakorn C: Group B streptococcal endocarditis: Report of seven cases and review of the literature. *Rev Infect Dis* 1986;8:175.
15. Banks T, Fletcher, R, Nayab A: Infective endocarditis in heroin addicts. *Am J Med* 1973;55:444.
16. Cherubim CE, Baden M, Kavaler F: Infective endocarditis in narcotic addicts. *Ann Intern Med* 1968;69:1091.
17. Neufiel GK, Branson CG, Marshall LW: Infective endocarditis as a complication of heroin use. *South Med J* 1976;69:1148.
18. El-Khatib MR, Wilson FM, Lerner AM: Characteristics of bacterial endocarditis in heroin addicts in Detroit. *Am J Med Sci* 1976;271:197.

19. Menda KB, Gorbach SL: Favorable experience with bacterial endocarditis in heroin addicts. *Ann Intern Med* 1973;78:25.
20. Graham DY, Reul GJ, Martin R, et al: Infective endocarditis in drug addicts: Experiences with medical and surgical treatment. *Circulation* 1973;48:S37.
21. Stimmel B, Donoso E, Dack S: Comparison of infective endocarditis in drug addicts and nondrug users. *Am J Cardiol* 1973;32:924.
22. Lange M, Salaki JS, Middleton JR: Infective endocarditis in heroin addicts: Epidemiological observation and some unusual cases. *Am Heart J* 1978;86:144.
23. Archer G, Fekety FR, Supena R: *Pseudomonas aeruginosa* endocarditis in drug addicts. *Am Heart J* 1974;88:570.
24. Shekad R, Rice TW, Zierdt CH, et al: Outbreak of endocarditis caused by *Pseudomonas aeruginosa* serotype 011 among pentazocine and tripelennamine abusers in Chicago. *J Infect Dis* 1985;151:203.
25. Louria DB, Hensle T, Rose J: The major medical complications of heroin addiction. *Ann Intern Med* 1967;67:1.
26. Stimmel B, Donoso E, Dack S: Comparison of infective endocarditis in drug addicts and nondrug users. *Am J Cardiol* 1973;32:924.
27. Weens J Jr: *Candida parapsilosis* pathogenicity: Clinical manifestations and antimicrobial susceptibility. *Clin Infect Dis* 1992;14:756.
28. Rubinstein E, Noreiga EB, Simberkoff MS, et al: Fungal endocarditis: Analysis of 24 cases and review of the literature. *Medicine* 1975;54:331.
29. Dreyer NP, Fields BN: Heroin-associated infective endocarditis. A report of 28 cases. *Ann Intern Med* 1973;78:699.
30. Pollack S, Mogtader A, Lange M: *Neisseria subflava* endocarditis. Case report and review of the literature. *Am J Med* 1984;76:752.
31. Thornhill-Joynes M, Li MW, Canawati HN, et al: *Neisseria sicca* endocarditis in intravenous drug abusers. *West J Med* 1985;142:255.
32. Davis CL, Towns M, Henrich WL, et al: *Neisseria mucosa* endocarditis following drug abuse. Case report and review of the literature. *Arch Intern Med* 1983;143:583.
33. Yu VL, Rumans LW, Wing EJ, et al: *Pseudomonas maltophilia* causing heroin-associated infective endocarditis. *Arch Intern Med* 1978;138:1667.
34. Sobel JD, Carrizosa J, Ziobrowski TF, et al: Case report. Polymicrobial endocarditis involving *Eikenella corrodens*. *Am J Med Sci* 1981;282:41.
35. Brooks GF, O'Donoghue JM, Rissing JP: *Eikenella corrodens*, a recently recognized pathogen: Infection in medical-surgical patients and in association with methylphenidate abuse. *Medicine* 1974;53:325.
36. Saravolatz LD, Burch KH, Quinn EL, et al: Polymicrobial infective endocarditis: An increasing clinical entity. *Am Heart J* 1978;95:163.
37. Olle-Goig JE, Mildvan D: Possible pathogenic implications of right-sided polymicrobial endocarditis in a heroin abuser. *Eur J Clin Microbiol* 1986;5:449.
38. Olsson RA, Romansky MF: Staphylococcal tricuspid endocarditis in heroin addicts. *Ann Intern Med* 1962;57:755.
39. Simberkoff MS: Narcotic-associated infective endocarditis, in Kaplan EL, Taranta AV (eds): *Infective Endocarditis*. Dallas, American Heart Association, 1977, p 46.
40. Levine D: Infectious endocarditis in intravenous drug abusers, in Levine D, Sobel J (eds): *Infections in Intravenous Drug Abusers*. New York, Oxford University Press, 1991, p 258.
41. Niebel J: Infective endocarditis in immune-compromised patients, in Horstkotte D, Bodnar E (eds): *Current Heart Valve Disease: Infective Endocarditis*. London, ICR Publishers, 1991, p 156.
42. Kozel NJ, Adams EH: Epidemiology of drug abuse: An overview. *Science* 1986;234:970.
43. Chambers HF, Korzeniowski OM, Sande MA, et al: *Staphylococcus aureus* endocarditis: Clinical manifestations in addicts and nonaddicts. *Medicine* 1983;62:170.
44. Sande J, Lee B, Mills J, et al: Endocarditis in intravenous drug abusers, in Kaye D (ed): *Infective Endocarditis*, ed 2. New York, Raven Press, 1992, p 345.
45. Levine E: Infectious endocarditis in intravenous drug abusers, Levine D, Sobel J (eds):

Infections in Intravenous Drug Abusers. New York, Oxford University Press, 1991, p 259.

46. Niebel J, Held E: Endokarditis bei Drogenabhangigen. Fortschr. der antimikr. und antineopl. *Chemotherapie* 1987;6:781.

47. Watanakunakorn C: Changing epidemiology and newer aspects of infective endocarditis. *Adv Intern Med* 1977;22:21.

48. Baddour LM: Twelve year review of recurrent native valve infective endocarditis: A disease of the modern antibiotic era. *Rev Infect Dis* 1988;10:1163.

49. Eichacker PQ, Miller K, Robbins M: Echocardiographic evaluation of heart valves in IV drug abusers without a previous history of endocarditis. *Clin Res* 1984;32:670A.

50. Hussey HH, Keliher TF, Schaefer BF, et al: Septicemia and bacterial endocarditis resulting from heroin addiction. *JAMA* 1944;125:535.

51. Wilhelm F, Hirsh HL, Hussey HH, et al: The treatment of acute bacterial endocarditis with penicillin. *Ann Intern Med* 1947;26:221.

52. Haverkos H, Lange W: Serious infections other than human immunodeficiency virus among intravenous drug abusers. *J Infect Dis* 1990;161:894.

53. Dressler FA, Roberts WC: Infective endocarditis in opiate addicts: Analysis of 80 cases studied at necropsy. *Am J Cardiol* 1989;63:1240.

54. Roberts WC, Buchbinder NA: Right-sided valvular infective endocarditis: A clinicopathologic study of twelve necropsy patients. *Am J Med* 1972;53:7.

55. Buchbinder NA, Roberts WC: Left-sided valvular active infective endocarditis; a study of forty-five necropsy patients. *Am J Med* 1972;53:20.

56. Cannon NJ, Cobbs NG: Infective endocarditis in drug addicts, in Kaye D (ed): *Infective Endocarditis.* Baltimore, University Park Press, 1976, p 11.

57. McGeown MG: Bacterial endocarditis: An experimental study of healing. *J Pathol Bacteriol* 1954;67:179.

58. Angrist AA, Oka M, Nakao K, et al: Studies in experimental endocarditis. I. Production of valvular lesions by mechanisms not involving infection or sensitivity factors. *Am J Pathol* 1960;36:181.

59. Highman B, Altland PD: Effect of exposure and acclimatization to cold on susceptibility of rats to bacterial endocarditis. *Proc Soc Exp Biol Med* 1962;110:663.

60. Tuburo E, Borell G, Croce C, et al: Effect of morphine on resistance to infection. *J Infect Dis* 148; 1983: p 656.

61. Tuazon CU, Sheagren JN: Staphylococcal endocarditis in parenteral drug abusers: Source of the organism. *Ann Intern Med* 1975;82:790.

62. Botsford KB, Weinstein RA, Nathan CR, et al: Selective survival in pentazocine and tripelennamine of *Pseudomonas aeruginosa* serotype 011 from drug addicts. *J Infect Dis* 1985;151:209.

63. Sheagren J: Endocarditis complicating parental drug abuse, in Remington J, Suartz M (ed): *Current Clinical Topics in Infectious Disease,* Vol 2. New York, McGraw-Hill, 1981, p 211.

64. Klaver A, Hoffman J, Greenman R: Staphylococcal endocarditis in addicts. *South Med J* 1978;71:638.

65. Thadepalli H, Francis C: Diagnostic clues in metastatic lesions of endocarditis in addicts. *West J Med* 1978;128:1.

66. Hussey H, Katz S: Infections resulting from narcotic addictions. *Am J Med* 1980;9:260.

67. Duma R, Weinberg A, Medrick T, et al: Streptococcal infections: A bacteriologic and clinical study of streptococcal bacteremia. *Medicine* 1969;48:87.

68. Stimmel B, Dack S: Infective endocarditis in narcotic addicts, in Rahimtoola SH (ed): *Infective Endocarditis.* San Francisco, Grune and Stratton, 1978, p 195.

69. Craven D, Rininger A, Goulart T, et al: Methicillin resistant *Staphylococcus aureus* bacteremia limited to intravenous drug abusers using a shooting gallery. *Am J Med* 1989;80:770.

70. Levine DP, Cushing RD, Jui J, et al: Community-acquired methicillin resistant *Staphylococcus aureus* endocarditis in the Detroit Medical Center. *Ann Intern Med* 1982;97:330.

71. Joseph WL, Fletcher HS, Giordano JM, et al: Pulmonary and cardiovascular implications of drug addiction. *Ann Thorac Surg* 1973;69:1148.

72. Neufeld GK, Branson CG, Marshall LW, et al: Infective endocarditis as a complication of heroin use. *South Med J* 1976;69:1148.

73. Tuazon CU, Cardella TA, Sheagren JN: Staphylococcal endocarditis in drug users. *Arch Intern Med* 1975;135:1555.

74. White A: Medical disorders in drug addicts: 200 consecutive admissions. *JAMA* 1973;223:1469.

75. SanDretto MA, Scanlon GT: Multiple mycotic pulmonary artery aneurysms secondary to intravenous drug abuse. *Am J Radiol* 1984;142:89.

75. Dreyer NP, Fields BN: Heroin-associated infective endocarditis. A report of 28 cases. *Ann Intern Med* 1973;78:699.

77. Chambers H, Mills J: Endocarditis associated with intravenous drug abusers, in Sande J, Kaye D (eds): *Contemporary Issues Infectious Disease*, Vol 2: *Endocarditis.* New York, Churchill Livingstone, 1984, p 186.

78. Cohen PS, Maguire JH, Weinstein L: Infective endocarditis caused by gram-negative bacteria: A review of the literature 1945–1977. *Prog Cardiovasc Dis* 1980;22:205.

79. Chandrasekar P, Narule A: Bone and joint infections in intravenous drug abusers. *Rev Infect Dis* 1969;8:909.

80. Scheidegger C, Zimmerli W: Infectious complications in drug addicts: Seven year review of 269 hospitalized narcotics abusers in Switzerland. *Rev Infect Dis* 1989;11:486.

81. Banks T, Fletcher R, Ali N: Infective endocarditis in heroin addicts. *Am J Med* 1973;55:444.

82. Marantz P, Lanzer M, Finer C, et al: Inability to predict diagnosis in febrile intravenous drug abusers. *Ann Intern Med* 1987;106:823.

83. Pazin GJ, Saul S, Thompson ME: Blood culture positivity. Suppression by outpatient antibiotic therapy in patients with bacterial endocarditis. *Arch Intern Med* 1982;142:263.

84. Ferguson R, Feeney C, Chirurgi L: Enterobacter agglomerans-associated cotton fever. *Arch Intern Med* 1993;153:381.

85. Levine D: Infectious endocarditis in intravenous drug abusers, in Levine D, Sobel J (eds): New York, Oxford University Press, 1991, p 270.

86. Chambers H, Mills J: Endocarditis associated with intravenous drug abusers, in Sande J, Kaye D (eds): *Contemporary Issues in Infectious Disease*, Vol 2: *Endocarditis.* New York, Churchill Livingstone, 1984, p 191.

87. Infective valvulitis in drug addicts. Editorial. *Lancet* 1983;2:1180.

88. Nahass R, Weinstein M, Bartels A: Infective endocarditis in intravenous drug users. A comparison of human immunodeficiency virus type I negative and positive patients. *J Infect Dis* 1990;162:967.

89. Gusenhoven EJ, Taams MA, Roelandt JRTC, et al: Transesophageal two dimensional echocardiography: Its role in solving clinical problems. *J Am Coll Cardiol* 1986;8:975.

90. Daniel WG, Schroeder E, Nonnast-Daniel B, et al: Conventional and transesophageal echocardiography in the diagnosis of infective endocarditis. *Eur Heart J* 1987;8(Suppl 3):287.

91. Meyer J: Daignostic value of two-dimensional transesophageal versus transthoracic echocardiography in patients with infective endocarditis. *Eur Heart J* 1987;8(Suppl 1):303.

92. Daniel WG, Schroeder E, Muegge A, et al: Transesophageal echocardiography in infective endocarditis. *Am J Cardiac Imaging* 1988;2:78.

93. Polak PE, Gussenhoven WJ, Roelandt JRTC: Transesophageal cross-sectional echocardiographic recognition of an aortic valve ring abscess and a subannular mycotic aneurysm. *Eur Heart J* 1987;8:664.

94. Stechberg J, Murphy S, Ballard D: Emboli in infective endocarditis prognostic value of echocardiography. *Ann Intern Med* 1991;119:635.

95. Freedman LR, Valone J: Experimental infective endocarditis. *Prog Cardiovasc Dis* 1979;27:169.

96. Borrow KM, Alpert JS, Pennington J: Transient *Pseudomonas* bacteremia in a heroin addict. Resemblance to right-sided endocarditis. *JAMA* 1978; 240.

97. Levine D: Infectious endocarditis in intravenous drug abusers, in Levine D, Sobel J (eds): *Infections in Intravenous Drug Abusers.* New York, Oxford University Press, 1991, p 372.

98. Brumfitt W, Hamilton JM: Methicillin resistant *Staphylococcus albus. N Engl J Med* 1989;320:1188.

99. Watanakunakorn C, Guerriero JC: Interaction between vancomycin and rifampin against *Staphylococcus aureus. Antimicrob Agents Chemother* 1981;19:1089.

100. Deum T, Schaberz D, Terpenning M: Increasing resistance of *Staphylococcus aureus* to ciprofloxacin antimicrobial agents. *J Chemother* 1990;34:1862.

101. Saravolatz LD: Methicillin-resistant *Staphylococcus aureus,* in Magilligan DJ Jr, Quinn EL (eds): *Endocarditis—Medical and Surgical Management.* New York, Marcel Dekker, 1986, p 30.

102. Korzeniowski O, Sande M: The normal collaborative endocarditis study group. Combination antimicrobial therapy for *Staphylococcus aureus* endocarditis in patients addicted to parenteral drugs and non-addicts: A prospective study. *Ann Intern Med* 1982;97:466.

103. Chambers H, Miller RT, Newman MD: Right-sided *Staphylococcus aureus* endocarditis in intravenous drug abusers: Two-week combination therapy. *Ann Intern Med* 1988;109:609.

104. Hecht S, Berger M: Right-sided endocarditis in intravenous drug abusers. Prognostic features in 102 episodes. *Ann Intern Med* 1992;117:560.

105. Reyes MP, El-Khatib MR, Brown WJ, et al: Synergy between carbenicillin and an aminoglycoside (tentamicin or tobramycin) against *Pseudomonas aeruginosa* isolated from patients with endocarditis and sensitivity of isolates to normal human serum. *J Infect Dis* 1979;140:192.

106. Rubinstein E, Noreiga ER, Simberkoff MS, et al: Tissue penetration of amphotericin B in candida endocarditis. *Chest* 1974;66:376.

107. Robbins MJ, Soeiro R, Frishman WH, et al: Right-sided valvular endocarditis: Etiology diagnosis and an approach to therapy. *Am Heart J* 1986;111:128.

108. Robbins MJ, Frater RWM, Soeiro R, et al: Influence of vegetation size on clinical outcome of right-sided infective endocarditis. *Am J Med* 1986;80:165.

109. Wann LS, Dillon JC, Weyman AE, et al: Echocardiography in bacterial endocarditis. *N Engl J Med* 1976;295:135.

110. Stewart JA, Silimperi D, Harris P, et al: Echocardiographic documentation of vegetative lesions in infective endocarditis: Clinical implications. *Circulation* 1980;61:374.

111. Davis RS, Strom JA, Frishman W, et al: The demonstration of vegetations by echocardiography in bacterial endocarditis, an indication for early surgical intervention. *Am J Med* 1980;69:57.

112. Kunis RL, Sherrid MV, McCabe JB, et al: Successful medical therapy for mitral annular abscess complicating infective endocarditis. *J Am Coll Cardiol* 1986;7:953.

113. DiNubile M: Surgery for addiction-related tricuspid valve endocarditis: Caveat emptor. *Am J Med* 1987;82:811.

114. Hubbell G, Cheitlin MD, Rapaport E: Presentation, management, and follow-up evaluation of infective endocarditis in drug addicts. *Am Heart J* 1981;102:85.

115. Barbour DJ, Roberts WC: Valve excision only versus valve excision plus replacement for active infective endocarditis involving the tricuspid valve. *Am J Cardiol* 1986;57:475.

116. Arbulu A, Asfaw I: Tricuspid valvulectomy without prosthetic replacement, ten years of clinical experience. *J Thorac Cardiovasc Surg* 1981;82:684.

117. Wilson WR, Danielson GK, Giuliani ER, et al: Valve replacement in patients with active infective endocarditis. *Circulation* 1978;58:585.

118. Okies JE, Bradshaw MW, Williams TW Jr: Valve replacement in bacterial endocarditis. *Chest* 1973;63:898.

119. Jung JY, Saab SB, Almond CH: The case for early surgical treatment of left-sided primary infective endocarditis, a collective review. *J Thorac Cardiovasc Surg* 1975;70:509.

10

Prosthetic Valve Endocarditis

The first successful replacements of aortic and mitral valves were performed by Starr and Edwards[1] and Harkness et al.[2] in 1960. This procedure has been limited by two major problems: infection and thrombosis. About 50,000 mechanical and prosthetic valves have been implanted yearly in the United States; 1–4% eventually become infected.[3,4] A relatively small number of native cardiac valves have been reconstructed. Infection of prosthetic valves accounts for about 10–20% of all instances of infective endocarditis.

Primary prosthetic valvular endocarditis (*PVE*) refers to valves that were uninfected when they were replaced. *Secondary PVE* is a situation in which valvular infection is present at the time of surgery.[3]

The criteria on which the diagnosis of PVE has been established have led to differences in the results of clinical investigations that appear to be compatible with respect to the population of patients studied and the type of prosthetic valve infected.[5–7] The incidence of PVE ranges from 0.65 to 2.16 events per 100 patient-years.

Infection of prosthetic valves that develops within 60 days of implantation is considered *early PVE*. Disease that appears after this point is labeled *late PVE*. This difference is based on the change in pathogens that occurs 2 months following cardiac surgery. *S. aureus*, gram-negative aerobes, and fungi predominate in early PVE. The bacteria responsible for late PVE are the same as those responsible for infection of native valves. The validity of using a 60-day cutoff to distinguish early from late PVE should be reexamined. When the infection is caused by coagulase-negative staphylococci (CONS), an interval of 12 months appears to be a better basis on which to distinguish early from late disease. This is based on the results of several studies[8–16] indicating that in PVE produced by CONS, 84–87% of the organisms recovered within a year after surgery were resistant to methicillin compared to only 20–30% of CONS recovered later. Resistance of this group of organisms to methicillin is considered a marker for nosocomially acquired infection. The incidence of PVE produced by these bacteria decreases significantly after the second year.

The cumulative risk of PVE, based on actuarial data derived from a study of 1,597 patients by Rutledge et al.[17], indicated that it was 3.2% at 5 years and 5% at 10 years. Five to 6 months after surgery, the incidence of infection decreased significantly and remained constant after 1 year. It must be emphasized that implanted valves are at risk of infection throughout life.

A major reason for the decrease in incidence of PVE is the availability of antimicrobial prophylaxis.[18] In 1963, before it was standard practice, Geraci et al.[12] reported an incidence of 10% of infective endocarditis in patients who underwent open cardiac surgery but were not given prophylaxis.

PVE is on the increase. This is probably related to advances in cardiac surgery and the techniques that permit more patients to undergo replacement of natural valves.[19,20]

There appears to be a relationship between the type of model and placement of a prosthetic valve and the incidence of PVE.[17] A mechanical prosthetic valve may be more vulnerable to infection than a bioprosthetic one.[16] Ivert et al.[11] and Calderwood et al.[9] pointed out that there was an increase in the incidence of infection of mechanical valves during the first 3 months after surgery. After 12 months, porcine valves were involved more often than mechanical ones.[20]

Pathogenesis

A sterile thrombus referred to as a *vegetation* that contains fibrin and platelets is the nidus infected by organisms invading native or prosthetic valves. The forces leading to the development of this lesion are (1) the impact of blood flow on the endocardium and (2) a variety of localized or systemic hypercoaguable states.[21] Nonlaminar flow of blood over the endocardium may be adequate to alter the interaction between endothelial cells and platelets. In lining cells over which blood flows, the ability to prevent aggregation of platelets decreases markedly. The pattern of blood flow is markedly altered by the location and type of the prosthetic valve.[22,23] There is a marked difference in the pathogenetic potential of mechanical and bioprosthetic valves. Microorganisms do not adhere to artificial materials from which valves are constructed. Once a foreign body is implanted on the surface of the heart, it undergoes a reaction called *conditioning*.[24,25] An inflammatory reaction that varies with the shape and physicochemical composition of a prosthesis, various body fluids, and other substances present in the surrounding tissues are absorbed on the surface of the prosthesis independently of the inflammatory reaction.[26] Biofilm is a layer of biological materials attached to a prosthetic valve. This may serve as a receptor for attachment of circulating organisms. The second phase of conditioning is the thrombotic response of the patient to the foreign body. The fibrin-platelet matrix is another location where bacteria attach.[27,28]

The sewing cuff of a mechanical valve is the site of a sterile thrombus in the early postoperative period. Prior to this time, the valve is covered by endothelial cells that play a role in the pathogenesis of nonbacterial thrombotic endocarditis. Because the layering cells function abnormally, their ability to minimize clumping of platelets and the development of thrombosis are decreased. These events explain, in part, the fact that infection usually starts in the cuff and progresses to produce paravalvular leaks and to invade the myocardium, leading to the development of ring abscesses.[29,30]

In contrast to mechanical valves, bioprosthetic ones are very vulnerable to infection of the leaflets alone.[31] Glutaraldehyde increases the resistance of porcine valvular leaflets or bovine pericardial tissue to microbial invasion. Intracardial flow of blood injures the surface of bioprosthetic valves and leads to the formation of microthrombi that serve as a target for bacterial adhesion and eventual invasion of the valvular cusps.[32–36] As the thrombi enlarge, they produce increasing disturbances in the rheology of the cardiac chamber that amplifies the thrombotic process. The importance of hemodynamic trauma is emphasized by the observation that mitral bioprosthetic valves are more likely to be infected than aortic ones. This is probably related to the level of mechanical stress to which mitral valves are exposed.[37,38] The difference in the portal entry of organisms into mechanical and bioprosthetic valves (sewing cuffs versus valvular leaflets) explains the fact that the former are more prone to infection that occurs during the first 30–60 days after surgery. However, bioprosthetic valves are at increasing risk of endocarditis.[9] The unendothelialized sewing cuff of a mechanical valve is the major risk factor up to 60 days after it has been implanted. Many years of hemodynamic stress are required for the valvular cusp to sustain a level of trauma sufficient to develop calcification and thrombosis.

Pathology

The incidence of ring abscesses in patients with PVE ranges from 10% to 100%[33]; most of them develop in persons with mechanical valves.[39] Dehiscence occurs in 64% of individuals with an abscess of the valvular bed[11]; 6% develop significant valvular obstruction due to thrombosis. Ring abscesses are present in all patients with PVE who succumb to the disease.[40–44] Nine percent develop pericarditis secondary to abscesses involving the cuff.

A study by Cortina et al.[44] indicated that the incidence of infection of adjacent tissues was identical for mechanical and bioprosthetic valves. An important determinant of the clinical course of complicated valvular disease is the time of onset. Infections that develop early are often associated with extensive penetration of cardiac tissue. This is not a common problem in patients with PVE that occurs more than 1 year after surgery.[45]

Bacterial growth is not restricted to the surface of bioprosthetic valves. Peripheral embolization is a major cause of morbidity, and the organisms eventually penetrate the valve. This invasion accelerates the inflammatory process that may result in a valve that requires replacement because of severe stenosis produced by fusion of its leaflets.

Embolization is a major cause of morbidity and mortality in patients with

PVE.[39,40] Ninety-five percent of those who die in the course of treatment have had an embolic episode; about 15 percent of these have involved the central nervous system. As in infective endocarditis of native valves, septic emboli may affect the kidneys and produce mycotic aneurysms of medium-sized and large arteries.

Microbiology

The microbiology of PVE emphasizes the fundamental differences between early and late disease. Studies by Karchmer et al.[10] and Calderwood et al.[9] have indicated that the incidence of PVE caused by CONS is almost identical in patients whose disease began within 2 months, 2–6 months, and 6–12 months after surgery (Table 10.1). It may be more appropriate to consider 12 months as the point separating early and late PVE. Infections that occur up to this time have developed during or about the time of surgery.[46–63]

CONS are the most frequent cause of PVE.[17,29,64] Infection by *S. aureus* is responsible for 17% of early and 12% of late PVE (Table 10.1). *S. viridans* and other streptococcal species produce 5% of early and 19% of late disease. Enterococci are involved in less than 4% of early disease; they are more common in late disease.

The organisms involved in the pathogenesis of late PVE are similar to those responsible for infective endocarditis of native valves. An exception is the diminished but significant role played by CONS. Prior to 1975, gram-negative bacteria were more often involved in early disease.[6] Later their role decreased, probably because of improved cardiac surgical proce-

Table 10.1. Microbiology of PVE

Organism	No. of Cases from 1975 to 1982		
	<2 mo	>2–12 mo	>12 mo
CONS	22	19	10
S. aureus	2	3	5
Gram-negative bacilli	2	1	1
Streptococci (nonenterococcal)	0	1	12
Enterococci	0	2	4
Pneumococci	0	0	0
Diphtheroids	4	0	1
Fungi	2	2	1
Fastidious gram-negative coccobacilli	0	1	7
Other	3	2	1
Culture negative	3	3	2

Source: Adapted from Karchmer AW, Bisno AL: Infections of prosthetic heart valves and vascular grafts, in Bisno AL, Waldvogel FA (eds): *Infections Associated with Indwelling Medical Devices.* Washington, DC, American Society for Microbiology, 1989, p 133.

dures.[65,66] Overall, these organisms account for fewer nosocomial infections. More recently, the fastidious members of the HACEK group have begun to play a small but significant etiological role.[67]

Many different genera and species of microorganisms, especially group JK corynebacteria, have been involved in the pathogenesis of PVE.[68–71] (Table 10.1). These organisms are difficult to culture because of their strict nutritional requirements. They are resistant to a number of antimicrobial agents, especially the cephalosporins.

Fungal PVE is increasing in incidence. This is probably related to the large number of IVDA, immunosuppressed patients and more frequent invasive vascular manipulations.[72–76] *C. albicans* and *C. stellatoidea* are involved in 32% and *Aspergillus* in 27%. Other species have been implicated in sporadic cases of PVE.[77–81]

Cases of culture-negative PVE do not occur until about 6 months after a prosthetic valve has been placed. Cultures of the blood are generally sterile in patients with PVE caused by species of *Legionella* and *Coxiella burnetii*.[82–84]

Sources of Infecting Organisms

Block et al.[85] have suggested that infection of prosthetic valves developing within 60 days after surgery is associated with a number of nosocomial factors.[85] Other studies have confirmed this use of the elegant techniques of plasmid pattern analysis. Archer et al.[86] documented the possibility of a prolonged incubation period for PVE originating during surgery.

Organisms involved in the pathogenesis of early PVE have been recovered from operating rooms and surgical equipment. Blakemore et al.[87] reported that the bypass pump was contaminated in 75% of the procedures. The organisms recovered from the equipment were CONS, some species of streptococci, gram-negative aerobes, fungi, and diphtheroids. The density of organisms present in the air appeared to be directly related to the number of individuals present in the operating room. Ankeney and Parket [88] have reported that 19% of cultures of blood drawn from several sites during surgery yielded a variety of bacteria; diphtheroids and CONS were most common.[55,88] When the bypass pump was removed, there was a striking decrease in the incidence of positive blood cultures. The results of a study by Kluge et al.[89] indicated that the valve and its bed were often contaminated when cultures were obtained prior to closing the sternal wound (71% positive cultures). Diphtheroids and CONS were recovered most often. It has been suggested that the ambient air is the source of the bacteria. The results of several studies have supported the theory that perioperative implantation of organisms is the source of early PVE.[90] Restrictive DNA analysis has demonstrated an association between some species of *Legionella* (*L. pneumophila*, *L. dumoffi*) and PVE.[91]

Many early infections have been caused by pacing wires,[92] endotracheal tubes, and a variety of wounds and soft tissues.[93,94] Prosthetic valves are rarely the source of infection. An exception is contamination of porcine valves by *Mycobacterium chelonei* during manufacture.[95,96]

Physicians are rarely the source of infection of these devices. However, one well-documented case has been reported. This involved a surgeon colonized by CONS who transmitted the organism to the patient's valve; the source was a tear in his surgical glove.[97]

Infections that develop sometime after a prosthetic valve has been implanted involve the same mechanisms that operate in the pathogenesis of infection of native valves.[98–100] An important risk factor in the development of PVE is a prior episode of infective endocarditis that requires replacement of the infected valve. This is necessary in 38% of patients due to persistent or relapsing infections.[101–104] PVE is five times more likely to occur when a prosthetic valve is inserted during active endocarditis.[49,105–108] The organism that infects the artificial valve is often different from the one responsible for the original infection.

Clinical Manifestations

The clinical features of PVE are similar to those present in infected natural valves[93,100,109,110] (Table 10.2, Fig. 10.1). Because PVE usually involves an injured heart, congestive cardiac failure develops earlier and is more severe than it is in native valvular disease.[111] Cardiac failure occurs in 30–100% of patients with PVE. Valvular regurgitation caused by infection of the sewing

Table 10.2. Clinical Manifestation of Prosthetic Endocarditis

Symptom/Sign	Early PVE (%)	Late PVE (%)
Fever	95–100	95–100
New/changing murmur	50–70	40–60
Congestive cardiac failure	30–100	30
Shock	33	0–10
Conduction abnormality	15–20	5–10
Splenomegaly	20–30	15–40
Emboli	5–30	10–40
Petechiae	30–60	40–50
Osler's nodes Janeway lesions Roth's spots	5	15
Anemia	75	75
Leukocytosis	40	30–50
Hematuria		65

Source: Adapted from Burckhardt D, Stulz P, Follath F, et al: Prosthetic valve endocarditis: Conservative therapy and indications for reoperation, in Horstkotte D, and Bodnar E (eds): *Infective Endocarditis.* London, ICR Publishers, 1991, p 262.

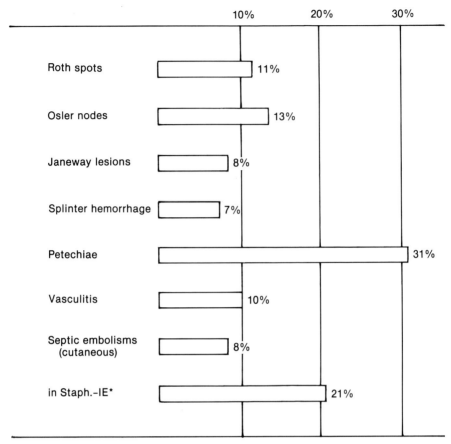

*infective endocarditis

Fig. 10.1. Frequency of retinal and cutaneous manifestations of PVE. (Adapted from Ref. 16, p 242)

cuff or destruction of the leaflets of a bioprosthetic valve are the main reasons for the development of cardiac decompensation.

Valvular leaks are the most common complication of infection of mechanical valves. Thrombosis of a prosthetic valves impairs ventricular function, impedes the outflow tract, or interferes with the function of mechanical valves in 10% of patients with PVE.[112–114] Myocarditis or pericarditis may develop. All the primary cardiac complications develop in the early stages of the infection.[115] Fever is present in almost all patients.[6,15,29,65,116–121]

The murmur of valvular regurgitation is present in about 50% of patients with PVE.[122] This may not develop until late in the course of an infection caused by relatively noninvasive organisms (e.g., *S. viridans*). It is important to distinguish the murmur of regurgitation caused by a paravalvular leak due to infection from one associated with a noninflammatory disorder. The latter develops immediately after surgery in about 1% of patients whose valves have been replaced.[123] Hepatosplenomegaly is present in 30% of individuals with PVE. This is more common in those infected by *S. viridans*.[124]

The dermal and ocular manifestations of PVE are increasing in frequency.[125] Janeway lesions, splinter hemorrhages, Osler's nodes, and Roth's spots are present in 15–20% of patients. These are most common in late disease. Large septic emboli that involve the skin occur in 20% of individuals with disease caused by *S. aureus*.[126] Several clinical studies have reported a high incidence of embolic stroke in the first 3 days after the onset of PVE. Treatment with coumadin protects against the development of neurological disorders.[127]

Diagnosis

The diagnosis of PVE is based on the presence both of bacteremia and of a prosthetic valve that has developed a paravalvular leak or thrombus. However, leaks and clots can be absent early in the disease. Unlike endocardial infection that involves native valves, bacteremia may be discontinuous.[128] The primary lesion may be an abscess of the sewing cuff not in direct communication with the intravascular space in 85–90% of patients (Table 10.3).

Table 10.3. Retrospectively Elaborated Point System for Diagnosing PVE

	PVE After Valve Replacement	
	Within 1 Year	Beyond 1 Year
Septicemia plus cultured		
Streptococci or enterococci	1	3
Staphylococci	1	3
Gram-negative bacteria	3	3
Mixed infections	3	3
Fungi	2	1
Other germs	1	1
Clinical signs and symptoms of endocarditis	2	3
Thromboembolic phenomena	1	1
First manifestation of conduction disturbances	1	2
Echocardiography showing		
Vegetations (no baseline examination available)	2	2
Vegetation or abscesses		
(baseline examination available)	4	4
Newly developed		
stenosis or insufficiency	4	4
Demonstration of prosthetic valve malfunction	2	4
Diagnostic criteria	>8 points	>10 points

Source: Adapted from Ref. 16, p 244.

The diagnosis of PVE is based on the recovery of the organism from cultures of blood incubated at 37°C for a minimum of 1 month. This is required for the detection of fungi and other fastidious organisms. Cultures of blood should be obtained several days after treatment has been discontinued.[129]

The presence of bacteremia may be related to causes other than PVE. Among these are infections of the mediastinum or contamination of vascular catheters. The situations in which uncomplicated bacteremia occurs [130] include (1) the onset of infection within 25 days of surgery; (2) a proved or strongly suspected point of origin; (3) failure to develop a new murmur; and (4) bacteremia with gram-negative organisms.[131]

Although the results of a physical examination and laboratory studies may establish the diagnosis of PVE, other approaches are necessary. Cinefluoroscopy is presently considered the procedure of choice for documenting the presence of valvular dysfunction.[132–134] This technique identifies abnormalities in the excursion of the valvular cage and the occluder component of the valve. However, this approach does not distinguish infections from noninfectious disease.

Because the availability of cinefluoroscopy is limited in the United States, more reliance has been placed on echochardiography. Ultrasonography may define the severity of cardiac failure by measuring left ventricular end-diastolic volume and by detecting premature closure of the mitral valve.[135] Doppler echocardiography may estimate the degree of valvular regurgitation.[136]

Transthoracic echocardiography (TTE) is useful in establishing the diagnosis of PVE in 30–80% of patients, and in identifying the presence of valvular dysfunction and myocardial abscesses.[137–140] Transesophageal echocardiography (TEE) is more specific and sensitive than TTE.[141–146] Prosthetic materials interfere with TTE and TEE.[147] Two-dimensional TEE combined with Doppler studies detects the presence of valvular abscesses in about 80% of infected patients.[148] Despite its limitations, echocardiography is the best approach to the diagnosis of PVE.[149] When TEE fails to disclose direct or indirect evidence of PVE, biplane TEE is recommended.[150,151] This is rapidly becoming the diagnostic standard. Serial electrocardiography identifies new atrial or ventricular blocks and supplements echocardiography in identifying the presence of myocardial abscesses[143,148,151–153] in patients with PVE.[154] The P-R interval may be prolonged when the aortic valves are infected.

Nuclear imaging technics (gallium 67 or indium 111 leukocyte scans) have been used to supplement the diagnostic procedures described above.[155,156] Cardiac catheterization is required when all other approaches have failed to establish the diagnosis of PVE. This may also be helpful in ruling out the presence of significant disease of the coronary arteries.[157] Hemolytic anemia may develop in patients with valvular leaks.[158]

Treatment

The treatment of PVE differs from that employed in the management of infected native valves in the following respects: (1) the anticoagulation required throughout life, which involves a high risk of bleeding; (2) the need to replace an infected valve with another prosthesis; (3) a greater incidence of embolic infarction; (4) the frequent development of mycotic aneurysms; and (5) complications involving the central nervous system when anticoagulation is terminated. It has been suggested that heparin be substituted when the patient is unstable since its effects can be reversed quickly. Standard anticoagulation is resumed as soon as any bleeding has ceased.[159–162]

A significant number of cases of infective endocarditis are caused by CONS. Many strains of this organism are resistant to methicillin, other penicillins, and the cephalosporins [163,164] but are usually sensitive to the aminoglycosides, rifampin, and vancomycin. A combination of vancomycin, rifampin, and gentamicin has been noted to be most effective in the management of PVE.[165] A trial that compared the effectiveness of vancomycin plus rifampin, or vancomycin and rifampin administered for 6 weeks plus gentamicin for the first 2 weeks, has been effective in eradicating CONS.[166] However, 33% of those treated with vancomycin and rifampin harbored organisms that developed resistasnce to rifampin. Treatment with gentamicin for 2 weeks prevented the development of bacterial resistance.

CONS are slowly becoming resistsant to gentamicin. This is not true for all of the aminoglycosides. Amikacin may be effective against those that are resistant to gentamicin.[167,168] If all isolates appear to be unresponsive to all members of this class of drugs, administration of another antibiotic to which CONS is sensitive (e.g., clindamycin) should be considered.

The basic principles for the treatment of PVE caused by penicillin-sensitive streptococci are the same as those for infection of native valves. It has been recommended that patients with PVE caused by nonenterococcal streptococci be treated with gentamicin for the first 2 weeks and with penicillin for 4 weeks.[169] Although animal models have indicated that this combination of drugs rapidly sterilizes vegetations, trials in humans have not supported this approach.[170] A retrospective study of infective endocarditis in hospitalized patients has indicated that penicillin administered for 4 weeks is as effective as penicillin plus an aminoglycoside administered for 2 weeks.[171] These regimens are indicated for the management of disease that involves native valves. The Committee on Rheumatic Fever, Endocarditis and Kawasaki Disease has recommended treatment of PVE with penicillin. Infection produced by nonenterococcal streptococci resistant to penicillin (MIC$\geq$ 1 μg/ml) mandates therapy with penicillin plus gentamicin.[172]

Successful therapy of enterococcal PVE rests on the administration of a combination of a cell wall–active drug and an aminoglycoside.[173]

Not all diphtheroids are sensitive to the beta-lactam drugs. When an organism is sensitive to gentamicin, the addition of penicillin produces a synergistic effect.[174] Vancomycin appears to be the drug of choice for the management of infection caused by strains resistant to gentamicin.

Therapy with vancomycin plus gentamicin for infection caused by gentamicin-sensitive isolates appears to be superior to treatment with penicillin plus gentamicin.[175]

When the clinical status of a patient is precarious, treatment must not be delayed until the results of cultures of the blood become available. Immediate therapy with vancomycin and gentamicin is indicated. This combination of drugs is effective in eradicating most of the organisms involved in the pathogenesis of PVE.

PVE produced by fungi requires surgery, as well as treatment with an antifungal agent. This is so because amphotericin penetrates valvular vegetations poorly. Medical therapy prior to surgery is probably unnecessary.[176–178] Suprainfection caused by fungi may develop during the therapy of PVE bacterial caused by fungi.[179] It may be eliminated by prophylaxis with mycostatin.

Despite advances in antimicrobial therapy, the fatality rate of early and late PVE has not declined. This holds true in patients with congestive cardiac failure. Death occurs in about 88% of individuals with severe cardiac failure; 29% of infected valves develop little or no dysfunction.[180]

An analysis of the complications and outcome of PVE by Calderwood et al.[64] disclosed the following: (1) complicated disease is associated with a high fatality rate; (2) damage to cardiac tissue is extensive; (3) striking disturbances in conduction frequently occur; (4) perivalvular abscesses are common; (5) fever persists after 10 days of therapy; (6) the greatest incidence of endocarditis is within a year after replacement of a valve; and (7) 50% of patients with PVE treated medically and/or surgically survive and are free of the complications described above.

The indications for surgery are thoroughly presented in a later chapter (Surgical Management).[181–183] About 30% of patients with PVE do not require surgery. It is usually not required for individuals with late PVE caused by methicillin-sensitive or -resistant strains of *S. aureus*. CONS usually require therapy with more than one antimicrobial agent, especially when isolates are nosocomially acquired. This is necessary less often in individuals with late PVE caused by *S. viridans* or the HACEK group of organisms.[181,184,185] The presence of significant renal failure early in the course of PVE mandates surgery.[44] Bacteremia clears in about a week after therapy is initiated; surgery should be considered when this fails.

Among the surgical methods employed to treat patients with complicated PVE are aortic ventriculoplasty and reconstruction of the root of the annulus by inserting a tube graft.[186–190] The timing of surgery is critical. Antimicrobial therapy for 10–14 days prior to and following such cardiac surgery is mandatory.[186]

References

1. Starr A, Edwards ML: Mitral replacement: Clinical experience with a ball valve prosthesis. *Ann Surg* 1960;154:726.

2. Harkness JE, Soroff M, Taylor MC: Prostheses in aoritc insufficiency. *J Thorac Cardiovasc Surg* 1960;40:744.
3. Cowgill LD, Addonizio VP, Hopeman AR, et al: Prosthetic valve endocarditis. *Curr Probl Cardiol* 1986;11:617.
4. Heimburger TS, Suma RJ: Infections of prosthetic heart valves and cardiac pacemakers. *Infect Dis Clin North Am* 1989;3:221.
5. Gonzales-Lavin L, Chi S, Lewis B: An 8-year experience with the Standard Ionescu-Shiley pericardial valve in the aortic position, in Bodnar E, Yacoub M (eds): *Biologic and Bioprosthetic Valves.* New York, Medical Books, 1986, p 199.
6. Garcia-Benogochia JB, Rubio Alvarez J, Gil de la Pena M: Long-term results with the Ionescu-Shiley pericardial xenograph valve, in Bodnar E, Yacoub M (eds): *Biologic and Bioprosthetic Valves.* New York, Medical Books, 1986, p 205.
7. Ionescu MJ, Tandon AP, Silverton NP: Long-term durability of the pericardial valve, in Bodnar E, Yacoub M (eds): *Biologic and Bioprosthetic Valves.* New York, Medical Books, 1986, p 166.
8. Hammond GW, Stiver G: Combination antibiotic therapy in an outbreak of prosthetic endocarditis caused by *Staphylococcus epidermidis. J Can Med Assoc* 1978;118:524.
9. Calderwood S, Swinski L, Waternaus C, et al: Risk factors for the development of prosthetic valve endocarditis. *Circulation* 1985;72:31.
10. Karchmer AW, Archer GL, Dismukes WE: *Staphylococcus epidermidis* causing prosthetic valve endocarditis: Microbiologic and clinical observations as guides to therapy. *Ann Intern Med* 1983;98:447.
11. Ivert T, Dismukes W, Cobbs G, et al: Prosthetic valve endocarditis. *Circulation* 1984; 69:223.
12. Geraci JE, Dale AJD, McGoon DC: Bacterial endocarditis following cardiac operation. *Wis Med J* 1963;62:302.
13. Baumgartner WA, Miller DC, Reitz BA, et al: Surgical treatment of prosthetic valve endocarditis. *Ann Thorac Surg* 1983;35:87.
14. Schulte HD, Horstkotte D, Evangelopoulos N, et al: Reoperations for malfunction of heart valve prostheses, especially with endocarditis. *Thorac Cardiovasc Surg* 1987; 35:16.
15. Watanakunakorn C: Prosthetic valve infective endocarditis: A review. *Prog Cardiovasc Dis* 1979;22:181.
16. Horstkotte D: Prosthetic valve endocarditis, in Horstkotte D, Bodnar E (eds): *Infective Endocarditis.* London, ICR Publishers, 1991, p 233.
17. Rutledge RR, Leim BJ, Applebaum RE: Actuarial analysis of the risk of prosthetic valve endocarditis in 1598 patients with mechanical and bioprosthetic valves. *Arch Surg* 1985;120:469.
18. Talkington CM, Thompson JE: Prevention and management of infected prostheses. *Surg Clin North Am* 1982;62:515.
19. Wilson WR, Danielson GK, Giuliani E, et al: Prosthetic valve endocarditis. *Mayo Clin Proc* 1982;57:155.
20. Dismukes WE, Karchmer AW, Buckley MJ, et al: Prosthetic valve endocarditis: Analysis of 38 cases. *Circulation* 1973;48:365.
21. Carpenter JL: Perivalvular extension of infection in patients with infectious endocarditis. *Rev Infect Dis* 1991;13:127.
22. Blackstone EH, Kirklin JW: Death and other time related events after valve replacement. *Circulation* 1985;72:753.
23. Horstkotte D, Haerten K, Seipel L, et al: Central haemodynamics at rest and during exercise after mitral valve replacement with different prostheses. *Circulation* 1983; 68(Suppl 2):161.
24. Christensen GD, Simpson WA, Bisno AL, et al: Adherence on slime-producing strains of *Staphylococcus epidermidis* to smooth surfaces. *Infect Immun* 1982;37:318.
25. Christensen GD, Simpson WA, Beachey EH: The adhesion of bacteria to animal tissues: Complex mechanisms, in Salvage DC, Fletcher M (eds): *Bacterial Adhesion.* New York, Plenum, 1985, p 279.

26. Gristina AG: Biomaterial-centered infection: Microbial adhesion versus tissue integration. *Science* 1987;237:1588.

27. Chen SC, Sorrell TC, Dwyer DE: Endocarditis associated with prosthetic cardiac valves. *Med J Aust* 1990;152:458.

28. Arnet E, Roberts WC: Valve ring abscess in active infective endocarditis: Frequency, location, and clues to clinical diagnosis from the study of 95 autopsy patients. *Circulation* 1976;54:140.

29. Karchmer AW, Dismukes WE, Buckley MJ, et al: Late prosthetic valve endocarditis: Clinical features influencing therapy. *Am J Med* 1978;64:199.

30. Richardson JV, Karp RB, Kirklin JW, et al: Treatment of infective endocarditis: A 10 year comparative analysis. *Circulation* 1978;58:589.

31. Zussa C, Galloni MR, Zattera CF: Endocarditis in patients with bioprostheses: Pathology and clinical correlations. *Int J Cardiol* 1984;6:719.

32. Lakler JB, Khaja F, Magilligan DJ, et al: Porcine xenograft valves. Long-term (60–89 months) follow-up. *Circulation* 1980;62:313.

33. Gavin JB, Herdson PB, Monro JC: Pathology of antibiotic-treated human heart valve allografts. *Thorax* 1973;28:473.

34. Reichenbach DD, Mohri H, Merendino KA: Pathological changes in human aortic valve homografts. *Circulation* 1969;33(Suppl 1):4.

35. Camilleri JP, Pornin B, Carpentier A: Structural changes of glutaraldehyde-treated porcine bioprosthetic valves. *Arch Pathol Lab Med* 1982;106:490.

36. Reul GJ, Cooley DA, Duncan JM: Valve failure with the Ionescu-Shiley bovine pericardial bioprothesis: Analysis of 2680 patients. *J Vasc Surg* 1985;2:192.

37. Broom ND: Fatigue-induced damage in glutaraldehyde-preserved heart valve tissue. *J Thorac Cardiovasc Surg* 1978;76:202.

38. Sabbah HN, Hamid MS, Stein PD: Mechanical stresses on closed cusps of porcine bioprosthetic valves: Correlation with sites of calcification. *Ann Thorac Surg* 1986;42:93.

39. Anderson DJ, Bulkley BH, Hutchins GM: A clinicopathologic study of prosthetic valve endocarditis in 22 patients: Morphologic basis for diagnosis and therapy. *Am Heart J* 1977;94:325.

40. Arnett EN, Roberts WC: Prosthetic valve endocarditis. Clinicopathologic analysis of 22 necropsy patients with comparison of observations in 74 necropsy patients with active infective endocarditis involving left-sided cardiac valve. *Am J Cardiol* 1976;38:281.

41. Magilligan DJ Jr, Quinn EL, Davila JC: Bacteremia, endocarditis, and the Hancock valve. *Ann Thorac Surg* 1977;24:508.

42. Nunez L, de la Llana R, Aguado MG, et al: Bioprosthetic valve endocarditis: Indicators for surgical intervention. *Ann Thorac Surg* 1983;35:262.

43. Baumgartner WA, Miller DC, Reitz BA, et al: Surgical treatment of prosthetic valve endocarditis. *Ann Thorac Surg* 1983;35:87.

44. Cortina JM, Martinelli J, Artiz V, et al: Surgical treatment of active prosthetic valve endocarditis. Results in 66 patients. *Thorac Cardiovasc Surg* 1987;35:209.

45. Madison J, Wang K, Gobel FL, et al: Prosthetic aortic valvular endocarditis. *Circulation* 1975;51:940.

46. Masur H, Johnson WD: Prosthetic valve endocarditis. *J Thorac Cardiovasc Surg* 1980; 80:31.

47. Horstkotte D, Loogen F, Kleikamp G, et al: The influence of heart valve replacement on the natural history of isolated mitral aortic and multivalvular disease. Clinical results in 783 patients up to 8 years after implantation of Bjork-Shiley tilting-disc prostheses. *Z Kardiol* 1983;72:494.

48. Baumgartner WA, Miller DC, Reitz BA: Surgical treatment of prosthetic valve endocarditis. *Ann Thorac Surg* 1983;35:87.

49. Slaughter L, Morris JE, Starr A: Prosthetic valvular endocarditis: A 12 year review. *Circulation* 1973;47:1319.

50. Karchmer AW: Prosthetic valve endocarditis: Mechanical valves, in Magilligan DJ, Quinn EL (eds): *Endocarditis: Medical and Surgical Management*. New York, Marcel Dekker, 1986, p 241.

51. Klosters FE: Infective prosthetic valve endocarditis, in Rahimtoola SH (ed): *Infective Endocarditis.* New York, Grune and Stratton, 1978, p 291.
52. Anger P, Marquis G, Dyrda I: Infective endocarditis update experience from a heart hospital. *Acta Cardiol* 1981;36:105.
53. Grignon A, Spencer H, Robson HG: Prosthetic valve infections. *Can J Surg* 1981;24:625.
54. Paneth M: Native and prosthetic valve endocarditis. *Thorac Cardiovasc Surg* 1982; 30:302.
55. Ben Ismail M, Hannachi N, Abib F: Prosthetic valve endocarditis—a survey. *Br Heart J* 1987;5778:72.
56. Schulte HD, Horstkotte D, Evangelopoulos N: Reoperations for malfunction of heart valve prostheses, especially with endocarditis. *Thorac Cardiovasc Surg* 1987;35:16.
57. Watanakunakorn IC: Changing epidemiology and new aspects of infective endocarditis. *Adv Intern Med* 1977;22:21.
58. Moore-Gillon J, Eykyn SJ, Phillips I: Prosthetic valve endocarditis. *Br Med J* 1983;287:739.
59. Leport C, Vilde JI, Bricaire C: Fifty cases of late prosthetic valve endocarditis improvement in prognosis over a 15-year period. *Br Heart J* 1987;58:66.
60. Eisenberg FP, Lorber B, Suk B: Prosthetic valve endocarditis due to the nutritionally variant streptococcus. *Am J Med Sci* 1985;289:249.
61. Torbjorns S, Ivert A, Dismukes W: Prosthetic valve endocarditis. *Circulation* 1984;69:223.
62. Magilligan DJ Jr: Bioprosthetic valve endocarditis, in Magilligan DJ Jr, Quinn EL (eds): *Endocarditis: Medical and Surgical Management.* New York, Marcel Dekker, 1986, p 217.
63. Malone JM, Moore WS, Campagna G, et al: Bacteremic infectability of vascular grafts: The influence of pseudointimal integrity and duration of graft function. *Surgery* 1975;78:211.
64. Calderwood SB, Swinshi LA, Karchmer AW: Prosthetic valve endocarditis: Analysis of factors affecting the outcome of therapy. *J Thorac Cardiovasc Surg* 1986;92:776.
65. Mayer KH, Schoenbaum SC: Evaluation and management of prosthetic valve endocarditis. *Prog Cardiovasc Dis* 1982;25:43.
66. Karchmer AW, Swartz MN: Infective endocarditis in patients with prosthetic heart valves, in Kaplan EL, Taranta AV (eds): *Infective Endocarditis.* American Heart Association Symposium monograph No. 52. Dallas, American Heart Association, 1977, p 58.
67. Meyer DJ, Gerding DN: Favorable prognosis of patients with prosthetic valve endocarditis caused by gram-negative bacilli of the HACEK group. *Am J Med* 1988;85:104.
68. Anger P, Marquis G, Dyrda I: Infective endocarditis update: Experience from a heart hospital. *Acta Cardiol* 1981;36:105.
69. Grignon A, Spencer H, Robson HG: Prosthetic valve infections. *Can J Surg* 1981;24:625.
70. Murray BS, Karchmer AW, Moellering RC Jr: Diphtheroid prosthetic valve endocarditis: A study of clinical features and infecting organisms. *Am J Med* 1980;69:838.
71. Vanbosterhaut B, Surmont I, Vandeven J, et al: *Corynebacterium jeikeium* (group JK diphtheroids) endocarditis: A report of five cases. *Diagn Microbiol Infect Dis* 1989;12:265.
72. Thomas TV, Heilbrunn A: Prosthetic aortic valve replacement complicated by diphtheroid endocarditis and aortopulmonary fistula. *Chest* 1971;59:679.
73. Watanakunakorn C: Prosthetic valve infective endocarditis. *Prog Cardiovasc Dis* 1979;22:181.
74. McLeod R, Remington JS: Postoperative fungal endocarditis, in Duma RJ (ed): *Infections of Prosthetic Heart Valves and Vascular Grafts.* Baltimore, University Park Press, 1977, p 163.
75. Seelig MS, Speth CP, Kozinn PJ, et al: Patterns of *Candida* endocarditis following cardiac surgery: Importance of early diagnosis and therapy (an analysis of 91 patients). *Prog Cardiovasc Dis* 1974;18:125.
76. Norenberg RG, Sethi GK, Scott SM, et al: Opportunistic endocarditis following open-heart surgery. *Ann Thorac Surg* 1575;19:592.
77. Aslam PA, Gourley R, Eastridge CE: Aspergillus endocarditis after aortic valve replacement. *Int Surg* 1970;53:91.
78. Carrizosa J, Levison ME, Lawrence T: Cure of *Aspergillus ustus* endocarditis on a prosthetic valve. *Arch Intern Med* 1974;133:486.

79. Chandhuri MR: Fungal endocarditis after valve replacement. *J Thorac Cardiovasc Surg* 1970;60:207.

80. Kahn TH, Kane EG, Dean DC: Aspergillus endocarditis of mitral prosthesis. *Am J Cardiol* 1968;277:280.

81. Kicha GJ, Berroya RB, Escano FB, et al: Mucormycosis in a mitral prosthesis. *J Thorac Cardiovasc Surg* 1972;63:903.

82. Tompkins LS, Roessler BJ, Redd SC, et al: Legionella prosthetic valve endocarditis. *N Engl J Med* 1988;318:530.

83. Fernandez-Guerrero ML, Muelas JM, Aguado JM, et al: Q fever endocarditis on porcine bioprosthetic valves: Clinicopathologic features and microbiologic findings in three patients treated with doxycycline, cotrimoxazole, and valve replacement. *Ann Intern Med* 1988;108:209.

84. Stein PD, Folkens AT, Hruska KA: *Saccharomyces* fungaemia. *Chest* 1970;58:173.

85. Block PC, DeSanctis RW, Weinberg AN, et al: Prosthetic valve endocarditis. *J Thorac Cardiovasc Surg* 1970;60:540.

86. Archer GL, Vishniavsky N, Stiver HG: Plasmid pattern analysis of *Staphylococcus epidermidis* isolates from patients with prosthetic valve endocarditis. *Infect Immun* 1982;35:627.

87. Blackemore WE, McGarrity GJ, Turer RJ: Infection by airborne bacteria with cardiopulmonary bypass. *Surgery* 1971;70:830.

88. Ankeney JL, Parker RF: Staphylococcal endocarditis following open heart surgery related to positive intraoperative blood cultures, in Brewer LA III, Cooley DA, Davila JA (eds): *Prosthetic Heart Valves.* Springfield, IL, Charles C Thomas, 1969, p 719.

89. Kluge RM, Calia FM, McLaughlin JS: Sources of contamination in open heart surgery. *JAMA* 1974;230:1415.

90. Wilson W, Danielson G, Giuliani E, Geraci J: Prosthetic valve endocarditis. *Mayo Clin Proc* 1982;57:155.

91. Tompkins LS, Roessler BJ, Redd SC, et al: Legionella prosthetic valve endocarditis. *N Engl J Med* 1988;318:530.

92. Freeman R, King D: Analysis of results of catheter tip cultures in open heart surgery patients. *Thorax* 1975;30:26.

93. Dismukes WE, Karchmer AW: The diagnosis of infected prosthetic heart valves: Bacteremia versus endocarditis, in Duma RJ (ed): *Infections of Prosthetic Heart Valves and Vascular Grafts.* Baltimore, University Park Press, 1977, p 61.

94. Mayer KH, Schoenbaum SC: Evaluation and management of prosthetic valve endocarditis. *Prog Cardiovasc Dis* 1982;25:43.

95. Wallace RJ Jr, Musser JM, Huss SI: Diversity and sources of rapidly growing mycobacteria associated with infections following cardiac surgery. *J Infect Dis* 1989;159:708.

96. Rumisek JD, Albus RA, Clarke JS: Late *Mycobacterium chelonei* bioprosthetic valve endocarditis activation of implanted contaminant? *Ann Thorac Surg* 1985;39:277.

97. Van den Broek PJ, Lampe AS, Berbee GAM: Epidemic of prosthetic valve endocarditis caused by *Staphylococcus epidermidis. Br Med J* 1985;291:949.

98. Ismail MB, Hannachi N, Abid F, et al: Prosthetic valve endocarditis: A survey. *Br Heart J* 1987;58:72.

99. Meyer DJ, Gerding DN: Favorable prognosis of patients with prosthetic valve endocarditis caused by gram-negative bacilli of the HACEK group. *Am J Med* 1988;85:104.

100. Hortskotte D, Rosin H, Friedrichs W, et al: Contribution for choosing the optimal prophylaxis of bacterial endocarditis. *Eur Heart J* 1987;8(Suppl J):379.

101. Arnett EN, Roberts WC: Prosthetic valve endocarditis. Clinicopathologic analysis of 22 necropsy patients with comparison of observations in 74 necropsy patients with active infective endocarditis involving natural left-sided cardiac valves. *Am J Cardiol* 1976;38:281.

102. Horstkotte D, Schulte HD, Bircks W: Factors influencing prognosis and indication for surgical intervention in acute native-valve endocarditis, in Horstkotte D, Bodnar E (eds): *Current Issues in Heart Valve Disease: Infective Endocarditis.* London, ICR Publisher, 1991, p 171.

103. Rechmann P, Seewald M, Thomas I, et al: Untersuchungen zur Bakteriamie bei zahnarzlichen Eingriffen. *Dtsch Zahnarztl Z* 1986;41:996.

104. Arvay A, Lengyel M: Early operation for infective endocarditis and the activity of infection. *Z Kardiol* 1986;75(Suppl 2):186.

105. Angrist AA, Oka M, Nakoa K: Vegetative endocarditis. *Pathol Ann* 1967;2:155.

106. Muffe A: Prognose der infefktiosen Endokarditis. *FAC* 1987;6:839.

107. Jung JY, Saab SB, Almond CH: The case for early surgical treatment of left-sided primary infective endocarditis: A collective review. *J Thorac Cardiovasc Surg* 1975; 70:509.

108. Madison J, Wang K, Gobel FL, et al: Prosthetic aortic valvular endocarditis. *Circulation* 1975;51:940.

109. Dismukes WE, Karchmer AW: The diagnosis of infected prosthetic heart valves: Bacteremia versus endocarditis, in Duma RJ (ed): *Infections of Prosthetic Heart Valves and Vascular Grafts*. Baltimore, University Park Press, 1976, p 61.

110. Kobasa WD, Kaye KL, Shapiro T, et al: Therapy for experimental endocarditis due to *Staphylococcus epidermidis*. *Rev Infect Dis* 1983;5(Suppl):S533–S537.

111. Crawford HH, Badke FR, Amon KW: Effect of the undisturbed pericardium on left ventricular size and performance during acute volume loading. *Am Heart J* 1983; 105:267.

112. Reeve R, Reeve FJS, Matula G, et al: Mitral obstruction by vegetations of staphylococcal endocarditis. *JAMA* 1974;228:75.

113. Ghosh PK, Miller HJ, Vidne BA: Mitral obstruction in bacterial endocarditis. *Br Heart J* 1985;53:341.

114. Copeland JG, Salomon NW, Stinson EG: Acute mitral valvular obstruction from infective endocarditis: Echocardiographic diagnosis and report of the second successfully treated case. *J Thorac Cardiovasc Surg* 1979;78:128.

115. Wilson WR, Jaumin PM, Danielson GK, et al: Prosthetic valve endocarditis. *Ann Intern Med* 1975;82:751.

116. Petheram IS, Boyce JMH: Prosthetic valve endocarditis: A review of 24 cases. *Thorax* 1977;32:478.

117. Cogwill LD, Addonizio VP, Hopeman AR: Prosthetic valve endocarditis. *Curr Probl Cardiol* 1986;11:623.

118. Horstkotte D, Bircks W, Loogen F: Infective endocarditis of native and prosthetic valves—the case for prompt surgical intervention? A retrospective analysis of factors affecting survival. *Z Kardiol* 1986;75(Suppl 2):168.

119. Anderson DJ, Bulkley BH, Hutchins GM: A clinicopathologic study of prosthetic valve endocarditis in 22 patients: Morphologic basis for diagnosis and therapy. *Am Heart J* 1977;94:325.

120. Cowgill LD, Addonizio P, Hopeman AR, et al: A practical approach to prosthetic valve endocarditis. *Ann Thorac Surg* 1987;43:450.

121. Douglas JL, Cobbs CG: Prosthetic valve endocarditis, in Kaye D (ed): *Infective Endocarditis*, ed 2. New York, Raven Press, 1992, p 301.

122. Quenzer RW, Edwards LD, Levin S: A comparative study of 48 host valves and 24 prosthetic valve endocarditis cases. *Am Heart J* 1976;92:18.

123. Horstkotte D: Prosthetic valve endocarditis, in Horstkotte D, Bodnar E (eds): *Current Issues in Heart Valve Disease: Infective Endocarditis*. London, ICR Publishers, 1991, p 238.

124. Horstkotte D: Prosthetic valve endocarditis, in Horstkotte D, Bodnar E (eds): *Current Issues in Heart Valve Disease: Infective Endocarditis*. London, ICR Publishers, 1991, p 241.

125. Horstkotte D: Prosthetic valve endocarditis, in Horstkotte D, Bodnar E (eds): *Current Issues in Heart Valve Disease: Infective Endocarditis*. London, ICR Publishers, 1991, p 242.

126. Horstkotte D: Prosthetic valve endocarditis, in Horstkotte D, Bodnar E (eds): *Current Issues in Heart Valve Disease: Infective Endocarditis*. London, ICR Publishers, 1991, p 243.

127. Davenport J, Hart RG: Prosthetic valve endocarditis 1976–1987. Antibiotics, anticoagulation, and stroke. *Stroke* 1990;21:993.

128. Heimberger T, Duma R: Infections of prosthetic heart valves and cardiac pacemakers, in Westenfelder GO (ed): Infectious Disease Clin of North America: Infections of prosthetic devices. Philadelphia, WB Saunders, 1989, p 228.

129. Rossiter S, Stinson E, Oyer P: Prosthetic valve endocarditis: Comparison of heterograft tissue valves and mechanical valves. *J Thorac Cardiovasc Surg* 1978;76:795.

130. Sande MA, Johnson WD, Hook EW: Sustained bacteremia in patients with prosthetic cardiac valves. *N Engl Med* 1972;286:1067.

131. Parker FB, Greiner-Hayes C, Tomar RH: Bacteremia following prosthetic valve replacement. *Ann Surg* 1983;197:147.

132. Sands MJ, Lachman AS, O'Reilly DJ: Diagnostic value of cinefluoroscopy in the evaluation of prosthetic heart valve dysfunction. *Am Heart J* 1982;104:622.

133. White AF, Dinsmore RE, Buckley MJ: Cineradiographic evaluation of prosthetic cardiac valves. *Circulation* 1973;48:882.

134. Ellis K, Jaffe C, Malm JR: Infective endocarditis: Roentgenographic considerations. *Radiol Clin North Am* 1973;11:415.

135. Mann T, McLaurin L, Grossman W, et al: Assessing the hemodynamic severity of acute aortic regurgitation due to infective endocarditis. *N Engl J Med* 1975;293:108.

136. Panidis IP, Ross J, Mintz GS: Normal and abnormal prosthetic valve function as seen by Doppler echocardiography. *J Am Coll Cardiol* 1986;8:317.

137. McFadden M, Gonzalez-Lavin L, Remington JS: Limited reliability of the "negative" two-dimensional echocardiogram in the evaluation of infective vegetative endocarditis: Diagnostic and surgical implications. *J Cardiovasc Surg* 1985;26:59.

138. Chesler E, Korns ME, Porter GE, et al: False aneurysm of the left ventricle secondary to bacterial endocarditis with perforation of the mitral-aortic intervalvular fibrosa. *Circulation* 1968;37:518.

139. Come PC, Riley MF: Echocardiographic recognition of perivalvular infection complicating aortic bacterial endocarditis. *Am Heart J* 1984;108:166.

140. Ellis SG, Goldstein J, Popp RL: Detection of endocarditis associated perivalvular abscess by two-dimensional echocardiography. *J Am Coll Cardiol* 1985;5:647.

141. Mugge A: Prognose der infektiösen Endokarditis. *FAC* 1987;6:839.

142. Stafford WJ, Petch J, Raford DJ: Vegetations in infective endocarditis. *Br Heart J* 1985;53:310.

143. Erbel R, Rohmann S, Drexler M: Improved diagnostic value of echocardiography in patients with infective endocarditis by transesophageal approach. A prospective study. *Eur Heart J* 1988;9:43.

144. Gussenhoven EJ, Taams MA, Roelundt JRT: Transesophageal two-dimensional echocardiography: Its role in solving clinical problems. *J Am Coll Cardiol* 1986;8:975.

145. Mugge A, Daniel WG, Frank G, et al: Echocardiography in infective endocarditis: Reassessment of prognostic implications of vegetation size determined by the transthoracic and the transesophageal approach. *J Am Coll Cardiol* 1989;14:631.

146. Carnier B, Vitoux B, Starkman C: Value of transesophageal echocardiography. From a preliminary experience of 532 cases. *Arch Mal Coeur* 1990;82:23.

147. Daniel WG, Mugge A, Martin RP: Improvement in the diagnosis of abscesses associated with endocarditis by transesophageal echocardiography. *N Engl J Med* 1991;324:795.

148. Gonzalez Vilchez FJ, Martin Duran R, Delgado Ramis C, et al: Endocarditis infecciosa activa complicada con absceso paravavular. *Rev Esp Cardiol* 1991;44:648.

149. Khan SS, Gray RJ: Valvular emergencies. University of California, School of Medicine, Los Angeles. *Cardiol Clin* 1991;9:689.

150. Lengyel M, Temesvari A: Clinical use of biplane transesophageal endocardiography. *Orszagos Kardiologiai Intezet Budapest Ory Hetil* 1992;133:1029.

151. Kalish SB, Goldschmidt R, Li C, et al: Infective endocarditis caused by *Paecilomyces varioti. Am J Clin Pathol* 1982;78:249.

152. Lichtlen PR, Gahl K, Daniel WG: Infectious endocarditis: Clinical aspects and diagnosis. *Schweiz Med Wochenschr* 1984;114:1566.

153. DeMaria AN, King JF, Salel AF: Echography and phonography of acute aortic regurgitation in bacterial endocarditis. *Ann Intern Med* 1975;82:329.

154. King ME, Weyman AR: Echocardiographic findings in infective endocarditis. *Cardiovasc Clin* 1983;13:147.

155. Thivolle P, Varenne L, Heyden Y, et al: Gallium-67 citrate whole body scanning for localization of infected vascular synthetic grafts. *Clin Nucl Med* 1985;19:330.

156. Cerqueira MD, Jacobson AF: Indium 111 leukocyte scientigraphic detection of myocardial abscess formation in patients with endocarditis. *J Nucl Med* 1989;30:703.

157. Nunez L, de la Llana R, Aguado MG, et al: Bioprosthetic valve endocarditis: Indicators for surgical intervention. *Ann Thorac Surg* 1983;35:262.

158. Horstkotte D, Aul C, Seipel L: Einfluß von Klappentyp und Klappenfunktion auf die chronische intravasale Hamolyse nach Mitral und Aortenklappenersatz. *Z Kardiol* 1983;72:119.

159. Wilson WR, Geraci JE, Danielson GU: Anticoagulant therapy and central nervous system complications in patients with prosthetic valve endocarditis. *Circulation* 1978; 57:1004.

160. Carpenter JC, McAllister CU, US Army Collaborative Group: Anticoagulation in prosthetic valve endocarditis. *South Med J* 1983;76:1372.

161. Davenport J, Hart RG: Prosthetic valve endocarditis 1976–1986. Antibiotics, anticoagulation and stroke. *Stroke* 1990;21:993.

162. Durack DT, Beeson PB: Pathogenesis of infective endocarditis, in Rahimtoola SH (ed): *Infective Endocarditis.* New York, Grune and Stratton, 1978, p 33.

163. Archer GL: Antimicrobial susceptibility and selection of resistance among *Staphylococcus epidermidis* isolates recovered from patients with infections of indwelling foreign devices. *Antimicrob Agents Chemother* 1978;14:353.

164. Karchmer AW, Archer GL, Dismukes WE: *Staphylococcus epidermidis* causing prosthetic valve endocarditis; microbiologic and clinical observations as guides to therapy. *Ann Intern Med* 1983;98:447.

165. Archer GL, Johnston JL, Vazquez GJ, et al: Efficacy of antibiotic combinations including rifampin against methicillin-resistant *Staphylococcus epidermidis:* In vitro and in vivo studies. *Rev Infect Dis* 1983;5(Suppl):S538.

166. Karchmer AW: Treatment of prosthetic valve endocarditis, in Sande MA, Root R (eds): *Endocarditis.* New York, Churchill Livingstone, 1985, p 163.

167. Karchmer AW, Archer GA, the Endocarditis Study Group: Methicillin-resistant *Staphylococcus epidermidis* prosthetic valve endocarditis: A therapeutic trial (476). In *Programs and Abstracts of the Twenty-Fourth Interscience Conference on Antimicrobial Agents and Chemotherapy,* Washington, DC, 1984.

168. Karchmer AW, Archer GL, Dismukes WE: *Staphylococcus epidermidis* causing prosthetic valve endocarditis: Microbiologic and clinical observations as guides to therapy. *Ann Intern Med* 1983;98:447.

169. Bisno AL, Dismukes WE, Durack DT: Antimicrobial treatment of infective endocarditis due to viridans streptococci, enterococci, and staphylococci. *JAMA* 1989;261:1471.

170. Tuazon CU, Gill V, Gill F: Streptococcal endocarditis: Single vs. combination antibiotic therapy and role of various species. *Rev Infect Dis* 1986;8:54.

171. Wilson WR, Giuliani ER, Geraci JR: Treatment of penicillin-sensitive streptococcal infective endocarditis. *Mayo Clin Proc* 1982;57:95.

172. Moellering RC, Korzeniowski OM, Sande MA: Species specific: resistance to antomicrobial synergism in *Streptococcus faecium* and *Streptococcus faecalis. J Infect Dis* 1979; 140:203.

173. Harwick HJ, Halmanson GN, Guze LB: In vitro activity of ampicillin or vancomycin combined with gentamicin or streptomycin against enterococci. *Antimicrob Agents Chemother* 1973;4:383.

174. Oster HS, Kong TQ: *Bacillus cereus* endocarditis involving a prosthetic valve. *South Med J* 1982;75:508.

175. Murry BS, Karchmer AW, Moellering RC Jr: Diphtheroid prosthetic valve endocarditis: A study of clinical features and infecting organisms. *Am J Med* 1980;69:838.

176. Rubinstein E, Noriega ER, Simberkoff MS, et al: Tissue penetration of amphotericin B in *Candida* endocarditis. *Chest* 1974;66:376.

177. Utley JR, Mills J, Roe BB: The role of valve replacement in the treatment of fungal endocarditis. *J Thorac Cardiovasc Surg* 1975;69:255.

178. Nathwani D, Reid TM, Gould IM, et al: An open study of teicoplanin in the treatment of gram-positive infections. Infection Unit, City Hospital, Aberdeen Scotland. *J Chemother* 1991;3:315.

179. Tingleff J, Arendrup H, Pettersson G: Surgical repair of a postendocarditis abscess cavity in the heart guided by intraoperative transesophageal echocardiography. *Eur J Cardiothorac Surg* 1992;6:106.

180. Oakley C: Treatment of prosthetic valve endocarditis. *J Antimicrob Chemother* 1987; 20:181.

181. Skehan JD, Murray M, Mills PG: Infective endocarditis: Incidence and mortality in the North East Thames Region. *Br Heart J* 1988;59:62.

182. Leport C, Vilde JL, Bricaire F, et al: Fifty cases of late prosthetic valve endocarditis: Improvement in prognosis over a 15 year period. *Br Heart J* 1987;58:66.

183. Horstkotte D, Korfer R, Loogen F, et al: Prosthetic valve endocarditis: Clinical findings and management. *Eur Heart J* 1984;5(Suppl C):117.

184. Alsip SG, Blackstone EH, Kirklin JW: Indications for cardiac surgery in patients with infective endocarditis. *Am J Med* 1985;78(6B):138.

185. Saffle JR, Gardner P, Schoenbaum SC, et al: Prosthetic valve endocarditis: A case for prompt valve replacement. *J Thorac Cardiovasc Surg* 1977;73:416.

186. Gagliardi C, Di Tommaso L, Mastroroberto P, et al: Bioprosthetic valve endocarditis: Factors affecting bad outcome. *J Cardiovasc Surg* 1991;32:800.

187. Murayama H, Takahara Y, Nakada I, et al: A case report of early prosthetic valve endocarditis due to methicillin resistant *Staphylococcus aureus* infection—an experience of intraatrial implantation of mitral prostheses with a Gore-Tex flange. *Nippon Kyobu Geka Gaddai Zasshi* 1991;39:1803.

188. Ketosugbo AD, Basu S, Greengart A, et al: Aortoventriculoplasty in the management of an infected Cabrol graft. *Ann Thorac Surg* 1992;53:892.

189. Tingleff J, Arendrup H, Pettersson G: Surgical repair of a postendocarditis abscess cavity in the heart guided by intraoperative transesophageal echocardiography. *Eur J Cardiothorac Surg* 1992;6:106.

190. Glazier JJ, Verwilghen J, Donaldson RM, et al: Treatment of complicated aortic valve endocarditis with annular abscess formation by homograft aortic root replacement. *J Am Coll Cardiol* 1991;17:1177.

11

Pediatric Endocarditis

The surgical treatment of congenital cardiac disease has led to an increase in the frequency of infective endocarditis in young children. Although the disease is more common in adults, its incidence in youngsters was about 1 in 4,500 admissions to hospitals prior to 1963.[1,2] Since then, it has increased among hospitalized children to 1 per 2,000.[3–6] The frequency of this disease continues to trend upward among the pediatric age group.[7] In the last two decades the average age of children with endocardial infection has increased from 5 to 13 years.[3,4,8,9]

Although still relatively uncommon, infective endocarditis also appears to be increasing in incidence among neonates.[10–14] Autopsy studies have indicated that the frequency of the disease in newborns is about 3%.[15] The clinical presentation is often atypical. Postmortem examination is the most reliable approach to establishing the diagnosis of endocardial disease in these patients.

Although any structural cardiac abnormality may predispose children to the development of infective endocarditis, congenital heart disease is presently the most common cause (80% of cases)[4,6,9,16–19] (Table 11.1). This is in sharp contrast to the experience over the first four decades of the present century, when acute or chronic rheumatic fever was the disease on which

Table 11.1. Underlying Heart Disease in 266 Children with Infective Heart Disease

Congenital heart disease		78%
Tetralogy of Fallot	24%	
Ventricular septal defect	16%	
Congenital aortic stenosis	8%	
Patent ductus arteriosus	7%	
Transposition of the great vessels	4%	
Other causes	19%	
Rheumatic heart disease		14%
No heart disease		8%

Source: Adapted from Ref. 4.

infective endocarditis was superimposed in 50% of patients. Although presently uncommon, rheumatic fever continues to play a role in the pathogenesis of infective endocarditis in about 3–4% of youngsters.

Cyanotic cardiac disease, for example the tetralogy of Fallot, is becoming a more frequent contributing factor.[20] This predisposes babies with systemic pulmonary shunts to the development of infective endocarditis. Eight of 12 youngsters who were operated on for a shunt developed endocardial infection postoperatively.[21] Eight percent of children with the tetralogy of Fallot who received a Potts shunt became infected.[22] Since 1972, less than 1% of those who underwent surgery for correction of the tetralogy have been affected by infective endocarditis. Abut 10% of those with a ventricular septal defect (VSD) developed endocardial disease before they were 30 years old. This was the case in less than 2% of those who had undergone cardiac surgery.[23] However operative intervention may increase the risk of infective valvular disease in patients who undergo valvulotomy for aortic stenosis: 1.4% without surgery compared to 7.4% postoperatively.

Mitral valve prolapse appears to play a role in the pathogenesis of infective endocarditis in children[24,25]; surgery may increase the risk. Over 50% of pediatric patients with prolapsed mitral valves have undergone cardiac catheterization or a variety of surgical procedures.[9,18,26,27]

From 8% to 12% of children with infective endocarditis are free of underlying cardiac disease[2,17]; this is a more common situation in neonates.[11,12–14] The presence of intravascular devices (e.g., ventriculoatrial shunts and cental lines) may be responsible for the infection of a normal valve especially the tricuspid.[8,26–31]

A number of factors are involved in the pathogenesis of infective endocarditis in young children. The sequence of events is as follows: Initially, a sterile fibrin-platelet thrombus develops on the low-pressure side of the gradient across a septal defect or valve.[32] This is followed by an episode of bacteremia that can seed the matrix of fibrin. The surface of the pulmonary valve or the main pulmonary artery is the site of endocarditis in individuals with the tetralogy of Fallot. Infection develops on the pulmonary side of a systemic-pulmonary shunt or patent ductus arteriosus. Endocardial infection in individuals with a VSD is located on the right side of the ventricular defect or on the septal leaflet of the tricuspid or pulmonary valve. The smaller the defect, the higher the risk of developing endocardial infection. This is so because the pressure differential between the ventricles is highest when the hole in the septum is small. Aortic regurgitation increases significantly the risk of endocardial infection in the setting of a VSD.

The use of intravascular lines and catheters has led to an increase in the incidence of infective endocarditis in neonates. In this setting, the disease involves primarily the tricuspid or pulmonary valves. This is most likely related to the frequent use of umbilical or central venous catheters that traumatize valvular surfaces. It is important to distinguish infective endocardial disease from nonbacterial thrombotic endocarditis in newborn infants. Among the complications are (1) damage to the endothelium of the valvular leaflets; (2) irritation of the ventricular surfaces produced by intravascular lines; (3) hypoxia of the tissues; and (4) disseminated intravascular coagulation induced by hypoxia.[15]

A small number of sterile valvular thrombi are infected in the course of the bacteremia caused by *S. aureus* or *S. epidermidis*. Streptococcal species and other gram-positive organisms (e.g., *S. pneumoniae*, *S. aureus*, and *S. epidermidis*) account for about 90% of cases of infective endocarditis in children; 40% are caused by *S. viridans*, an incidence similar to that in adults. Infection by this organism is uncommon in patients younger than 4 years. This is probably related to the low incidence of periodontal disease, the primary source of bacteremia caused by *S. viridans*.[2,19,20,33–35,49]

Subacute and acute infective endocarditis are usually caused by the organisms described above.[36] The incidence of infection caused by *S. viridans* in children decreased during the 1980s.[21] It has been replaced by *S. aureus*. Enterococcal endocarditis is uncommon in children because infection of the urinary tract, the source of enterococcal bacteremia, is rare in this age group.[37]

Nutritionally variant streptococci (NVS)[38,39] have become important in the pathogenesis of infective endocarditis. These organisms now require consideration in the evaluation of children with culture-negative disease or infection that appears to be caused by *S. viridans* but fails to respond to therapy with adequate doses of penicillin.[39] Treatment with this agent plus an aminoglycoside is usually required to cure endocardial disease caused by NVS.

Since effective antimicrobial agents became available, group A and B beta-hemolytic streptococci have become rare causes of infective endocarditis. Although bacteremia with group B organisms is common in neonates, very few develop endocardial disease.[40–42]

S. pneumoniae caused 10–15% of cases of infective endocarditis in children before antimicrobial agents were available. This organism is presently responsible for only 1% of the disease in youngsters. However, it is responsible for about 6% of bacteremia in infants.

Infective endocarditis caused by the pneumococcus usually produces rapidly progressive disease that involves the aortic and mitral valves. It infects children with normal hearts. The fatality rate in youngsters infected by this organism is approximately 60%.[43–45] Concurrent meningitis or pneumonia has been well described.

S. aureus is the second most common cause of infective endocarditis in children.[2,17] It is also the organism most often involved in infections following cardiac surgery in youngsters. Disease caused by the staphylococci has been increasing in frequency as the use of invasive medical devices has increased. Infection by *S. epidermidis* has also become more common. This organism has a striking tendency to infect prolapsed mitral valves in children.[46]

Although *H. influenzae* is the second most common cause of bacteremia in youngsters, it is rarely involved in the development of infective endocarditis.[47–49] *H. parainfluenzae* and *H. aphrophilus* are more often responsible for the development of this disease in children.[50]

Clinical Features

The clinical presentation of infective endocarditis in children is determined by factors similar to those in adults (Table 11.2). These include (1) the nature of the organism involved; (2) the presence of metastatic infection; and (3) the development of immune complexes. Infective endocarditis may present as acute sepsis or as an indolent immunologically mediated disease.[5,9,18,20,51,52] The interval between the onset of symptoms and the establishment of the diagnosis ranges from 5 to 8 weeks.[2,21,52,53] Although fever is the cardinal manifestation of infective endocarditis in children, it may be absent in 10%. More often, it is intermittent or so low-grade that the severity of the disease is not appreciated.[54] Antimicrobial therapy for what appears to be an unimportant minor illness may delay the diagnosis of infective endocarditis.

Because most endocardial infections in children are superimposed on congenital cardiac disease, the presence of a murmur may not be diagnostic. Fewer than 40% of youngsters with endocarditis present with a new or changing murmur.[2] The central nervous system is involved in about 25%.[35] Among the disorders that complicate the clinical course of the disease are hemiplegia, seizures, and a variety of focal neurological defects. Splenomegaly is present in about 50%. Mucocutaneous manifestations include Osler's nodes, Janeway lesions, and Roth spots. These are less common in children than in adults and are absent in neonates.[55] About 20% of young-

Table 11.2. Clinical Manifestations of Bacterial Endocarditis in Children

Symptom	Average Percentage	Physical Findings	Average Percentage
Fever	90	Fever	90
Malaise	55	Splenomegaly	55
Anorexia/weight loss	31	Petechiae	33
Heart failure	30	Embolic phenomenoa	28
Arthralgia	24	New heart murmur or change in existing murmur	24
Neurological phenomena	18	Clubbing	14
Gastrointestinal phenomena	16	Osler nodes	7
Chest pain	9	Roth spots	5
		Janeway lesion	5
		Splinter hemorrhages	5

Source: Adapted from Ref. 4.

sters with infective endocarditis die; this incidence increases to 50% in neonates.[4,28]

References

1. Zakrewski T, Keith JD: Bacterial endocarditis in infants and children. *J Pediatr* 1965;67:1179.
2. Johnson DH, Rosenthal A, Nadas A: A forty-year review of bacterial endocarditis in infancy and childhood. *Circulation* 1975;51:581.
3. Parras F, Bouza A, Romero J: Infectious endocarditis in children. *Pediatr Cardiol* 1990;11:7.
4. Starke J: Infection of the heart: Infective endocarditis, in Feigin R, Cherry J (eds): *Pediatric Infectious Disease*, ed 3. Philadelphia, WB Saunders, 1992, p 326.
5. Sholler GF, Hawker RE, Celermajer JM: Infective endocarditis in childhood. *Pediatr Cardiol* 1986;6:183.
6. Coutlee F, Carceller A, Deschamps L, et al: The evolving pattern of pediatric endocarditis from 1960 to 1985. *Can J Cardiol* 1990;6:164.
7. Blumenthal S, Griffiths SP, Morgan BC: Bacterial endocarditis in children with heart disease: A review based on the literature and experience with 58 cases. *Pediatrics* 1960;26:993.
8. Geva T, Frand M: Infective endocarditis in children with congenital heart disease: The changing spectrum, 1965–85. *Eur Heart J* 1988;9:1244.
9. Stanton BF, Baltimore RS, Clemens JD: Changing spectrum of infective endocarditis in children. *Am J Dis Child* 1984;138:720.
10. Blieden LC, Morehead RR, Burke B: Bacterial endocarditis in the neonate. *Am J Dis Child* 1972;124:747.
11. Edwards K, Ingall D, Czapek E: Bacterial endocarditis in 4 young infants. Is this complication on the increase? *Clin Pediatr* 1977;16:607.
12. McGuinness GA, Schieken RM, Maguire GF: Endocarditis in the newborn. *Am J Dis Child* 1980;134:577.
13. Millard DD, Shulman ST: The changing spectrum of neonatal endocarditis. *Clin Perinatol* 1988;15:587.
14. O'Callaghan C, McDougall P: Infective endocarditis in neonates. *Arch Dis Child* 1988;63:53.
15. Symchych PS, Krauss AW, Winchester P: Endocarditis following intracardiac placement of umbilical venous catheters in neonates. *J Pediatr* 1977;90:287.
16. Schollin J, Bjarke B, Wesstrom G: Follow-up study on children with infective endocarditis. *Acta Paediatr Scand* 1989;78:615.
17. Kaplan EL, Rich H, Gersony W: A collaborative study of infective endocarditis in the 1970's. Emphasis on infections in patients who have undergone cardiovascular surgery. *Circulation* 1979;59:327.
18. Van Hare GF, Ben-Shachar G, Liebman J, et al: Infective endocarditis in infants and children during the past 10 years: A decade of change. *Am Heart J* 1984;107:1235.
19. Channer KS, Joffe HS, Jordan SC: Presentation of infective endocarditis in childhood and adolescence. *J R Coll Physicians London* 1989;23:152.
20. Blumenthal S, Griffith SP, Morgan BC: Bacterial endocarditis in children with congenital heart disease. *Pediatrics* 1960;26:993.
21. Kramer H, Horstkotte D, Rammos S: Bacterial endocarditis in infancy, childhood and adolescence, in Horstkotte D, Bodnar E (eds): *Infective Endocarditis*. London, ICR Publishers, 1991, p 137.
22. Kaplan S, Helmworth JA, Ahern EN: Results of palliative procedures for tetralogy of Fallot in infants and young children. *Ann Thorac Surg* 1968;5:489.
23. Gersony WM, Hayes CJ: Bacterial endocarditis in patients with pulmonary stenosis, aortic stenosis, or ventricular septal defect. *Circulation* 1977;56(Suppl 1):84.

24. Nolan CM, Kane JJ, Grunow WA: Infective endocarditis and mitral prolapse: A comparison with other types of endocarditis. *Arch Intern Med* 1981;141:447.

25. Clemens JO, Horwitz RI, Jaffee CC: A controlled evaluation of the risk of bacterial endocarditis in persons with mitral valve prolapse. *N Engl J Med* 1982;307:776.

26. Karl T, Wensley D, Stark J, et al: Infective endocarditis in children with congenital heart disease: Comparison of selected features in patients with surgical correction of palliation and those without. *Br Heart J* 1987;58:57.

27. Yu LC, Greene G, Sperling D, et al: Infective endocarditis following cardiac catheterization in infancy. *Clin Pediatr* 1986;25:222.

28. Oelberg DG, Fisher DJ, Gross DM, et al: Endocarditis in high-risk neonates. *Pediatrics* 1983;71:392.

29. Musewe N, Hecht B, Hesslin P: Tricuspid valve endocarditis in two children with normal hearts: Diagnosis and therapy of unusual clinical entity. *J Pediatr* 1987;110:733.

30. Wheeler JG, Weesner KM: *Staphylococcus aureus* endocarditis and pericarditis in an infant with a central venous catheter. *Clin Pediatr* 1984;23:46.

31. Noel GJ, L'Loughlin JE, Edelson PJ: Neonatal *Staphylococcus epidermidis* right-sided endocarditis: Description of five catheterized infants. *Pediatrics* 1988;82:234.

32. Roberts WC: Characteristics and consequences of infective endocarditis (active or healed or both) learned from morphologic studies, in Rahimtoola SH (ed): *Infective Endocarditis*. New York, Grune and Stratton, 1977, p 55.

33. Rosenthal A, Nadas AS: Infective endocarditis in infancy and childhood, in Rahimtoola SH (ed): *Infective Endocarditis*. New York, Grune and Stratton, 1977, p 149.

34. Johnson DH, Rosenthal A, Nadas A: Bacterial endocarditis in children under 2 years of age. *Am J Dis Child* 1975;129:183.

35. Mendelsohn G, Hutchins GM: Infective endocarditis during the first decade of life. *Am J Dis Child* 1979;133:619.

36. Hosea SW: Virulent *Streptococcus viridans* bacterial endocarditis. *Am Heart J* 1981; 101:174.

37. Teixeira OH, Carpenter B, Vlad P: Enterococcal endocarditis in early infancy. *Can Med Assoc J* 1982;127:612.

38. Narasimhan SL, Weinstein AJ: Infective endocarditis due to a nutritionally deficient streptococcus. *J Pediatr* 1980;96:61.

39. Stein DS, Nelson KE: Endocarditis due to nutritionally deficient streptococci: Therapeutic dilemma. *Rev Infect Dis* 1987;9:908.

40. Agarwala BN: Group B streptococcal endocarditis in a neonate. *Pediatr Cardiol* 1988;9:51.

41. Gallagher PG, Watanakunakorn C: Group B streptococcal endocarditis: Report of seven cases and review of the literature. *Rev Infect Dis* 1986;8:175.

42. Backes RJ, Wilson WR, Geraci JE: Group B streptococcal infective endocarditis. *Arch Intern Med* 1985;145:693.

43. Jackson MJ, Rutledge J: Pneumococcal endocarditis in children. *Pediatr Infect Dis* 1982;1:120.

44. Teele DW, Pelton SI, Grant MJA: Bacteremia in febrile children under 2 years of age: Results of cultures of blood of 600 consecutive febrile children seen in a "walk-in" clinic. *J Pediatr* 1975;87:227.

45. Elward K, Hruby N, Christy C: Pneumococcal endocarditis in infants and children: Report of a case and review of the literature. *Pediatr Infect Dis J* 1990;9:652.

46. Baddour LM, Phillips TN, Bisno AL: Coagulase-negative staphylococcal endocarditis: Occurrence in patients with mitral valve prolapse. *Arch Intern Med* 1986;146:119.

47. Callanan DL, Bermudez OB, Stull TL: Valvular insufficiency after bacteriologic cure of *Haemophilus influenzae* endocarditis in a child. *Pediatr Infect Dis J* 1987;6:865.

48. Danford DA, Kugler JD, Cheatham JP: *Hemophilus influenzae* endocarditis: Successful treatment with ampicillin and early valve replacement. *Neb Med J* 1984;38:88.

49. Marinell PV, Diana DJ, Todd WA: Survival of a child after *Hemophilus influenzae* B endocarditis. *Pediatr Infect Dis J* 1983;2:46.

50. Lynn DC, Kane JG, Parker RH: *Haemophilus parainfluenzae* endocarditis: A review of forty cases. *Medicine* 1977;56:115.

51. Cutler JG, Ongley PA, Schwachman H: Bacterial endocarditis in children with heart disease. *Pediatrics* 1958;22:706.
52. John CM, Rhodes KH: Pediatric endocarditis. *Mayo Clin Proc* 1982;57:86.
53. Schollin J, Bjarke B, Wesstrom G: Infective endocarditis in Swedish children. II. Location, major complications, laboratory findings, delay of treatment, treatment and outcome. *Acta Paediatr Scand* 1986;74:999.
54. Kramer HH, Bourgeois M, Liersch R, et al: Current clinical aspects of bacterial endocarditis in infancy, childhood and adolescence. *Eur M Pediatr* 1983;140:253.
55. Libman E, Friedberg C: *Subacute Bacterial Endocarditis,* ed 2. New York, Oxford University Press, 1948.

12

Diagnosis

Persistent bacteremia is the hallmark of infective endocarditis. The number of organisms present in the circulation is usually less than 30 cfu/ml.[1] Recovery of bacteria from the bloodstream suggests, but does not prove, the presence of endocardial infection because bacteremia may be a feature of many other infectious disorders.[2-5] Refinement of the diagnostic criteria for establishing the presence of infective endocarditis and improvement in the methods employed to culture blood have led to increased recognition of the disease.[6,7]

Among the disorders that resemble infective endocarditis, but in which the blood may be sterile, are (1) infections caused by *Brucella, Haemophilus,* and nutritionally variant streptococci (NVS); (2) disease that involves the right side of the heart; (3) mural endocarditis; (4) atral myxoma; and (5) nonbacterial thrombotic (marantic) endocardial disease.

The major reasons for the sterility of blood cultures in patients with endocardial infection are (1) the institution of treatment prior to obtaining cultures of blood and other sites; (2) therapy before a prosthetic valve is replaced; and (3) difficulty in identifying bacteria that are difficult to grow.

Although false-negative cultures of blood are presently infrequent, they may increase in number over time. This is so for the following reasons: (1) the indiscriminate use of antibiotics; (2) the increased placement of prosthetic cardiac valves; and (3) the increased number of immunosuppressed patients prone to develop infections caused by organisms difficult to culture.[8-17]

Treatment prior to obtaining cultures of the blood is responsible for the failure to recover organisms from the circulation in many cases. Pesanti and Smith[3] reported that about two-thirds of their patients with sterile blood had received an antibiotic. The bacteremia associated with streptococcal endocarditis is easily suppressed in the absence of treatment. A study of 789 cultures of blood drawn from 206 patients with streptococcal valvular infection was carried out by Werner et al.[18] in the mid-1960s. The initial culture of blood grew the organism in 96% of individuals. The first two cultures yielded streptococci in 98% of the patients.

Sixty-four percent of cultures of blood obtained from patients with endocardial infection pretreated with antibiotics failed to yield the infecting organism.[5] In those not given any antimicrobial agents, the incidence of positive cultures was 100%. Administration of an anti-infective agent led to sterility of the blood within 2–3 days. However, when treatment was discontinued, the cultures became positive within 48 hr. When treatment was continued over an extended period and then withdrawn, cultures remained sterile for several weeks.[19] Another study[3] disclosed that 62% of patients with endocarditis who had received an antibiotic had sterile specimens.

Inadequate therapy in terms of the duration, dose, and effectiveness of an antibiotic often masks the clinical activity of infective endocarditis. A suboptimal dose of an antibiotic inhibits the multiplication of bacteria in the bloodstream but not deep within cardiac vegetations. When therapy is discontinued, the organism makes its way to the surface of the vegetation and reappears in the blood.

Individuals with suspected endocarditis who have recently been given antibiotics must have cultures of the blood taken 48 hr after treatment has been discontinued. When this procedure fails to identify the infectious agent, a second group of cultures of blood must be obtained 7–10 days later. If these do not detect an organism, a disease other than infective endocarditis may be present (Table 12.1).

A delay of a week in initiating treatment is acceptable in individuals with subacute infective endocarditis because death is uncommon early in the course of the disease. Most likely, the patient by this time has been partially treated for most of the complications of the disease. The emboli that appear early in the course of infective endocarditis are not prevented by treatment with antimicrobial agents.

The addition of a resin to cultures of the blood makes it possible to retrieve organisms from patients receiving antimicrobial therapy.[20] This markedly increases the possibility of detecting bacteremia, especially that caused by *S. aureus*. The resin may remove up to 100 μg/ml of an antibiotic from the culture medium. However, the disadvantage is an increase in the turbidity of the medium to a level that interferes with visual inspection. Repeated subcultures present a small but important risk of contamination.

Sulfopolyanetholsulfonate (SPS), an anticoagulant, is usually added to media into which organisms have been inoculated.[21–24] SPS interferes with the antimicrobial activity of lysozyme and complement, disrupts phagocytosis, and blocks the activity of the aminoglycosides. However, this agent interferes with multiplication of some organisms (e.g., *Neisseria*). When both a resin and SPS are present in a medium, less than a 1 to 10 dilution of blood should be added.[23]

The lysis-centrifugation system is useful in detecting bacteria, mycobacteria, and fungi present in the blood. This technique disrupts red and white blood cells and the organisms they contain. The resulting lysate is concen-

Table 12.1. Laboratory Findings in Patients with Infective Endocarditis

Manifestation	Percent of Patients
Hematological	
Anemia	70–90
Leukocytosis	20–30
Leukopenia	5–15
Thrombocytopenia	5–15
Elevated erythrocyte sedimentation rate	90–100
Renal	
Red cell casts	12
Proteinuria	50–65
Microscopic hematuria	30–50
Elevated serum creatinine level	10–20
Immunological	
Hypergammaglobulinemia	20–30
Cryoglobulinemia	20–95
Positive rheumatoid factor	5–50
Circulating immune complexes	65–100
Low serum complement level	5–40
Positive blood cultures	80–100

Source: from Kaye K, Kaye D: Laboratory findings including blood cultures, in Kaye D (ed): *Infective Endocarditis,* ed 2. New York, Raven Press, 1992, p 20.

trated by centrifugation and cultured on appropriate media. This is especially helpful in detecting intracellular organisms such as *Legionella* species, *Brucella* species, various fungi, and *S. aureus*. It is less useful for retrieving *S. pneumoniae, Haemophilus* species, and other aerobic and anaerobic organisms.[21]

Cultures of blood may fail to detect the bacteremia of infective endocarditis. Among the reasons for this are (1) an inadequate volume of blood for culture; (2) too few cultures; (3) a shortened period of incubation; and (4) failure to recognize the need for incubation at a low concentration of oxygen for anaerobic organisms. Because the number of bacteria in the blood of patients with subacute infective endocarditis is low (less than 100 cfu in about 85% of patients),[1] at least 10 ml of blood is best used for culture. The 1:10 ratio of blood to broth may provide an optimal dilution because it inhibits the antibacterial activity of many antibiotics and preexisting antibodies. Trypticase soy or thioglycolate broth is used to grow aerobic and anaerobic organisms. With rare exceptions, all cultures must be incubated at 37°C, frequently subcultured, and examined macroscopically or by radionuclides that detect microbial growth very early. Routine subculture of anaerobes is required in some situations, especially when *H. influenzae* may be involved. Vented (aerobic) bottles must always be subcultured after 16–18 hr of incubation. The use of biphasic media eliminates the need for subculture.[25,26] Hypertonic media may be useful in detecting cell wall–deficient organisms. A difference of 35% between the concentration of bacteria in mixed venous and arterial blood has been reported by Beeson et al.[1] However, there is no evidence that blood drawn from an artery rather than a vein is a better source of organisms.

A single positive culture of blood may represent either a valid result or contamination. This is a problem in severely ill children in whom a single culture of blood grows *S. aureus* and in patients with a prosthetic valve in whom a single culture grows *S. epidermidis*.

There is considerable controversy concerning the optimal number and timing of blood cultures required to identify infective endocarditis. Belli and Waisbren[25] stated that at least five cultures of blood are required to detect infective endocarditis. This conclusion was based on their observation that only 82% of three cultures of blood contained the organism responsible for the disease. The time at which blood for culture is drawn is less important because the bacteremia associated with subacute disease is continuous.[1]

Because fever appears about 2 hr after bacteremia develops, the optimal time for obtaining cultures is before the temperature begins to rise. This lag represents the time required for the production of endogenous pyrogens by leukocytes and macrophages. When the temperature increases 1°C, blood for culture is drawn every 5–6 min until six cultures have been obtained; three cultures drawn in this fashion usually disclose the organism.[19]

Blood for culture must be obtained under strictly sterile conditions. The site of venipuncture must be cleansed, first with alcohol and then with iodine (2%) or an iodophor less irritating to the skin.[26] The disinfectant must remain on the skin for about 1 min before venipuncture is undertaken. Blood must not be drawn through intravascular lines because it may be contaminated.[26] Replacement of the needle first used to obtain the blood is not necessary before injection into the media.[27]

Neisseria species and members of the HACEK group multiply easily in a 5–10% atmosphere of CO_2. NVS grow in media that contain pyridoxal hydrochloride or 2-cystine. *Brucella* species require special methods for culture (e.g., the Castaneda technique) and incubation in an atmosphere of CO_2. Culture in buffered charcoal and yeast extract agar with added alpha-ketoglutarate is required for the growth of *Legionella*.

Too short a period of incubation is often responsible for failure to retrieve some organisms. Most grow well in blood cultures in less than 1 week; some require a significantly longer period. The HACEK group requires 3 weeks of incubation and *Brucella* species 6 weeks in an atmosphere of CO_2.

Cultures of the blood of patients with fungal infective endocarditis are often sterile.[28] About 50% of the disease caused by various species of *Candida* is associated with fungemia. *Aspergillus* and *Histoplasma* are rarely recovered from the bloodstream.[25] Fungal endocarditis must be considered in patients who present with many of the signs and symptoms of endocardial infection but whose cultures of the blood are sterile and who fail to respond to standard antimicrobial therapy. Cultures of the bone marrow may be the only source of fungi, mycobacteria, and brucellae.[4]

It has been estimated that about 50% of positive cultures of blood are contaminated.[29–32] Because it is difficult for clinicians to ignore a microorganism growing in the blood especially when severely ill patients are involved, antimicrobial therapy has been initiated unnecessarily. Bates and Lee[29] developed a method to aid the clinician in deciding whether or not an initial positive culture of the blood represented a true infection. They noted that the independent predicters of bacteremia are (1) the type of organism involved; (2) the period required for cultures to grow; (3) multiple positive cultures of blood; and (4) the severity of the illness. Examination of peripheral blood for intraleukocytic organisms has been helpful occasionally but cannot be accepted as a routine diagnostic procedure.[33] This should be considered in patients with culture-negative endocarditis.

Serological studies are useful in establishing the diagnosis of infective endocarditis caused by organisms difficult, if not impossible, to retrieve from routine cultures. Among these are *Coxiella burnetii, Chlamydia, Cryptococcus, Brucella, Candida,* and *Legionella*.[13] The available serological tests for *C. albicans* are of little clinical value. Increasing titers of precipitating and agglutinating antibodies do not always indicate infection in a recently implanted prosthetic valve.[34–36] For a more complete review of the diagnostic methods employed to identify fungal endocarditis, the reader is referred to an excellent review by McLeod and Remmington.[37]

The most often used serological tests detect antibody to teichoic acid, a major component of the cell wall of *S. aureus*.[38] Wheat et al.[39] found increased levels of IgG and IgM antibodies for teichoic acid in 50% of patients with infective endocarditis and complicated bacteremia caused by this organism. These antibodies are present in about 5% of localized staphylococcal infections and in about 3% of uninfected individuals. They may be elevated in disease caused by other gram-positive bacteria, and are often absent at the onset of endocarditis and appear several weeks later.[40–46]

Positive rheumatoid factor is present for weeks in 50% of patients with subacute infective endocarditis.[47] This represents a "poor man's" measurement of circulating immune complexes. Similar to aggregates of antibody and antigen, the level of rheumatoid factor declines and finally disappears when treatment has been successful. Table 12.1 summarizes the laboratory data in individuals with infective endocarditis.

Electrocardiographic studies are helpful in identifying heart block, bundle branch block, and premature ventricular contractions in patients with septal abscesses or myocarditis. Electrocardiography is required every 48 hr for at least 2 weeks in all individuals with acute endocardial infection, especially those with disease caused by *S. aureus*.

The "low-tech" electrocardiogram may identify septal abscesses that require surgical removal. About 9% of patients develop a new or changing unstable abnormality of conduction; an additional 7% have irregularity of unknown duration. The close proximity of the noncoronary cusp of the aortic valve and the mitral ring to the conduction system is thought to be responsible for changes in the electrocardiogram.[48]

A variety of radionuclide scans have been employed to establish the presence of infective endocarditis and its complications. Wiseman and his colleagues were among the first to inject gallium 67 into patients with suspected valvular infection.[49] Uptake of this radionuclide in the precordial region was confirmed at autopsy. Forty-eight hours after injection, scans were positive for 8 days. Scanning with gallium 67 detected the presence of ventricular abscesses.[50] The disadvantages of this method are (1) a level of resolution inadequate to locate the site of infection accurately; (2) the time (up to 48 hr) required for visualization of the pathology; and (3) false-negative results in about 40% of patients.

Injection of indium 111–labeled platelets and granulocytes has been employed to identify infective endocarditis.[51,52] This radionuclide appears to localize in areas with a high rate of turnover of the indium. Failure to visualize an infected area may be related to lessened cell flux associated with an indolent infection, a decrease in thrombotic activity in the vegetations, and prior treatment with antimicrobial agents. These methods are limited by the same disadvantages as those of gallium 67 scans.

Cardiac catheterization is seldom indicated in evaluating the treatment of infective endocarditis.[53] A study by DePace et al.[54] compared the effectiveness of catheterization and echocardiography in the evaluation of aortic regurgitation. Both methods were equally sensitive. The diagnosis was based on the detection of abscesses in the aortic root. Welton et al.[55] also compared the prognostic importance of these diagnostic procedures in 87 patients and found them quite comparable. Catheterization was noted to be more effective in identifying the morphological changes present in the left ventricle and aneurysms of the aortic annulus. Angiography was highly specific when compared with transthoracic two-dimensional echocardiography. Invasive procedures, cardiac catheterization for example, are relatively dangerous in patients with significant cardiac failure.[56]

Culture of blood remains the most valuable approach to establishing the diagnosis of infective endocarditis. However, the need for sensitive, specific, indirect methods is clear because the clinical presentation of valvular infections has undergone significant changes over the years.[57,58] The classical features of endocardial infection, Janeway spots, and Osler lesions are now less common. Even significant fever is present less often.

Accordingly clinicians must increase the use of the indirect diagnostic methods presently available. Various types of radionuclide scans have not fulfilled their promise. Echocardiography has become the indirect method of choice because it visualizes the valvular vegetations of infective endocarditis. M-mode examination provides a one-dimensional view that has been compared to an "ice pick"[59–66] (Figs. 12.1 to 12.3). This identifies the shaggy valvular vegetations that do not move synchronously with other cardiac landmarks.[62] The potential for delineating morphological features and spatial relationships is relatively low. However, its high-frequency waveform permits M-mode to measure cardiac structures precisely and to time various cardiac events. The sensitivity of this type of echocardiography is relatively poor.[32]

In 1977, Gilbert[64] described the use of 2-D echochardiography for imag-

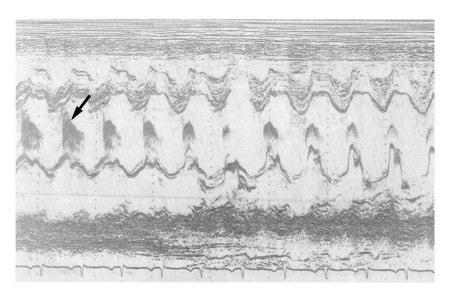

Fig. 12.1. Mitral echogram demonstrating a vegetation (arrow) prolapsing into the left ventricle in a 19-year-old man with alpha-hemolytic streptococcal endocarditis involving the aortic valve.

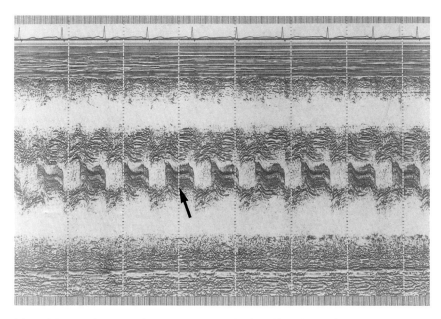

Fig. 12.2. Aortic vegetation (arrow) seen during diastole in a 74-year-old man with alpha-hemolytic streptococcal endocarditis.

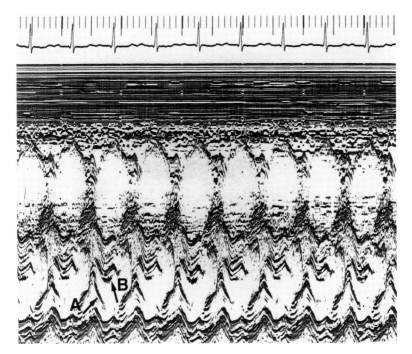

Fig. 12.3. Ruptured cusp (A) and vegetation (B) in the aortic valve of a 31-year-old man with acute, severe aortic insufficiency as the result of alpha-hemolytic streptococcal endocarditis.

ing the cardiac abnormalities associated with endocarditis (Fig. 12.4). This technique is superior to the M-mode method in defining spatial relationships and the configuration of various cardiac structures. It projects a cone-like beam that traverses a selected sector of the heart. The images produced by 2-D echocardiography are then processed by a microcomputer that produces a composite of the infected area. This method requires extended time and employs a lower frequency than the M-mode; the temporal resolution achieved is inferior.

Comparison of these methods by Winn et al.[65] indicated a major advantage of 2-D over the M-mode technique for visualizing valvular vegetations. Experience with the 2-D method proved to be superior because its power of resolution (1–2 mm) was high. In addition, it demonstrated spatial relationships in the heart accurately. The 2-D procedure clearly defines the shape of cardiac abnormalities and indicates whether a mass is pedunculated, sessile, a thickened valvular leaflet or a myocardial abscess.[68] The 2-D procedure visualizes the tricuspid valve and various types of prosthetic valves, especially those in the mitral position more effectively. The resolution of this method is about 2 mm. The M-mode detects vegetations in about 55 per cent of patients with infective endocarditis[67–72] The sensitivity of the two-dimensional echo to detect valvular vegetations, has been reported to range from 45% to 88%.[73–81] When both methods are employed simultaneously,

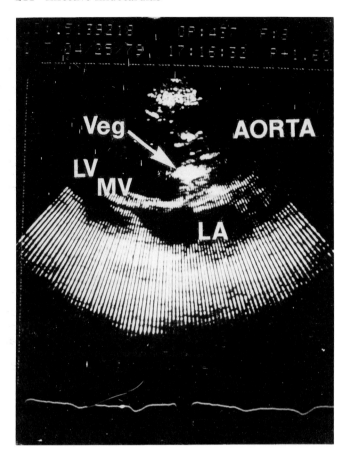

Fig. 12.4. Two-dimensional echogram demonstrating an aortic valve vegetation in a 19 year-old man with alpha-hemolytic streptococcal endocarditis involving the aortic valve.

70–80% of vegetations (average size, 3 mm in diameter) are visualized.[81,82]

In addition to size, other features related to the successful detection of valvular vegetations are (1) their location within the heart; (2) disease lasting for more than 2 weeks; and (3) abscess of a valvular ring or myocardium and an aneurysm of the sinus of Valsalva.[83] Echocardiography is not diagnostic in 10–15% of patients with misshaped chests due to pulmonary disease.[61] Injury to the mitral valve and aorta due to rheumatic fever or the sclerotic changes of old age may challenge echocardiographers. Small vegetations may be missed because the valvular surface is distorted. Mechanical prosthetic valves may disrupt the beam of a transducer to a degree that makes detection of a vegetation impossible, especially when it is present on the aortic valve.

Most patients with infective endocarditis have vegetations detectable by echocardiography. However, this is not always the case. Parker et al.[84] emphasized the fact that there is no gold standard on which the accuracy of echocardiography may be defined. The availability of more sophisticated ultrasonograms over the past few years has led to improved results. A study by Burger et al.[85] of 106 patients with the classical manifestations of infective endocarditis established two-dimensional echocardiography as a highly sensitive diagnostic tool.[85]

Transesophageal echocardiography (TEE) was developed in response to the limitations of transthoracic methods (Figs. 12.5 to 12.8). The shortcomings of the transthoracic methods were accentuated by the growing incidence of infection of prosthetic valves and endocarditis in drug abusers involving the right side of the heart. Placement of a transducer in the esophagus eliminates the need for an operator to find a window for adequate visualization. A decrease in the distance between the probe and the heart leads to a stronger signal, permits the use of higher frequencies, and results in marked improvement in resolution and detail. An increase in the number of imaging planes permits visualization of the posterior area of the heart, an area not detected by transthoracic echocardiography (TTE). In addition, the entire right side of the heart is better visualized. TEE is also more effective in detecting vegetations that involve previously damaged structures.[86–99] Improved imaging of the pulmonic valve by TEE has led to questioning of the long held belief that right-sided endocarditis in intravenous drug abusers involves the tricuspid but not the pulmonic valve.[95] The sensitivity of TEE ranges from 83% to 100%.[91–94] This procedure has identified valvular vegetations in 75% of patients with PVE; TTE visualizes only 35%.[98] TEE is markedly superior in identifying myocardial and perivalvular abscesses.[100–106] Daniel et al.[104] have reported that the sensitivity and specificity of TEE in detecting abscesses range from 87% to 95%.

Neither TEE nor TTE identifies the patterns of intracardiac flow of blood. They can define anatomical structures but not valvular function. Application of the Doppler principle, a shift in the frequency of a reflected wave by a moving object, permits ultrasonography to visualize the flow of blood through the cardiac valves and great vessels.[105,106] One of its most common uses is for serial determination of the degree of valvular insufficiency. Repeated measurements may permit a physician to decide that medical therapy has failed and that the damaged valve must be removed before irreversible myocardial damage develops.

Doppler echocardiography measures the flow of blood across some types of fistulas. This procedure may identify the presence of valvular vegetations because the movement of the valvular leaflets is abnormal. The Doppler method documents distorted flow of blood and cardiac pathology not identified by other methods.[107] Color Doppler technology identifies velocity gradients of the flow of blood. It produces excellent images of various abnormal "jet" lesions and differentiates perforation of the cusp of the mitral valve from valvular insufficiency.[108] Combined TEE and color Doppler is invaluable in determining the presence of intracardiac fistulas in patients who require surgery.[109]

A major issue in the treatment of infective endocarditis is determination of the clinical importance of vegetations. It is important to know that the

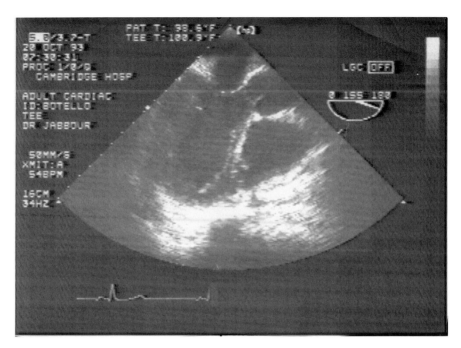

Fig. 12.5. Transesophageal two-dimensional echocardiogram of a normal aortic valve during diastole. (Courtesy of Dr. Salim Jabbour and Dr. Thomas Risser, Non-Invasive Cardiac Laboratory, Cambridge Hospital, Cambridge, MA)

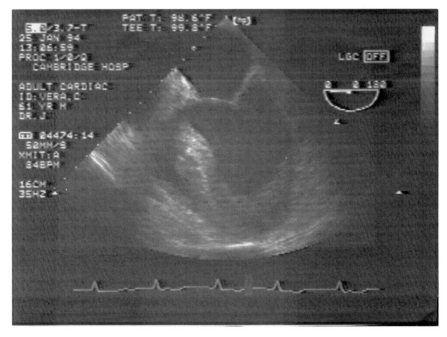

Fig. 12.6. Transesophageal two-dimensional echocardiogram of a normal mitral valve showing the anterior and posterior leaflets. (Courtesy of Dr. Salim Jabbour and Dr. Thomas Risser, Non-Invasive Cardiac Laboratory, Cambridge Hospital, Cambridge, MA)

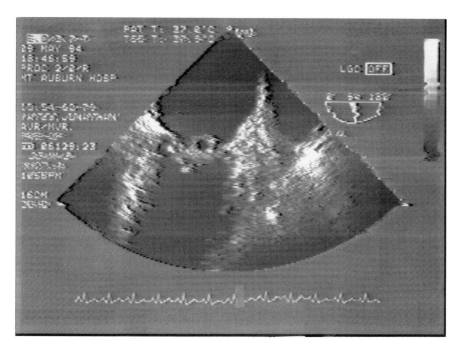

Fig. 12.7. Transesophageal two-dimensional echocardiogram showing the mitral valve with a large ring-like vegetation. (Courtesy of Dr. Panos Vonkydis, Non-Invasive Cardiac Laboratory, Mount Auburn Hospital, Cambridge, MA)

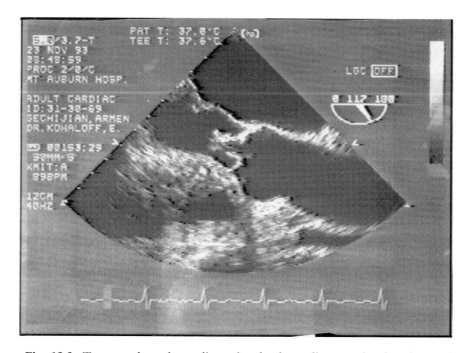

Fig. 12.8. Transesophageal two-dimensional echocardiogram showing the aortic valve with a vegetation during diastole. (Courtesy of Dr. Panos Vonkydis, Non-Invasive Cardiac Laboratory, Mount Auburn Hospital, Cambridge, MA)

results of all types of echocardiography are relatively nonspecific. The results of a study by Muggee et al.[91] indicated that 14 of 98 vegetations detected by echocardiography were areas of damaged valves with no thrombosis. Such diagnostic errors may fail to assess the risk of the development of valvular vegetations. Stewart et al.[68] pointed out that 30% of valvular vegetations remain stable for more than 16 months; about 8% disappear; some increased in size over this period.

Echocardiographic findings are unrelated to the response to treatment or the development of complications. No type of echocardiography differentiates sterile from infected vegetations.[110] Studies using the M-mode method have indicated that the presence of vegetations is associated with valvular disease, heart failure, and systemic embolization.[64,66,68,69,73,111]

The results of a study by Lutas et al.[70] indicated that neither the presence nor the site of a vegetation was related to the frequency of complications. The important prognostic factor was deterioration of cardiac function following the development of infection. They advanced the theory that vegetations identified only by the more sensitive two-dimensional method differed in behavior from those detectable by the M-mode technique. Some investigators have suggested that a vegetation more than 10 mm in diameter is more likely to embolize and produce cardiac failure.[74,75,78,91]

Steckelberg et al.[112] stated that the physical characteristics of a vegetation play no role in the risk of embolization in patients with infective endocarditis involving the left side of the heart. They suggested that the rate of embolization was related to the nature of the organism responsible for the disease. Infection caused by *S. viridans* appears to be associated with an average rank of embolization.[112]

Sanfilippo et al.[113] pointed out that the size and mobility of a vegetation beyond the valvular ring were associated with a high incidence of complications. They suggested that the organisms responsible for the infection played a minor role in the development of complications. They also developed a rating system that predicted the onset of complications.[113] The echocardiographic findings that predict the risk of embolization are presented in Table 12.2.

Rohmann et al.[114] studied the development of vegetations over 74 weeks. They found that an increase in the stability or size of a vegetation larger than 8 mm during antimicrobial therapy predicted prolonged healing. An increase in the size of a vegetation was related to a significant risk of complications but was not associated with bacteremia. Embolization occurred less often when vegetations were resolving quickly. Steckelberg et al.[112] and Sanfilippo et al.[113] stated that healing was rapid when the disease was caused by *S. viridans* and was slower to clear when produced by *S. aureus*.

All patients with proved or strongly suspected infective endocarditis should be evaluated by Doppler echocardiography. Follow-up studies are not required unless the clinical situation worsens (e.g., the development of congestive cardiac failure, embolization, the appearance of a new murmur, persistent bacteremia, or the development of abnormalities of conduction). The role of echocardiography in patients with a low level of suspicion of endocarditis is not clear (Table 12.3).

Table 12.2. Echocardiographic Characteristics for Predicting Risk of Embolus

Large vegetation

Multiple vegetations

Mobile-pedunculated vegetation

Possibly related to bacterial species

Noncalcified vegetations

Increasing size of vegetation

Prolapsing vegetation

Source: Ref. 63.

Table 12.3. When to Perform Echocardiography

Initial baseline study for diagnosis
  TTE
    Routine M-mode, two-dimensional, Doppler
  Transesophageal echocardiography
    Only if transthoracic echocardiography negative
    Clinical picture different from transthoracic echocardiographic findings
During therapy
  TTE or TEE, whichever serves as the baseline
    Evaluate vegetation during therapy
    Rule out new complications
During acute complications
  TEE is usually the most rewarding modality
Other studies usually not indicated if the clinical course is stable

Source: Adapted from Ref. 63.

About 10–20% of patients with infective endocarditis have no detectable vegetations.[115] All patients with bacteremia who have had vegetations are at risk of developing endocarditis. Individuals with echocardiographically detected valvular thrombi had several clear-cut risk factors or a clinical presentation consistent with endocardial infection. Echocardiography used to identify infective endocarditis should be restricted to the following situations: (1) persistent sterile cultures of blood together with striking signs and symptoms of infective endocarditis; (2) an unidentified source of bacteremia; and (3) bacteremia associated with the presence of intravascular devices.[116] Echocardiography may be useful for the study of fever of unknown origin, especially in patients with prosthetic valves.

The indications for ultrasonography of the heart are presented in Table 12.3. It must be emphasized that TEE should not be used for screening purposes. Most therapeutic decisions may be answered by two-dimensional and M-mode variations of TTE, with or without the need for a Doppler study. The use of TEE and Doppler scanning is limited to evaluation of high flow rates of blood caused by distortion of the signal aliasing.[117]

Although generally safe, TEE requires endoscopy. The need for antimicrobial prophylaxis of this procedure in patients with significant valvular lesions is unclear. Several instances of infective endocarditis following endoscopy have been reported.[118] Because aspiration, injury to the esophagus, and bronchospasm have been caused by TEE,[119] this procedure must be performed by experienced technicians.[120]

There is limited experience with other imaging techniques that are presently becoming available. Computed tomography (CT) scans may be useful in visualizing large aortic aneurysms and ring abscesses.[119–121] Magnetic resonance imaging is helpful in evaluating abcesses associated with endocarditis that involves a prosthetic valve.[122]

References

1. Beeson PE, Brannon ES, Warren JV: Observations on the sites of removal of bacteria from the blood of patients with bacterial endocarditis. *J Exp Med* 1945;81:9.
2. Tunkel A, Kaye D: Endocarditis with negative blood cultures. *N Engl J Med* 1992;326:1215.
3. Pesanti EL, Smith IM: Infective endocarditis with negative blood cultures: An analysis of 52 cases. *Am J Med* 1979;66:43.
4. Van Scoy RE: Culture-negative endocarditis. *Mayo Clin Proc* 1982;57:149.
5. Pazin GJ, Saul S, Thompson ME: Blood culture positivity: Suppression by outpatient antibiotic therapy in patients with bacterial endocarditis. *Arch Intern Med* 1982;142:263.
6. Von Reyn CF, Levy BS, Arbeit RD, et al: Infective endocarditis: An analysis based on strict case definitions. *Ann Intern Med* 1981;93(Part 1):505.
7. Washington JA II: The role of microbiology laboratory in the diagnosis and antimicrobial treatment of infective endocarditis. *Mayo Clin Proc* 1982;57:22.
8. Hall B, Dowling HF: Negative blood cultures in bacterial endocarditis: A decade's experience. *Med Clin North Am* 1966;50:159.
9. Hampton JR, Harrison MJ: Sterile blood cultures in bacterial endocarditis. *Q J Med* 1967;36:167.
10. Aronson MD, Bor DII: Blood cultures. *Ann Intern Med* 1987;106:246.
11. Cannaday PB, Sanford JP: Negative blood cultures in infective endocarditis: A review. *South Med J* 1976;69:1420.
12. Robbins MJ, Soeiro R, Frishman WH, et al: Right-sided valvular endocarditis: Etiology, diagnosis, and an approach to therapy. *Am Heart J* 1986;111:128.
13. Tompkins LS, Roessler BJ, Redd SC, et al: *Legionella* prosthetic valve endocarditis. *N Engl Med* 1988;318:530.
14. Rubenstein E, Noriega ER, Simberkoff MS, et al: Fungal endocarditis: Analysis of 24 cases and review of the literature. *Medicine (Baltimore)* 1975;54:331.
15. Turck WGP, Howitt G, Turnberg LA, et al: Chronic Q fever. *Q J Med* 1976;45:193.
16. Shapiro DS, Kenney SC, Johnson M, et al: *Chlamydia psittaci* endocarditis diagnosed by blood culture. *N Engl J Med* 1992;326:1192.
17. McKenzie R, Relmer L: Effect of antimicrobials on blood cultures in endocarditis. *Diagn Microbiol Infect Dis* 1987;8:165.
18. Werner AS, Cobbs CG, Kaye D, et al: Studies on the bacteremia of bacterial endocarditis. *JAMA* 1967;202:199.
19. Weinstein L: *Infective Endocarditis in Heart Disease: A Textbook of Cardiovascular Medicine*, ed 3. E Braunwald. Philadelphia, WB Saunders, 1988, p 1113.
20. Lichtlen P: General principles of conservative treatment of infective endocarditis, in Horstkotte D, Bodnar E (eds): *Infective Endocarditis*. London, ICR Publishers, 1991, p 85.

21. Washington JA: The microbiological diagnosis of infective endocarditis. *J Antimicrob Chemother* 1987;20(Suppl A):29.
22. Washington JA, Ilstrup DN: Blood cultures: Issues and controversies. *Rev Infect Dis* 1986;8:792.
23. Isenberg HD, Washington JA, Doern GV, et al: Specimen collection and handling, in Belows A, Herman KL, Hausler WJ, et al (eds): *Manual of Clinical Microbiology,* ed 5. Washington, DC, American Society for Microbiology, 1991, p 15.
24. Auckenthaler RW: Laboratory diagnosis of infective endocarditis. *Eur Heart J* 1984; 5(Suppl C):49.
25. Belli J, Waisgren B: The number of blood cultures necessary to diagnose most cases of bacterial endocarditis. *Am J Med Sci* 1956;232:289.
26. Miller M, Casey J: Infective endocarditis: New diagnostic techniques. *Am Heart J* 1978; 96:123.
27. Thamlikitkul V, Choklelkaew S, Tangtrukul T, et al: Blood culture: Comparison of outcome between switch-needle and no switch techniques. *Am J Infect Control* 1992;20:122.
28. Rubinstein E, Noriega ER, Simberkoff MS, et al: Fungal endocarditis: Analysis of 24 cases and review of the literature. *Medicine* 1975;54:331.
29. Bates D, Lee T: Rapid classification of positive blood cultures prospective validation of a multivariate algorithim. *JAMA* 1992;267:192.
30. Weinstein MP, Reller LB, Murphy JR, et al: The clinical significance of positive blood cultures: A comprehensive analysis of 500 episodes of bacteremia and fungemia in adults. I. Laboratory and epidemiologic observations. *Rev Infect Dis* 1983;5:35.
31. Bates DW, Goldman L, Lee TH: Contaminant blood cultures and resource utilization: The true consequences of false-positive results. *JAMA* 1991;265:365.
32. Bates DW, Cook EF, Goldman L, et al: Predicting bacteremia in hospitalized patients: A prospectively validated model. *Ann Intern Med* 1990;113:495.
33. Powers DL, Mandell GL: Intraleukocytic bacteria in endocarditis patients. *JAMA* 1974;227:312.
34. Reller LB: Laboratory procedures in the management of infective endocarditis, in *Treatment of Infective Endocarditis.* New York, Grune and Stratton, 1981, p 235.
35. Harford CH: Postoperative fungal endocarditis: Fungemia, embolism and therapy. *Arch Intern Med* 1974;134:116.
36. Seelig MS, Speth CP, Kozinn PJ, et al: Patterns of candida endocarditis following cardiac surgery: Importance of early diagnosis and therapy (an analysis of 91 cases). *Prog Cardiovasc Dis* 1974;17:125.
37. McLeod R, Remington J: Fungal endocarditis, in Rahimtoola SH (ed): *Infective Endocarditis.* New York, Grune and Stratton, 1977, p 119.
38. Nagel J, Tuazon D, Cordella T, et al: Teichoic acid. Serologic diagnosis of staphylococcal endocarditis. Use of gel diffusion and counterimmunoelectrophoretic methods. *Ann Intern Med* 1975;82:13.
39. Wheat L, Kohler R, Tabarah Q, et al: IgM antibody response to staphylococcal infection. *J Infect Dis* 1981;144:307.
40. Christensson B, Hedstrom S, Kronvall G: Clinical significance of serological methods in the diagnosis of staphylococcal septicemia and endocarditis. *Scand J Infect Dis* 1983;41(Suppl 140):140.
41. Wheat L, Wilkonson B, Kohler R, et al: Antibody response to peptidoglycan during staphylococcal infections. *J Infect Dis* 1983;147:16.
42. Bayer AS, Tillman DB, Concepcion N, et al: Clinical value of teichoic acid antibody titers in the diagnosis and management of staphylococcemias. *West J Med* 1980;132:294.
43. Bayer AS, Lam K, Ginzton L, et al: *Staphylococcus aureus* bacteremia: Clinical, serologic and echocardiographic findings in patients with and without endocarditis. *Arch Intern Med* 1987;147:457.
44. Kaplan JE, Palmer DL, Tung KSK: Teichoic acid antibody and circulating immune complexes in the management of *Staphylococcus aureus* bacteremia. *Am J Med* 1981;70:769.
45. Tuazon CU, Sheagren JN: Teichoic acid antibodies in the diagnosis of serious infections with *Staphylococcus aureus. Ann Intern Med* 1976;84:543.

46. Tuazon CU, Sheagren JN, Choa MS, et al: *Staphylococcus aureus* bacteremia: Relationship between formation of antibodies to teichoic acid and the development of metastatic abscesses. *J Infect Dis* 1978;137:57.

47. Weinstein L, Schlesinger J: Pathoanatomic, pathophysiologic and clinical correlates in endocarditis. *N Engl J Med* 1979;291:832.

48. Dinubile M, Calderwood S, Steinhaus DA, et al: Cardiac conduction abnormalities complicating native valve active infective endocarditis. *Am J Cardiol* 1986;58:1213.

49. Wiseman J, Rouleau J, Rigo P: Gallium-67 myocardial imaging for detection of bacterial endocarditis. *Pathology* 1979;120:135.

50. Spies SM, Mayers SN, Barresi V, et al: A case of myocardial abscess evaluated by radionuclide techniques: Case report. *J Nucl Med* 1977;18:1089.

51. Oates E, Sarno RC: Detection of bacterial endocarditis with indium-111 labeled leukocytes. *Clin Nucl Med* 1988;13:691.

52. Machac J, Vallabhajosula S, Goldman ME: Value of blood-pool subtraction in cardiac indium-11 labeled platelet imaging. *J Nucl Med* 1989;30:1445.

53. Hosenpud JD, Greenberg BH: The preoperative evaluation in patients with endocarditis. Is cardiac catheterization necessary? *Chest* 1983;84:690.

54. DePace NL, Nestico PF, Kotler MN: Comparison of echocardiography and angiography in determining the cause of severe aortic regurgitation. *Br Heart J* 1984;51:36.

55. Welton D, Young J, Raizner A: Value and safety of cardiac catheterization during active infective endocarditis. *Am J Cardiol* 1979;44:1306.

56. Bain RJ, Geddes AM, Littler WA, et al: The clinical and echocardiographic diagnosis of infective endocarditis. *J Antomicrob Chemother* 1987;20(Suppl A):17.

57. McKinsey DS, Ratts TE, Bisno AL: Underlying cardiac lesions in adults with infective endocarditis. The changing spectrum. *Am J Med* 1987;82:681.

58. Kaye D: Changing pattern of infective endocarditis. *Am J Med* 1985;78(Suppl 6B):157.

59. Dillon JC, Feigenbaum H, Konecke I, et al: Echocardiographic manifestations of valvular vegetations. *Am Heart J* 1973;86:698.

60. Spangler RD, Johnson MC, Holmes J, et al: Echocardiographic demonstration of bacterial vegetations in active infective endocarditis. *J Clin Ultrasound* 1973;1:126.

61. Kochar G, Maniet A: Echocardiographic findings in infective endocarditis. Current opinion. *J Infect Dis* 1992;5:642.

62. Gilbert BW, Haney RS, Crawford F: Two dimensional echocardiographic assessment of vegetative endocarditis. *Circulation* 1977;55:346.

63. Wann L, Hallam C, Dillon J, et al: Comparison of M-mode and cross-sectional echocardiography in infective endocarditis. *Circulation* 1979;60:728.

64. Berger M, Gallerstein PE, Benhuri P, et al: Evaluation of aortic valve endocarditis by two-dimensional echocardiography. *Chest* 1981;80:61.

65. Martin RP, Melzer RS, Chia BI, et al: Clinical uility of two-dimensional echocardiography in infective endocarditis. *Am J Cardiol* 1980;46:369.

66. Croney D, Chandraratna PN, Wishnow R, et al: Clinical implications of large vegetations in infective endocarditis. *Arch Int Med* 1983;143:1874.

67. Roy P, Tajik AJ, Giuliani ER, et al: Spectrum of echocardiographic findings in bacterial endocarditis. *Circulation* 1976;53:474.

68. Stewart JA, Silimperi D, Harris P, et al: Echocardiographic documentation of vegetative lesions in infective endocarditis: Clinical implications. *Circulation* 1980;61:274.

69. Buda AJ, Zotz RJ, LeMire MS, et al: Prognostic significance of vegetations detected by two-dimensional echocardiography in infective endocarditis. *Am Heart J* 1986; 112:1291.

70. Lutas EM, Roberts RB, Devereux RB, et al: Relation between the presence of echocardiographic vegetations and the complication rate in infective endocarditis. *Am Heart J* 1986;112:107.

71. Stafford WJ, Petch J, Radford DJ: Vegetations in infective endocarditis. Clinical relevance and diagnosis by cross-sectional echocardiography. *Br Heart J* 1985;53:310.

72. Melvin ET, Berger M, Lutzker LG, et al: Noninvasive methods for detection of valve vegetations in infective endocarditis. *Am J Cardiol* 1981;47:271.

73. Wong D, Chandraratna PAN, Wishnow RM, et al: Clinical implications of large vegetations in infective endocarditis. *Arch Intern Med* 1983;143:1874.

74. Davis RS, Strom JA, Frishman W: The demonstration of vegetations by echocardiography in bacterial endocarditis. *Am J Med* 1980;69:57.

75. Come PC, Isaacs RE, Riley MF: Diagnostic accuracy of M-mode echocardiography in active infective endocarditis and prognostic implications of ultrasound-detectable vegetations. *Am Heart J* 1982;103:839.

76. Sheikh MD, Covarrubias EA, Ali N, et al: M-mode echocardiographic observations during and after healing of active bacterial endocarditis limited to the mitral valve. *Am J Med* 1981;101:37.

77. Sheikh MU, Covarrubias EA, Ali N, et al: M-mode echocardiographic observations in active bacterial endocarditis limited to the aortic valve. *Am Heart J* 1981;101:66.

78. Hickey AJ, Wolfers J, Wilcken DE: Reliability and clinical relevance of detection of vegetations by echocardiography in bacterial endocarditis. *Br Heart J* 1981;46:624.

79. Mintz GS, Kotler MN, Segal BL, et al: A comparison of two-dimensional and M-mode echocardiography in the evaluation of patients with endocarditis. *Am J Cardiol* 1979;43:738.

80. Gintzon LE, Siegel RJ, Criley JM: Natural history of tricuspid valve endocarditis: A two-dimensional echocardiographic study. *Am J Cardiol* 1982;49:1853.

81. Berger M, Delfin LA, Jelveh M, et al: Two-dimensional echocardiographic findings in right-sided infective endocarditis. *Circulation* 1980;61:855.

82. Strom J, Becker R, Davis R, et al: Echocardiographic and surgical correlation in bacterial endocarditis. *Circulation* 1980;62(Suppl I):1.

83. Amsterdam E: Value and limitations of echocardiography in endocarditis. *Cardiology* 1989;71:229.

84. Parker J, St John Sutton M, Karchmer A: Echocardiography in the management of patients with suspected or proven endocarditis, in Remington J, Wurtz MS (eds): *Current Clinical Topics in Infectious Disease,* Vol II. Cambridge, MA, Blackwell Scientific, 1991, p 248.

85. Burger AJ, Peart B, Jabi H, et al: The role of two-dimensional echocardiography in the diagnosis of infectious endocarditis. *Angiology* 1991;42:552.

86. Daniel WG, Schroeder E, Muegge A, et al: Transesophageal echocardiography in infective endocarditis. *Am J Cardiac Imag* 1988;2:78.

87. Polak PE, Gussenhoven WJ, Roelandt JRTC: Transesophageal cross-sectional echocardiographic recognition of an aortic valve ring abscess and a subannular mycotic aneurysm. *Eur Heart J* 1987;8:664.

88. Daniel WJ, Schroeder E, Nonnast-Daniel B, et al: Conventional and transesophageal echocardiography in the diagnosis of infective endocarditis. *Eur Heart J* 1987;8(Suppl 3):287.

89. Drexler M, Erbel R, Rohmann S, et al: Diagnostic value of two-dimensional transesophageal versus transthoracic echocardiography in patients with infective endocarditis. *Eur Heart J* 1987;8(Suppl 1):303.

90. Erbel R, Rohmann S, Drexler M: Improved diagnostic value of echocardiography in patients with infective endocarditis by transesophageal approach. A prospective study. *Eur Heart J* 1988;9:43.

91. Muggee A, Daniel WG, Frank G, et al: Echocardiography in infective endocarditis: Reassessment of prognostic implications of vegetation size determined by the transthoracic and the transesophageal approach. *J Am Coll Cardiol* 1989;14:631.

92. Taams MA, Gussenhoven EJ, Bos E: Enhanced morphologic diagnosis in infective endocarditis by transesophageal echocardiography. *Br Heart J* 1990;63:109.

93. Remetz MS, Quagliarello V: Endovascular infections arising from right-sided heart structures. *Cardiol Clin* 1992;10:137.

94. Allen MD, Slachman F, Eddu AC, et al: Tricuspid valve repair for tricuspid valve endocarditis: Tricuspid valve "recycling." *Ann Thorac Surg* 1991;51:593.

95. Shapiro SM, Young E, Ginzton LE, et al: Pulmonic valve endocarditis as an underdiag-

nosed disease: Role of transesophageal echocardiography. *J Am Soc Echocardiogr* 1991;5:48.

96. Omoto R, Yokote Y, Takamoto S, et al: The development of real-time two-dimensional Doppler echocardiography and its clinical significance in acquired valvular regurgitation. *Jpn Heart J* 1984;25:325.

97. Shively BK, Gurule FT, Roldan CA, et al: Diagnostic valve of transesophageal compared with transthoracic echocardiography in infective endocarditis. *J Am Coll Cardiol* 1991;18:391.

98. Birmingham GD, Rahko PS, Ballantyne F: Improved detection of infective endocarditis with transesophageal echocardiography. *Am Heart J* 1992;23:774.

99. Pedersen WR, Walker M, Olson JD, et al: Value of transesophageal echocardiography as an adjunct to transthoracic echocardiography in evaluation of native and prosthetic valve endocarditis. *Chest* 1991;100:351.

100. McKenney PA, Shemin RJ, Wiegers SE: Role of transesophageal echocardiography in sinus of Valsalva aneurysm. *Am Heart J* 1992;123:228.

101. Northbridge DB, Gnanapragasam P, Houston AB: Diagnosis of mitral valve aneurysm by transesophageal echocardiography. *Br Heart J* 1991;65:227.

102. Rohmann S, Erbel R, Darius H, et al: Prediction of rapid versus prolonged healing of infective endocarditis by monitoring vegetation size. *J Am Soc Echocardiogr* 1991; 4:465.

103. Giannoccaro P, Ascah KJ, Sochowski RA, et al: Spontaneous drainage of paravalvular abscess diagnosed by transesophageal echocardiography. *J Am Soc Echocardiogr* 1991;4:397.

104. Daniel WG, Mugge A, Martin RP, et al: Improvement in the diagnosis of abscesses associated with endocarditis by transesophageal echocardiography. *N Engl J Med* 1991;324:795.

105. Pons-Llado G, Carreras F, Borras X, et al: Findings on Doppler echocardiography in asymptomatic intravenous heroin users. *Am J Cardiol* 1992;69:238.

106. Shapiro SM, Bayer AS: Transesophageal and Doppler echocardiography in the diagnosis and management of infective endocarditis. *Chest* 1991;100:1125.

107. Spreckler DL, Adamick R, Adams D, et al: In virtro colour flow, pulsed and continuous wave Doppler ultrasound masking of flow by prosthetic valves. *J Am Coll Cardiol* 1987;9:1306.

108. Miyatake K, Yamamoto K, Park YD, et al: Diagnosis of mitral valve perforation by real-time two-dimensional Doppler flow imaging technique. *J Am Cardiol* 1986;8:1235.

109. Fisher EA, Estioko MR, Stern EH, et al: Left ventricular to left atrial communication secondary to a para-aortic abscess: Colour flow Doppler documentation. *J Am Coll Cardiol* 1987;10:222.

110. Neimann J, Fischer M, Kownator S, et al: Echocardiographic follow-up of vegetations in infectious endocarditis. *Arch Mal Coeur* 1982;75:1329.

111. Pratt C, Whitcomb C, Neumann A, et al: Relationship of vegetations on echocardiograms to the clinical course and systemic emboli in bacterial endocarditis. *Am J Cardiol* 1978;41:384.

112. Steckelberg JM, Murphy JG, Ballard D, et al: Emboli in infective endocarditis: The prognostic value of echocardiography. *Ann Intern Med* 1991;114:635.

113. Sanfilippo AJ, Picard MH, Newell JB, et al: Echocardiographic assessment of patients with infectious endocarditis: Prediction of risk for complications. *J Am Coll Cardiol* 1991;18:1181.

114. Rohmann S, Seiffert T, Erbel R, et al: Identification of abscess formation in native-valve infective endocarditis using transesophageal echocardiography: Implications for surgical treatment. *Thorac Cardiovasc Surg* 1991;39:273.

115. Stratton JR, Werner JA, Pearlman AS, et al: Bacteremia and the heart: Serial echocardiographic findings in 80 patients with documented or suspected bacteremia. *Am J Med* 1982;73:851.

116. White H, Wynne J: Clinical utility of echocardiography in suspected infective endocarditis. *Circulation* 1982;66(Suppl 2):103.

117. Rubenson DS, Tucker CR, Stinson EG: The use of echocardiography in diagnosing culture-negative endocarditis. *Circulation* 1981;64:641.

118. Pearlman A: Transesophageal echocardiography—sound diagnostic technique or two edge sword? *N Engl J Med* 1991;324:841.

119. Pritchard TM, Foust RT, Cantey JR, et al: Prosthetic valve endocarditis due to *Cardiobacterium hominis* occurring after upper gastrointestinal endoscopy. *Am J Med* 1991;90:516.

120. Daniel WG, Erbel R, Kasper W: Safety of transesophageal echocardiography: A multicenter survey of 10,419 examinations. *Circulation* 1991;83:817.

121. Cowan JC, Patrick D, Reid DS: Aortic root abscess complicating bacterial endocarditis, demonstration by computed tomography. *Br Heart J* 1984;52:591.

122. Akins EW, Limacher M, Slone RM, et al: Evaluation of an aortic annular pseudoaneurysm by MRI: Comparison with echocardiography, angiography and surgery. *Cardiovasc Intervent Radiol* 1987;10:188.

13

Medical Management

The availability of effective antimicrobial agents as well as advances in cardiac surgery, have played critical roles in the successful management of infective endocarditis. This is in sharp contrast to the experiences with this disease prior to the availability of effective therapy, when most patients with subacute and acute disease died.

Physicians were limited to observation of the natural history of an invariably fatal disease before treatment with antibiotics became available. The use of vaccines and the parenteral administration of dyes, such as gentian violet, was popular but was abandoned when it became clear that they were ineffective. However, the use of antibiotics and the employment of various surgical techniques have, themselves, created a number of difficult and, at times, insoluble problems.

The information required prior to initiating treatment of patients with infective endocarditis includes (1) the nature of the organism responsible for the disease; (2) determination of the minimal inhibitory concentration (MIC) and minimal bactericidal concentration (MBC) of the agent active against the involved organism; (3) the route of administration of the selected drug; and (4) the incidence and types of reactions provoked by treatment.

The choice of a potentially effective antimicrobial drug is determined by the nature of the organism recovered from the blood and its susceptibility to a variety of drugs. With rare exceptions, immediate treatment is not mandatory when subacute endocardial infection is suspected because the disease has usually been present for about 1–2 months. Death that occurs before initiation of treatment is usually due to the development of complications of the disease (e.g., rupture of a cerebral aneurysm) that occur early in the course of the disease and are not prevented by treatment.[1]

Delay in the therapy of acute infective endocarditis is never justified because of the risk of rapid valvular destruction. The choice of antibacterial agents in this situation is empirical and is based on the clinical history and physical examination, not on the definitive results of microbiological studies.

Sterilization of an infected thrombus on a valve requires therapy with a bactericidal agent. This conclusion is based on the results of studies in animals, in vitro experiments, and clinical experience. For example, therapy with clindamycin, a bacteriostatic drug, has led to a high incidence of relapse in patients with endocarditis caused by *S. aureus*.[2,3] Analysis of the time-kill curves in rabbits has indicated that chloramphenicol decreases the rate of killing of *S. viridans* by interfering with the bactericidal activity of penicillin G.[4]

Several factors are involved in the diminished capacity of antibiotics to sterilize an infected thrombus. The density of organisms in an infected vegetation is quite high 10^9 to 10^{10} cfu/g. In this environment the organisms have a reduced metabolic rate and decreased replicative activity. Also, very few leukocytes are present. The fibrin meshwork interferes with their functioning. In this situation, bactericidal agents have significant advantages over those that are bacteriostatic.[5-7]

Cremieux and Carbon[8] have pointed out that there are major differences in the pharmacokinetics of several antibiotics when they are present in a vegetation.[8] Over the past 60 years, it has been recognized that the ability of antimicrobial agents to cure valvular infections is related to their capacity to achieve therapeutic levels in an infected fibrin thrombus (vegetation).[9] The failure of the sulfonamides to cure infective endocarditis is related to the fact that this group of drugs is bacteriostatic and fails to penetrate adequately the infected vegetations.[10]

In vivo models have been developed to investigate the entry of antimicrobial agents into the fibrin thrombus. Weinstein et al.[11-13] studied the entry of various antibiotics into fibrin plugs implanted subcutaneously in rabbits. They noted that there was a delay in the movement of a compound from the serum into the clot and that its penetration was indirectly proportional to its degree of binding to protein. One problem with this model was the fact that the distribution of the antibiotic was considered to be homogeneous throughout the clot; this was probably not a valid assumption. Because the concentration of the antibiotic was measured in an aliquot of the clot after it was dissolved in trypsin, it was impossible to detect any variation in the distribution of the agent.

Other models have been developed to study the pharmacokinetics of antibiotics in thrombi produced on the cardiac valves of rabbits. The results of these models differed from those reported by Weinstein et al.[11-13] The entry of antimicrobial agents into the vegetations was found to be quite rapid; infection of the vegetations (fibrin clots) appeared to facilitate this process.[14-17] The difficulty in sterilizing an infected clot was not related to inadequate penetration of the antibiotic.

Using autoradiographic methods, Cremieux and Carbon[8] identified three patterns of the entry of antibiotics into cardiac vegetations: (1) limitation of diffusion to the periphery of a fibrin plug; (2) progressive penetration from the periphery to the core of the thrombus; and (3) homogeneous diffusion throughout the vegetation. The determinants of these patterns were not defined. Ceftriaxone and teicoplanin are highly protein bound and exhibited limited penetration. However, daptomycin, a highly bound drug, entered fibrin masses readily, probably due to its preferential binding to protein within the fibrin matrix.[18–20]

Suppression of microbial multiplication may continue even after the level of the drug falls below the MIC of the agent administered. This phenomenon is related to the concentration of an antibiotic and the duration of exposure of an organism to it. This apparently is due to the sublethal effect of the antimicrobial agent.[21–23] Unlike the aminoglycosides and quinolones cell wall–active antibiotics do not exhibit this phenomenon among gram-negative bacteria. This postantibiotic effect (PAE) permits an antibiotic to be administered at longer intervals than would be based on its half-life in serum. Absence of this effect, as is the case when beta-lactams are used to treat infections caused by gram-negative bacteria, requires that the concentration of an antibiotic remain above its MIC continuously in order to suppress microbial growth. Whether there is a PAE for a specific antibiotic in an infected vegetation is determined by the concentration of the drug and by how long the organisms are exposed to it. For most beta-lactams except the carbapenems, the rate of bacterial killing is directly proportional to the growth of the organism. As pointed out by Durack and Beeson,[24] microorganisms lying deep within a vegetation exhibit markedly reduced metabolic activity. Morphological changes occur in some bacteria within the thrombus (vegetation).[25] In this setting, organisms produce exopolysaccharides that appear to act as a barrier to the movement of penicillin into the cellular wall.[26]

The MIC and MBC in serum or broth may not reflect the concentration of an antibiotic required to eradicate a pathogen. It has been reported that the cure of experimental endocarditis produced by *E. coli* requires a concentration of ceftriaxone in the cardiac vegetation 220 times higher than the MBC of the drug.[27]

It is probably not valid to transfer in vitro measurements of PAE to the clinical situation.[28] The PAE of imipenem for *Ps. aeruginosa* is markedly decreased in a vegetation by the very same mechanisms that affect the MIC. Limited evidence has indicated that the aminoglycosides may be less inhibited than the beta-lactams.[29]

There are no firm data on which to base the dosing schedules of the antibiotics used to treat infective endocarditis. The therapeutic goal is to produce an effective therapeutic level of a drug at the infected site—the cardiac valve—and to maximize the duration of contact of the organism with the drug.

It has been recommended that patients with infective endocarditis caused by an organism highly susceptible to penicillin be treated with doses of this drug ranging from 4–6 to 20–30 million units/day. The selection of antimicrobial agents for the management of fungal and other causes of infective endocarditis is discussed below.

Barza et al.[12] pointed out that the injection of a bolus of an antibiotic produces higher levels in a thrombus (vegetation) than does continuous infusion. The optimal interval between doses in patients with infective endocarditis and other infectious diseases is not well established. Six hours between doses appears appropriate in adults treated with beta-lactam antibiotics. Data derived from an experimental model of endocarditis caused by *S. aureus*[30] have indicated that an interval of 4–8 hr separating the doses of methicillin produced optimal therapeutic results. The same dose administered every 12 hr may be ineffective. The continuous infusion of methicillin yields poorer results than does intermittent injections. Studies by Gengo and Schentag[30] indicated that the optimal interval between doses is about equal to the sum of three factors: (1) the time at which serum levels of the antibiotic are higher than the MBC; (2) the duration of the PAE; and (3) the value of one "log growth time." For all the above reasons, we favor the intermittent method of administration. Its advantages over continuous infusion of an antibiotic in treating endocarditis remain controversial.

Because renal tubular function is decreased in elderly patients, the interval between doses of an antibiotic must be lengthened.

The total duration of therapy required for the cure of infective endocarditis is not clear. However, 4 weeks of treatment is considered adequate in most patients. There is an increasing tendency to treat for longer periods, but there is no evidence that this leads to a higher incidence of cure or a decrease in the frequency of relapse. Therapy may need to be prolonged in individuals infected by organisms less sensitive to antibiotics, in those infected by fungi, and in those with infection of prosthetic valves. Although it has been suggested that an extended course of treatment may not be dangerous, our experience has indicated that this is not always the case. A patient with streptococcal endocarditis treated for 1 month recovered but was suprainfected by *Ps. aeruginosa* and other gram-negative organisms when treatment with penicillin was administered for 6 weeks.[31]

Several trials of the treatment of endocarditis caused by penicillin-sensitive streptococci for 2 weeks have been reported. This regimen is not recommended by the authors.[32] In 1966, Lerner and Weinstein[33] reported that, prior to this time, there were only two groups of patients in whom the incidence of cure was 95% or higher and in whom there were no relapses. Penicillin had been administered intravenously for 4 weeks. Shorter courses of therapy resulted in no improvement in outcome. To be eligible for the 2-week course, patients had to meet several strict criteria (see below).

Orally administered penicillins plus streptomycin administered parenterally have cured infective endocarditis caused by streptococci.[32,34,35] In our opinion, the intravenous administration of antimicrobial agents is mandatory. This route reliably produces therapeutic levels. Oral therapy may produce concentrations in the serum too low to inhibit bacterial multiplication. This may be related to the inability of persons to adequately absorb orally administered antibiotics. Given by mouth, this may lead to gastrointestinal dysfunction, vomiting, diarrhea, and failure to comply with treatment. Oral therapy exposes patients to the risk of suprainfection similar to that induced by intravenous therapy.[36]

In 1949, Schlicter et al.[37] introduced the first in vitro method for evaluating the effectiveness of a therapeutic regimen for the management of infective endocarditis. The Schlicter test, the serum bactericidal titer (SBT), measures the highest dilution of serum that kills a standard concentration of the organism at the maximal or minimal concentration of the antibiotic present in the patient's bloodstream. An SBT of $^1/_8$ or higher predicts a favorable therapeutic outcome. Whether the measurement of the peak or trough SBT is more important has not been established due to lack of standardization of the inoculum and underestimation of the protein-binding capacity of an antibiotic diluted in broth or serum.[38] The results of a multicenter study has indicated that the SBT is a poor predicter of microbiological failure.[39] A peak SBT of $^1/_{64}$ and a trough SBT of $^1/_{32}$ predict therapeutic success. Lower titers do not always signify microbiological or clinical failure. The achievement of these levels of SBT may expose many patients to a significant risk of ototoxicity or nephrotoxicity. Cooper[40] noted that the outcome of right-sided endocarditis caused by *Serratia* was favorable in seven patients regardless of the level of SBT; 70% of those with left-sided infection died; 4 had high SBTs. Three individuals with high SBTs were cured but died of complications of endocarditis. These experiences indicate that the eventual outcome of infective endocarditis depends on a number of factors, not only on the concentration of a potentially effective antimicrobial agent in the blood.

Attempts to standardize the variables of the Schlicter test have been of little clinical benefit.[41] There appears to be no correlation between the SBT and the bactericidal concentration of an antibiotic in the valvular vegetations of experimental animals. This finding is consistent with the pharmacokinetics of an antibiotic present in a valvular vegetation.

Measurement of the SBT in patients treated with various combinations of antimicrobial agents may be misleading. For example, pairing of an aminoglycoside and another drug may decrease the concentration of the former to a level below that required to produce synergy; determination of "killing curves" is required to ascertain the level of synergism.[42]

The SBT is not required for all patients with infective endocarditis. It should be determined primarily in those with (1) a poor response to therapy; (2) disease caused by uncommon organisms; and (3) a change in the route of administration of a drug.[43–45]

Home Therapy of Infective Endocarditis

About 3–14% of patients with infective endocarditis are treated at home with drugs usually administered in the hospital. The development of various ambulatory infusion devices has contributed to this trend.[46–49] The pharmacokinetic properties of an antibiotic are more important than the hardware used to administer it. Drugs such as teicoplanin, the half-life of which permits dosing once a day, are very attractive in an ambulatory situation in which the problem of venous access is minimized.[50,51] Before the availability of antimicrobial agents with longer half-lives, outpatient therapy of infective endocarditis was based on the use of drugs that could be administered orally. One of the early clinical trials that documented the effectiveness of antibiotics administered parenterally for the therapy of infective endocarditis has been reported by Francioli and the BE Collaborative Study Group.[52]

The ability to administer antibiotics with long half-lives, such as ceftriaxone, precludes the necessity for intravenous access. However some infections, especially those caused by *S. aureus*, may not be suitable for treatment with a cephalosporin once a day.[53]

In general, it is our opinion that the aminoglycosides are not good candidates for home infusion.[54] Prompt reporting of the serum levels of these antibiotics to the physician is necessary for the prevention of nephrotoxicity. This is often difficult to achieve in an outpatient setting.

Candidates for any type of home therapy must have certain personal characteristics.[55,56] Among these are (1) stable physical and mental health; (2) the ability to learn self-administration of a drug; (3) the presence of another responsible person in the home; and (4) no past or present history of intravenous drug use.[57]

Clinical Response to Antimicrobial Therapy

It is important to monitor the temperature of the patient after treatment has been initiated. Fever that persists for more than 7–10 days after appropriate therapy has been initiated is a matter for concern.[58–63] Fifty percent of patients infected by *S. viridans* become afebrile within 7 days of treatment with penicillin and gentamicin; others do so in about 2–3 weeks. This indicates biphasic susceptibility of the organism to antimicrobial agents. Slow defervescence may indicate an organism, less sensitive than the average, to the agent being administered. Persistence of fever for more than 3 weeks does not mandate a change in treatment. Prolonged fever may be caused by extracardiac complications; "drug fever" must be ruled out. About 30% of individuals who initially defervesce during treatment redevelop fever.

Blumberg et al.[60] studied 36 patients with an extended febrile course despite favorable sensitivity tests of the prescribed antibiotic. They compared these patients to a matched group who responded to treatment. There appeared to be no relation between the pattern of fever and its cause. Nineteen percent of the individuals remained febrile for a number of reasons. This condition was related to a myocardial abscess and persistent infection in three individuals; there was no obvious cause in others. However, these patients defervesced when an infected valve was replaced. The presence of a large valvular vegetation (more than 1 cm in size) was associated with prolonged fever.

Mycotic aneurysms of the cerebral circulation present the most difficult diagnostic challenges. None were recognized prior to rupture. A larger number of complications occurred in individuals with persistent elevated temperature. Myocardial abscesses were present in two of seven patients studied by serial electrocardiography and TTE. These tests identified the lesions and led to surgery. The authors suggested that patients with persistent fever undergo TEE if transthoracic ultrasonography fails to disclose the cause of the prolonged elevation in temperature. MRI appears promising in detecting silent mycotic aneurysms.

Mansur et al.[64] reviewed 300 episodes of infective endocarditis that occurred in 227 patients between 1978 and 1986. Only one-third had no significant complications while being treated with antibiotics. There was an increased incidence of untoward events in those who died.[65] This was the finding in individuals with infection of prosthetic or native valves.[66,67] Mansur and his colleages suggested that the course of the disease was related to an increase in complications. They defined these complications as embolic, cardiac, and immunological and emphasized that they were not always associated with the clinical course of infective endocarditis. Cardiac failure developed in one-third of patients; other studies have indicated that this occurs in 15–65% of patients.[68,69] However, the studies of Mansur et al. have indicated that individuals with infective endocarditis die of congestive cardiac failure less often than they did in the past. Cardiac decompensation was the leading cause of death years ago.[70,71] The present situation may be related to aggressive surgery performed as soon as valvular destruction is identified. The central nervous system was the second most frequent site of infection. The frequency of cerebral embolism and intracerebral mycotic aneurysms was found to be identical in both native and prosthetic valve endocarditis. Forty-six patients suffered from the sepsis syndrome. *S. aureus* was the organism most often involved, especially in patients with cardiac pathology. Adverse reactions to antimicrobial agents occurred in 31 patients. Although cardiac complications occurred most often, the fatality rate was highest in patients with neurological syndromes or sepsis.

Relapse and Recurrence of Infective Endocarditis

Relapse of patients with infective endocarditis usually occurs about 2 months after apparently successful treatment.[63] The incidence of relapse is specific for the infecting organism. Lerner and Weinstein[72] and Karchmer et al.[73] identified no relapses caused by *S. viridans* in patients treated with penicillin G for 4 weeks. However, *S. aureus,* enterococci, and gram-negative organisms, especially *Ps. aeruginosa,* are associated with a high incidence of relapse.[74–76]

Patients with symptoms of infection for more than 3 months prior to the initiation of treatment are at high risk of a relapse. This is also the case in infections caused by *S. viridans* and enterococci.[77–79] Enterococcal infection of the mitral valve is most likely to recur.

Patients who have had infective endocarditis in the past are at risk of developing the disease in the future.[80] Fewer than 10% of infected prosthetic valves become reinfected.[81–83] Levinson et al.[84] have described the clinical features in patients who have had a second episode of infective endocarditis. Congenital heart disease was the most frequent underlying disorder. Welton et al.[85] emphasized the importance of intravenous drug abuse as a risk factor for the recurrence of the disease. Forty percent of individuals who used illicit drugs experienced a second episode of endocarditis.

A review of 281 cases of recurrent infective endocarditis that occurred over 10 years indicated that the incidence of reinfection was three times higher in men than in women; 43% of those reinfected had used intravenous drugs.[86] An increased frequency of the disease was indentified in patients with rheumatic heart disease and valvular prolapse. The interval between episodes of endocarditis was significantly shorter in individuals with drug-associated disease. Recurrences were produced by a variety of organisms. The fatality rate was less than 30%.

Streptococcal Endocarditis

Subacute infective endocrditis is caused by many types of streptococci. *S. viridans,* NVS, enterococci, hemolytic streptococci (groups A, E, C, and G), and *S. pneumoniae* cause about 40% of the cases of endocardial infection. Most strains of *S. viridans* and *S. bovis* are sensitive to penicillin; NVS are resistant to this antibiotic. Forty-eight percent of subacute infective endocarditis that occurs in the United States is caused by penicillin-sensitive bacteria.[87] An organism sensitive to penicillin is inhibited by 0.1 μg/ml of the antibiotic.[88] In the United Kingdom, streptococci with an MBC $\geq$ 1.0 mg/liter are classified as sensitive to penicillin.[89] Errors in determining the activity level of an antibiotic may lead to inadequate therapy.[90] Not all strains of *S. viridans* are inhibited or killed by exposure to penicillin.[91] Some isolates recovered from blood cultures of patients with active endocarditis are highly resistant to penicillin (MIC higher than 1 mg/ml); this appears to be related to changes in the penicillin-binding proteins.[92]

Therapeutic difficulties are often caused by NVS that are responsible for 5–10% of infective endocarditis produced by streptococci sensitive to penicillin in vitro.[93,94] The MIC of this antibiotic for these organisms has been found to be above 0.1 μg/ml in 17–33% of patients.[95–97] Roberts et al.[93] have reported that in 46 patients with valvular infection caused by NVS, 13% of the isolates were suppressed by penicillin with an MIC above 0.5 μg/ml. A high incidence of relapse and death may be due to infection caused by antibiotic-resistant organisms.[98–100] Failure to sterilize the blood of NVS occurred in 41% of patients; 56% had been treated with agents that appeared to be active in vitro.

Tolerance is a laboratory phenomenon in which the MBC of a drug exceeds its MIC by at least a factor of 10. All NVS are tolerant, if not highly resistant.[101] About 20% of strains of *S. viridans. S. mutans,* and *S. mitior* are tolerant. A combination of penicillin and an aminoglycoside eradicates tolerant strains of *S. viridans* more effectively than penicillin alone. There is no compelling evidence that the treatment of endocardial infections caused by *S. viridans* with two agents provides a therapeutic advantage. However, the use of dual therapy in patients with endocarditis caused by NVS reduces morbidity and mortality.

Strains of *S. viridans* are sensitive to penicillin, cephalothin, and vancomycin.[102] The cephalosporins are effective in the treatment of streptococcal endocarditis, especially in patients allergic to penicillin. The risk of significant cross-reactivity between penicillin and cephalothin is less than 1%.

Third-generation cephalosporins exhibit excellent in vitro activity against nonenterococcal streptococci.[103,104] Tolerance to penicillin indicates tolerance to the cephalosporins, ceftriaxone, vancomycin, and amoxicillin.[105,106] Isolates of *S. viridans* highly resistant to penicillin are resistant to ceftriaxone as well. Studies of the treatment of infective endocarditis caused by *S. viridans* have indicated that a daily dose of 1 g of ceftriaxone for 4 weeks or 2 g for 2 weeks, followed by amoxicillin taken orally for an additional 2 weeks, cures the disease in 98% of patients.[107,108]

The aminoglycosides do not inhibit the growth of *S. viridans*. However, the addition of gentamicin or streptomycin produces synergism in vitro and in vivo. When these antibiotics are combined with a beta-lactam, many streptococci, including sensitive, resistant, and tolerant strains and NVS, are killed.[109–112] Synergy has also been documented in an experimental model in which a combination of ceftriaxone and an aminoglycoside was studied.[108] Isolates of *S. viridans* resistant to streptomycin and kanamycin have been identified among strains that are highly resistant to penicillin. Gentamicin appears to be effective in the management of disease produced by *S. viridans* resistant to streptomycin and kanamycin but sensitive to penicillin.[112]

Treatment with bacteriostatic antibiotics such as erythromycin or clindamycin should be avoided because they produce variable results. Erythromycin appears to be a more effective bacteriostatic agent. Clindamycin must be considered a third-line drug for the management of nonenterococcal or streptococcal endocardial disease because it fails to sterilize infected valves and exposes patients to the risk of pseudomembranous colitis.[113]

It is important to note that the susceptibility of *S. bovis* to a number of antimicrobial agents is similar to that of *S. viridans*. Although *S. bovis* belongs in group D, it is usually much more sensitive to penicillin than are enterococci. The MBC of penicillin against *S. bovis* is 0.2 μg/ml or less. Recommendations for the treatment of endocarditis caused by *S. bovis* are essentially the same as those for disease produced by *S. viridans*.[114]

The principles that apply to the treatment of infective endocarditis caused by penicillin-susceptible streptococci were established in 1950.[115,116] It is clear that the dose of a drug and the time over which it is administered are vital in determining clinical and microbiological cure. The incidence of relapse has decreased as the dose of penicillin and the duration of treatment have been increased. Patients treated with 1 million units of penicillin daily for only 5 days had a relapse rate of 83%. This decreased to 50% when

500,000 units of the antibiotic were administered for 10 days. Twenty percent of individuals given only 250,000 units of the drug every day for 20 days were not cured.[117] Patients receiving 10–20 million units of penicillin G per day for 4 weeks responded; the incidence of relapse ranged from 0.6% to 5%.[118,119] However, when the same dose of penicillin was administered for only 2 weeks, 17% of patients relapsed.[120]

Treatment with penicillin plus an aminoglycoside is synergistic against penicillin sensitive streptococci.[104–109] In 1974, Wolfe and Johnson[109] reported their experiences with the therapy of 200 patients with infective endocarditis studied at the New York Hospital–Cornell Medical Center. Treatment involved the administration of 10–20 million units of penicillin intravenously per day or 1.2 million units intramuscularly every 6 hr for 4 weeks. All patients were given streptomycin (1 g) intramuscularly daily for the first 2 weeks of treatment. The incidence of relapse after treatment was discontinued was 1.4%.[121]

Infective endocarditis was treated with penicillin and streptomycin for 2 weeks during the 1950s.[122,123] This resulted in varying success. Wilson et al.[122] treated patients with 1.2 million units of penicillin every 6 hr plus streptomycin every 12 hr for 2 weeks. This regimen is preferred by many for the management of infective endocarditis caused by penicillin-sensitive streptococci.[124] Gentamicin has been substituted for streptomycin because of the ease of measuring serum levels of the former antibiotic. A recent recommendation has suggested treatment of penicillin-sensitive streptococci with ceftriaxone and gentamicin.[125]

A single daily dose of an aminoglycoside may be preferred. A high concentration of this antibiotic in serum maximizes the rate of killing of organisms and leads to a high level of the drug in the vegetation. This regimen permits washout of the aminoglycoside from the cortex of the kidney, which may decrease the risk of nephrotoxicity.[126]

Whether or not the treatment of infective endocarditis requires more than one drug has been questioned by Weinstein.[1] He treated a large number of patients with disease caused by streptococci with a single antimicrobial agent; all patients survived. No relapses occurred within 6 months after therapy was discontinued.

As a rule, patients with infective endocarditis caused by penicillin-sensitive streptococci require 4 weeks of therapy. Shorter periods, such as 2 weeks, may be feasible in the following situations: (1) infection by S. *viridans* or S. *bovis;* (2) infection of native valves; (3) symptoms of infective endocarditis for less than 3 months; (4) no complications of the disease, such as ring abscess; (5) absence of extracardiac infection; and (6) no risk of developing ototoxicity or nephrotoxicity when treated with an aminoglycoside. Symptoms of endocardial infection that persist for more than 3 months before treatment is initiated are associated with a high incidence of treatment failure.[124] Patients unsuitable for a short course of treatment require 10–20 million units of penicillin for 4 weeks. Ceftriaxone may be a promising alternative therapy, but it should not be considered standard treatment for endocardial infection caused by S. *viridans.*

Treatment of Penicillin-Resistant Streptococci

Strains of *S. viridans* sensitive to penicillin with an MIC of 0.2–0.4 μg/ml have been considered relatively resistant to this antibiotic by Roberts.[126] Those with an MIC above 0.5 μg/ml are totally resistant. However, Moellering[127] considered the breakpoint of MIC resistance to be 1.0 μg/ml; isolates with an MIC of 0.1–0.9 μg/ml are relatively resistant. Most cases of infective endocarditis caused by *S. viridans* are cured by treatment with penicillin.[72,73] High resistance to this agent develops in patients who have been given it prophylactically. Endocarditis caused by such isolates requires therapy with larger than standard doses of penicillin (36 million units per day for 4 weeks). The addition of an aminoglycoside provides no clinical advantage.

Tolerant streptococci generally are quite sensitive to penicillin. The major exceptions are NVS, the treatment of which requires 10–20 million units of penicillin plus streptomycin or gentamicin per day for 4 weeks. However, this regimen is associated with a high incidence of relapse or failure. Strains of *S. viridans* resistant to streptomycin do not respond to combined therapy. A short course of therapy with gentamicin may be effective.[128] A summary of the treatment regimens for *S. viridans* endocarditis is presented in Table 13.1.

Enterococcal Endocarditis

Although group D streptococci are now included in the genus *Enterococcus*, most clinicians consider them bona fide streptococci.[129] Of the 12 recognized species of enterococci, *E. faecalis* and *E. faecium* represent 90% of the clinically important organisms. They cause 87.5% and 12.5% respectively, of enterococcal endocarditis.[130] Not all streptococci that express the group D antigen are enterococci. *S. bovis,* an important major member of this group of bacteria, is quite sensitive to penicillin.

Enterococci have become resistant to penicillin and beta-lactam antibiotics over the past 10 years.[131,132] This is probably related to the presence of low-affinity binding proteins.[133] Changes in binding sites have been identified in populations that have never been exposed to any antimicrobial agents.[134] The MIC of penicillin and ampicillin for *E. faecalis* ranges from 1 to 4 μg/ml; for *E. faecium* it spans from 16 to 64 μg/ml.[133, 135–140] Bush et al.[141] noted that one-third of the strains of *E. faecium* had an MIC for penicillin above 200 μg/ml. *E. faecium* exhibited both a wider and a higher scope of resistance than *E. faecalis.*[142] This organism has been labeled the "nosocomial pathogen" of the 1990s.[143] All enterococci are tolerant to the beta-lactam drugs.[144] This fact is clinically important because it prevents the use of a single beta-lactam for the management of enterococcal endocarditis. Most enterococci are sensitive to vancomycin; the MBC for most strains is at least 10-fold higher than the MIC. These organisms are slightly susceptible to the fluroquinolones.

Table 13.1. Guidelines for Therapy of *S. viridans* Endocarditis

Antibiotic	Dosage Regimen*
1. Penicillin sensitive[†]	
Standard course	
Crystalline penicillin G	20 million units/day IV in four divided doses for 4 weeks
Short course	
Crystalline penicillin G	20 million units/day IV in four divided doses for 2 weeks
or	
procaine penicillin	1.2 million units every 6 hr
plus	IM for 2 weeks
streptomycin	7.5 mg/kg every 12 hr IM
or	
gentamicin	1.0 mg/kg every 8 hr IV
2. Relatively resistant to	
Penicillin[†]	20 million units/day IV in divided doses for 4 weeks
plus	
streptomycin	7.5 mg/kg every 12 hr IM
or	
gentamicin	1.0 mg/kg every 8 hr IV
3. Resistant to penicillin[†]	
Crystalline penicillin G	20 million units/day IV in divided doses for 6 weeks
plus	
streptomycin	7.5 mg/kg every 12 hr IM for 2 weeks
or	
gentamicin	1.0 mg/kg every 8 hr for 2 weeks IV
4. Tolerant to pencillin[†]	
Crystalline penicillin G	20 million units/day IV in four divided doses for 4 weeks
with or without	
streptomycin	7.5 mg/kg every 12 hr IM for 2 weeks
or	
gentamicin	1.0 mg/kg every 8 hr IV for 2 weeks
5. Nutrionally variant streptococci[†]	
Crystalline penicillin G	20 million units/day in divided IV doses for 6 weeks
plus	
streptomycin	7.5 mg/kg every 12 hr IM for 2 weeks
or	
gentamicin	1.0 mg/kg every 8 hr IV for 2 weeks

*Normal renal function.
†See text for definition.

Enterococci and other streptococci are resistant to the aminoglycosides. This resistance appears to be due to the failure of these antibiotics to penetrate the cellular wall of these organisms.[145] In 1947, Hunter[146] observed that treatment with penicillin and streptomycin was successful in the management of infective endocarditis caused by enterococci. Moellering and Weinberg[147] discovered the mechanism behind this effect. Penicillin and other antibiotics, such as vancomycin, that damage the integrity of the cell wall permit the penetration of aminoglycosides into the interior of bacteria. Aminoglycosides are lethal for the enterococci.[148] Vancomycin combined with streptomycin is synergistic for 80% of enterococci; streptomycin plus gentamicin is synergistic for 98% of these organisms.[149]

Although they appear to do so in vitro, neither the cephalosporins nor the antistaphylococcal penicillins are synergistic clincially when added to an aminoglycoside.[150–152] The reasons for this are (1) relatively poor intrinsic activity against the organism and (2) increased protein binding and in vivo production of inactive metabolites.[153,154] Not all combinations of aminoglycosides and cell wall–active antibiotics produce synergy. Gentamicin offers the best possibility for achieving synergistic activity when added to drugs active against microbial cell walls. Because of its increased activity against enterococci in vitro, ampicillin plus an aminoglycoside is most often used.[140] Antibiotics that interfere with the bacterial synthesis of proteins, such as erythromycin, chloramphenicol, or tetracyclines, when added to an aminoglycoside fail to produce synergy.[155]

Rifampin appears to be quite active against enterococci but these organisms develop resistance rapidly to this antibiotic. Since rifampin antagonizes the activity of ampicillin, the latter agent should not be used to decrease the development of resistance to rifampin.

The effectiveness of synergism is blunted as enterococci become resistant to more of the agents used in combination. The organisms are capable of developing resistance to a large number of antimicrobial agents. This phenomenon is not related to the mutation of preexisting DNA.[155–157]

The development of high-level resistance to the aminoglycosides (MIC above 2,000 μ/ml) and streptomycin is very important clinically.[158] This has been noted to be caused by a ribosomal mutation (infrequent) or by the presence of the gene that codes for streptomycin adenyl transferase. Despite a decrease in the use of streptomycin, resistance to this agent is a problem in about 50% of enterococcal disease. A plasmid that produces phosphotransferase is responsible for the development of resistance to kanamycin and amikacin.[159]

Strains of *E. faecalis* highly resistant to kanamycin amikacin, netilmicin, and gentamicin were first identified in 1979.[160] Organisms with similar antimicrobial patterns of susceptibility have been identified in the Far East, Europe, and the United States.[161,162] Enterococci resistant to gentamicin, on the basis of plasmid-induced production of both acetyltransferase and phosphotransferase, have been identified in about 50% of hospitals.[163] Fatal infective endocarditis has been caused by highly resistant enterococci.[164] Although these organisms are usualy resistant to all the aminoglycosides, 25% are susceptible to streptomycin.[165]

In 1983, Murray and Mederski-Samorap ascribed enterococcal resistance to the expression of beta-lactamases.[166] This is not as widespread as is resistance to the aminoglycosides[166] and appears to be similar to that produced by *S. aureus.*[167] Routine clinical studies may fail to detect their presence. Many organisms that produce beta-lactamase are also resistant to gentamicin. The results of several studies in animals have supported their clinical importance.[168] Enterococci are currently developing resistance to penicillin and ampicillin. This is not related to the production of these enzymes but is probably related to the acquisition of a gene that encodes for an altered penicillin-binding protein.[169]

Resistance of enterococci to vancomycin was first identified in 1988. These organisms have been considered resistant to this antibiotic when the MIC is above 64 μg/ml. A growing number of infections caused by isolates resistant to vancomycin and teicoplanin are being reported.[170,171] Enterococci resistant to teicoplanin are usually sensitive to daptomycin. Clinicians must rely on the microbiology laboratory to identify the presence of antibiotic resistance among clinical strains. An approach to screening of organisms and their response to vancomycin have been described by Murray.[131]

A synergistic combination of a cell wall–active antibiotic plus an aminoglycoside is required for the successful management of enterococcal endocarditis, although treatment with penicillin alone has cured the disease.[172] However, this treatment has not been successful in all cases.[120] For organisms sensitive to a combination of penicillin and an aminoglycoside, the addition of streptomycin increases the incidence of cures.[173]

Relapses occur in patients who have had symptoms for more than 3 months before treatment is initiated and in those with infected prosthetic valves.[125] Gentamicin is presently the drug of choice when the organism involved is sensitive to this agent. The specific dose required to produce synergy is unknown. Wilson[174] has advocated the use of a smaller dose of gentamicin (3 mg/kg/day) rather than 4–5 mg/kg/day. Synergy appears to develop at a level of 3 μg/ml of gentamicin in serum.

When there is evidence that infective endocarditis caused by an enterococcus is resistant to the newer aminoglycosides, a study of its sensitivity to streptomycin is indicated.[175] A strain may be resistant to gentamicin but sensitive to another aminoglycoside. We emphasize that there is no therapeutic reason for using an aminoglycoside in combination with cell-wall active antibiotics if the pathogen is resistant to the aminoglycoside.[176]

Ampicillin, administered by continuous infusion to produce a serum level of 16 μg/ml, appears to be the best therapy in the situation of aminoglycoside resistance.[131] Ampicillin is superior to vancomycin. Imipenem,[177] ciprofloxacin,[178] or ampicillin with sulbactam must be considered as alternative choices for the treatment of aminoglycoside-resistant enterococcal endocarditis.[179] Treatment with trimethoprim-sulfamethoxazole for resistant enterococcal disease is not recommended, although the organism may appear to be sensitive. Clinical studies have indicated that these organisms use exogenous folate and thus may bypass the antibacterial effect of this antibiotic.[180,181] Rifampin plays no role in the management of infection caused by multiple resistant enterococci. No firm recommendation can be made for treatment of isolates that are resistant to multiple antibiotics.[182,183] Usually the valve must be excised.

Treatment of A, B, C, and G Beta-Hemolytic Streptococci

All members of streptococcal groups A, B, C, and G are sensitive to penicillin G; the B, C and G strains are less so. The treatment of these organisms with penicillin plus gentamicin should be considered.[184–187] Infective endocarditis caused by these bacteria responds to treatment with 10–20 million units of penicillin G per day.[188]

The therapy of streptococcal endocarditis in patients allergic to penicillin presents a problem. Although potentially dangerous, desensitization can be carried out. We recommend, if at all possible, treatment with an agent other than penicillin. Vancomycin is the drug of choice in this situation.[189,190] However, when it is combined with an aminoglycoside, the dose of each agent must be monitored because the incidence of nephrotoxicity is increased.[191]

Staphylococcal Endocarditis

Staphylococci produce infective endocarditis in about 34% of patients. Ninety percent of the cases are caused by coagulase-positive *S. aureus*. About 25% of infections of native valves are due to this organism.[192,193] It is involved in 60% of IVDA.[194] Coagulase-positive *S. aureus* is responsible for 50% of endocarditis that involves prosthetic valves.[195] In contrast, coagulase-negative staphylococci (CONS) cause the disease in 50% of patients with newly implanted valves.[196] Infection of native valves by CONS is uncommon. Staphylococcal infection of native valves is fatal in 40% of individuals. This rate has not changed since penicillin became available.[193] Fifty percent of patients with endocarditis of prosthetic valves, due to *S. aureus*, die.[195] About 22% of those with prosthetic valves infected by CONS succumb to the disease despite aggresssive medical and surgical therapy.[197] Infections of native valves by CONS are much less resistant to therapy than are those caused by coagulase-positive staphylococci.[198] The therapy of tricuspid valvular disease caused by *S. aureus* in IVDA has been successful in more than 90% of cases treated with antimicrobial agents alone.[199] The outcome of infection of the left side of the heart in the same population has been similar to that in those who did not use drugs.[200]

Infective endocarditis caused by CONS may be complicated by the appearance of metastatic suppurative lesions and the development of resistance to a number of anticrobial agents, especially the beta-lactam drugs.

The present therapy of staphylococcal endocarditis often requires the administration of a cell wall–active antibiotic plus an aminoglycoside. This leads to more rapid sterilization of the vegetations. Surgery may be required to manage the complications of the disease.

Most strains of *S. aureus* were very responsive to penicillin when this antibiotic first became available; only 10% are presently sensitive to it.[201] Clinicians must now assume that a strain of *S. aureus* recovered from the blood or from an infected site is resistant to penicillin G. In our experience, the Kirby-Bauer disk sensitivity test is not always reliable in identifying penicillin-resistant *S. aureus*. Susceptibility to penicillin must be confirmed by determination of the MIC and MBC of this and other drugs.

Resistance of *S. aureus* to penicillin involves three mechanisms: (1) the production of penicillinase by bacteria; (2) altered penicillin-binding proteins (methicillin-resistant *S. aureus* [MRSA]); and (3) tolerance. Because most strains of this organism produce beta-lactamases, the semisynthetic, penicillinase-resistant penicillins, oxacillin or nafcillin, must be used to treat valvular disease produced by *S. aureus*. Animal models and clinical studies have proved the therapeutic equivalence of these antimicrobial agents.[202–204] Oxacillin may result in abnormal hepatic function; this is rarely important clinically.[205] Nafcillin may produce leukopenia.[206] However, a major advantage of this agent is the fact that it is excreted via the biliary tract.[207,208] This makes nafcillin the preferred choice for the treatment of infective endocarditis in patients with significant renal failure.

Treatment with oxacillin eradicates sensitive strains of *S. aureus* in 2–6 days.[209] Failure to sterilize the blood is a problem in only 1% of cases. This is usually related to the presence of an abscess within or outside the heart. The incidence of relapse following treatment in about 5%.[210] First-generation cephalosporins are a substitute for the semisynthetic penicillins, especially in individuals with a history of a relatively minor reaction to these agents, such as a maculopapular rash. The semisynthetic penicillins are preferred because they are not affected by the lactamases produced by *S. aureus* (the inoculum effect.).[211] Studies in animals have indicated that cefazolin is the most susceptible to the beta-lactamases.[212–217] This explains the increased incidence of treatment failure with the cephalosporins. Kaye[218] has pointed out that the half-life of cefazolin inactivation by the beta-lactamase produced by *S. aureus* ranges from 2 to 4 hr; the half-life of the drug in serum is only 2 hr. The discrepancy between the fate of degradation and the interval between doses of cefazolin (6–8 hr) makes it unlikely that a significant quantity of the antibiotic is destroyed. Intramuscular management of infection caused by *S. aureus* has been useful in patients with inadequate intravenous access.

Two incidations for the use of vancomycin for the treatment of infective endocarditis caused by *S. aureus* are (1) allergy to the beta-lactam antibiotics and (2) the presence of MRSA. Treatment with this agent must be closely monitored because it produces otoxicity and nephrotoxicity. This is primarily a problem when an aminoglycoside is added to vancomycin.[219,220] Peak levels of this agent in serum are reached 1–2 hr after infusion and range from 20 to 40 μg/ml; trough levels are 5 to 15 mg/ml. The dose of vancomycin must be adjusted in patients with decreased renal function. This antibiotic must be administered over at least 1 hr in order to avoid the generalized flushing reaction produced by the very large quantities of histamine released by most cells (red man's syndrome).

Vancomycin has been considered the therapeutic equivalent of the penicillinase-resistant penicillins. However, this conclusion has been questioned since the 1970s.[221] The suboptimal response of methicillin-sensitive *S. aureus* (MSSA) to vancomycin has been documented in the 1980s and 1990s.[222,223] Small and Chambers[223] reviewed 13 cases of infective endocarditis caused by MSSA treated with vancomycin. Despite adequate treatment, the incidence of failure was 35%. A study by Harstein et al.[224] indicated that 7 of 10 episodes of bacteremia with *S. aureus* following treatment with vancomycin were relapses. A similar incidence of failure was noted in endocardial infection caused by MRSA.

Teicoplanin, a glycopeptide, is presently being considered for approval by the U.S. Food and Drug Administration. Treatment with this antibiotic has been associated with a significant incidence of failure in patients with either infective endocarditis or other deep-seated infections caused by *S. aureus*.[225–227] Several theories have been advanced to explain the inconsistent effectiveness of this glycopeptide. Because the renal clearance of this agent is increased in febrile patients, its concentration in serum is low and its penetration of tissues is poor.[228,229] A recent report has documented the development in *S. aureus* of resistance to teicoplanin during the therapy of infective endocarditis.[230]

Combined Therapy of Staphylococcal Endocarditis

Several studies in animal models have indicated that the addition of an aminoglycoside to a penicillin or vancomycin often produces a synergistic effect. This leads to clearing of *S. aureus* from the bloodstream much more rapidly than is the case when a single drug is administered.[231–234] Three studies have failed to reach a definite conclusion with regard to the clinical relevance of these experimental observations. A retrospective review of the therapy of infective endocarditis caused by *S. viridans* in IVDA treated with a beta-lactam agent or an aminoglycoside has indicated no difference in the fatality rate in each group.[235] A study by Watanakunakorn and Baird[236] focused attention on staphylocccal endocarditis in individuals not addicted to drugs. Except for a much higher incidence of death (40%), the findings were similar to those reported by Abrams et al.[235] Infection of the mitral or aortic valve was associated with a fatality rate higher than that occurring when the right side of the heart was infected. In this situation, the outcome depended on the incidence of metastatic infection and on the presence of diabetes mellitus, alcoholism, and cardiac disease. A multicenter study of individuals with or without addiction to drugs has indicated that there was no difference in the fatality rate in those treated with nafcillin alone for 6 weeks or this antibiotic plus gentamicin for the first 2 weeks. Treatment with both agents decreased the duration of bacteremia in patients with infected tricuspid valves.[237] The median duration of fever decreased from 5 days in individuals treated with nafcillin alone to 3 days in those receiving combined therapy. The duration of bacteremia was shorter in nonaddicts who received combined therapy. The incidence of azotemia was much higher in individuals treated with penicillin and gentamicin.

In 1988, Chambers et al.[238] treated staphylococcal endocarditis involving the tricuspid valve in IVDA with nafcillin plus tobramycin for 2 weeks; 94% of the patients survived. It is important to note that most of these individuals had a small number of valvular vegetations and a very low incidence of metastatic infections. The original design of the study included therapy with vancomycin plus tobramycin. This combination was abandoned when two of three patients failed to respond to treatment.

The studies described above have not answered a number of questions regarding the importance of combined therapy for the management of infective endocarditis caused by *S. aureus*. All have had problems in design because the population studied has been relatively small and there have been difficulties in randomizing patients with multiple significant underlying disorders. Because *S. aureus* is a very aggressive organism, the valvular vegetations it produces must be sterilized rapidly in order to limit cardiac injury. With this in mind, it is reasonable to treat with a penicillinase-resistant penicillin plus gentamicin or tobramycin unless a complication, such as renal failure, is present. When combined therapy is not employed initially, an aminoglycoside must be added when patients fail to respond. The addition of tobramycin to nafcillin may decrease the duration of treatment of infected tricuspid valves to 2 weeks in IVDA. Combined therapy may be effective in individuals infected by tolerant strains of *S. aureus*.

Rifampin has two distinctive characteristics that make it an interesting agent for the treatment of infective endocarditis caused by *S. aureus*. One is its ability to penetrate phagocytes. The other is its capacity to sterilize staphylococcal abscesses more rapidly than other antimicrobial agents.[239,240] However, resistance develops quickly when rifampin alone is administered; this is prevented by the addition of a penicillin. There is conflicting evidence that rifampin decreases the bactericidal activity of the penicillinase-resistant penicillins. In vitro studies by Sande and Johnson[241] and Zinner et al.[242] have indicated that this agent interferes with the antistaphylococcal activity of the penicillins. Studies in rabbits have demonstrated that the addition of rifampin to cloxacillin produces more rapid sterilization of vegetations than does cloxacillin alone.[243] Although rifampin has been reported to increase the bactericidal activity of the beta-lactam antibiotics in the serum of patients undergoing treatment of endocarditis caused by *S. aureus*,[244] other clinical studies have not confirmed this finding.[245] On the basis of the data presented above, the routine use of rifampin to treat staphylococcal infections is presently not recommended.

Other drugs, including the quinolones, are active against MRSA in vitro and in a rabbit model of infective endocarditis.[246,247] Because these agents are well absorbed when administered orally, they may be effective in the management of infective endocarditis in patients with very limited venous access, such as IVDA. Chambers et al.[238] reported the successful treatment of infective endocarditis involving the right side of the heart in addicts treated with ciprofloxacin and rifampin. However, there is some evidence that the addition of rifampin may decrease the activity of ciprofloxacin and promote resistance to all of the quinolones.[248] The increasing resistance of MRSA to the fluroquinolones is disturbing.[249]

The treatment of infective endocarditis with trimethoprim-sulfamethoxazole has led to success, total failure, or relapse.[250] This combination of drugs appears to produce better clinical results in patients with infections that involve the valves or the right side of the heart. A study of IVDA by Markowitz et al.[251] indicated that the treatment of infective endocarditis caused by S. aureus failed when trimethoprim-sulfamethoxazole was administered but was effective when vancomycin was infused. However, failure of trimethoprim-sulfamethoxazole occurred only in patients infected by MSSA.

Therapy with bacteriostatic agents, such as clindamycin and erythromycin, has led to a significant incidence of relapse in patients with infective endocarditis caused by S. aureus. These drugs are not substitutes for the semisynthetic penicillins.[252]

Strains of S. aureus sensitive to a MBC of cell wall–active antibiotics much greater than their MIC were first recovered in the 1970s.[253] These organisms appear to contain inadequate levels of autolytic enzymes and are possibly responsible for the failure to treat some infections caused by S. aureus.[254] Up to 40% of isolates have been considered tolerant. However, only 7% of the members of a single bacterial colony may exhibit tolerance. This heterogeneity interferes with the identification of these strains, especially when the inoculum is small. There is evidence that infection by tolerant organisms often produces a complicated clinical course.[255] The approach to the treatment of disease caused by these isolates is unclear. Some investigators have identified no difference in the rate of killing of typical and tolerant strains of S. aureus by beta-lactam drugs.[256,257] Both types are susceptible to low concentrations of gentamicin. Unless there is a contraindication to its use, gentamicin should be administered over the first week of treatment. In addition to increasing the rate of sterilization of vegetations, this combination of drugs inhibits tolerant organisms but does not produce an improved clinical outcome.[255] If monotherapy does not produce an adequate clinical response, gentamicin must be added because the organism responsible for the disease may be tolerant. It must be emphasized that an inadequate response to treatment of endocarditis caused by S. aureus is usually due to an unidentified focus of infection that eventually requires drainage.[258]

Methicillin-resistant *S. aureus*

Endocarditis caused by MRSA poses unique problems. It is difficult to detect the presence of methicillin resistance because only a single bacterial cell among 10^4 to 10^5 organisms may be resistant. The expression of S. aureus resistance to methicillin may be improved by[259] growing the organism at 30°C, increasing the osmolality of the medium, and exposing cultures to subtherapeutic levels of a beta-lactam antibiotic.[260] Microtiter methods are not very sensitive in detecting MRSA. When there is a high level of suspicion of MRSA, more sensitive screening tests must be employed. Most helpful is Mueller-Hinton agar containing sodium chloride incubated at 35°C.

An organism resistant to oxacillin is resistant to all the beta-lactam agents, including the cephalosporins.

A major problem in the management of infective endocarditis caused by MRSA is the limited number of effective antimicrobial agents. Vancomycin is the mainstay of treatment. Although teicoplanin appears to be effective in animals,[261] therapy with this agent has failed in 75% of patients treated with 6 mg/kg/day.[262] However, when 24 mg/kg/day was administered, the incidence of cure increased to 78%, a result comparable to that achieved by vancomycin.[263]

Disease caused by MRSA responds more slowly to treatment with vancomycin than does that produced by MSSA. Patients with endocardial disease due to MRSA have persistent bacteremia for 9 days and remain febrile for 7 days after initiation of treatment with vancomycin. The addition of rifampin appears to make no difference in the clinical outcome.[264] Individuals with infective endocarditis caused by MSSA clear the bacteremia within 6 days of initiation of treatment with oxacillin.

The quinolones have been very effective in the management of experimental endocarditis caused by MRSA.[265] However, the rapid increase in resistance of MRSA to these antibiotics is a matter for concern.

There has been an increase in the use of trimethoprim-sulfamethoxazole for the treatment of endocarditis caused by MRSA. The results of a study by Markowitz et al.[266] have indicated that the therapy of infected tricuspid valves with this agent is highly successful. This approach must not be applied in non-IVDA with valvular infection.

A recently described type of resistance expressed by *S. aureus* appears to be related to the massive production of beta-lactamase by this organism. This is probably a laboratory phenomenon with little clinical significance because disease caused by this organism responds well to treatment with penicillinase-resistant penicillins or ampicillin plus sulbactam.[267]

The therapy of PVE caused by MSRA or MSSA requires the administration of penicillinase-resistant semisynthetic penicillins or vancomycin for 6–8 weeks; gentamicin is given for the first 2 weeks.[93] The treatment of endocarditis due to *S. aureus* is summarized in Table 13.2.

Coagulase-Negative *S. aureus*

Although 11 species of CONS [268] have been involved in human infections, most of the clinically important strains are *S. epidermidis*. This organism has become important in the pathogenesis of nosocomial infections that involve implantable materials.[269] *S. epidermidis* is responsible for about 50% of infections of prosthetic valves.[270,271] Several factors are involved in the propensity of *S. epidermidis* to infect various medical devices. Among these are (1) the production of extracellular glycocalyx or slime; (2) the widespread distribution of organisms on human skin; and (3) resistance to many antibiotics. While many strains of *S. epidermidis* that cause community-acquired infections are sensitive to the beta-lactam drugs, 58% of those

Table 13.2. Therapy of *S. aureus* Endocarditis*†

Valve Type	Antibiotic	Dose in Adults	Comments
		METHICILLIN-SENSITIVE *S. AUREUS*	
Native	Oxacillin‡	2 g IV every 4 hr for 4–6 weeks	
	Nafcillin‡§	3 g IV every 4 hr for 4–6 weeks	Larger doses than for oxacillin required because of greater volume of distribution
	Cefazolin‡	1.5 g IV every 6 hr for 4–6 weeks	For use in patients without minor allergies to penicillin but not anaphylaxtis
	Vancomycin‡	1.0 g IV every 12 hr for 4–6 weeks	For use in patients with no history of severe penicillin reactions
		METHICILLIN-RESISTANT *S. AUREUS*	
	Vancomycin	1.0 g IV every 12 hr for 4–6 weeks	
		METHICILLIN-SENSITIVE *S. AUREUS*	
Prosthetic	Nafcillin or oxacillin or cefazolin or vancomycin	In doses as described for native valve endocarditis for 6 weeks	Cefazolin or vancomycin in penicillin allergic patients above as described
	plus rifampin	300 mg PO every 8 hr for 6 weeks	
	Plus gentamicin	1.0 mg/kg 1M or IV every 8 hr for 2 weeks 1.5 mg/kg 1M or IV every 12 hr for 2 weeks	See text for gentamicin dosage intervals
		METHICILLIN-RESISTANT *S. AUREUS*	
Prosthetic	Vancomycin plus	1.0 g IV every 12 hr	
	rifampin plus	300 mg PO every 8 hr for 6 weeks	
	gentamicin	1.0 mg/kg every 8 hr IV for 6 weeks *or* 1.5 mg/kg every 12 hr for >6 weeks	See text for gentamicin dosing intervals

*For patients with normal renal function.
†See text for alternative regiments.
‡May be combined with gentamicin for first 3–7 days of therapy (see text).
§Preferred beta-lactam drug in patients with renal failure (see text).

involved in nosocomial infections are resistant to the penicillins and cephalosporins.[272] With few exceptions, all strains of *S. epidermidis* are sensitive to rifampin but may become resistant to this agent in a one-step process.[273] Many CONS recovered from patients with infected prosthetic valves are resistant to several antibiotics, including tetracycline, erythromycin, chloramphenicol, and clindamycin.[274,275] Resistance of *S. epidermidis* to penicillins is mediated by beta-lactamases; these enzymes are not inducible. The mechanism involved in the development of resistance to oxacillin among strains of *S. epidermidis* is similar to that in MRSA.[260] This property is heterogeneous and is screened by methods employed in the diagnosis of MRSA. It is important to note that a significant minority of MRSA may, despite appropriate testing, appear susceptible to the beta-lactam antibiotics.[276–279]

The aminoglycosides, especially gentamicin, are bactericidal for CONS. However, they are gradually becoming inactive against these organisms. Karchmer et al.[279] noted that 30% of strains of *S. epidermidis* are presently resistant to gentamicin, tobramycin, and amikacin.[279,280]

All CONS are sensitive to vancomycin and teicoplanin[281]; the latter appears to be the drug of choice. The development of resistance to both glycopeptides has been identified in *S. haemolyticus*.[282,283]

Infective endocarditis caused by *S. epidermidis* is associated with a high incidence of complications, including abscesses and leaks of paravalvular rings, dehiscence of prosthetic valves, and congestive cardiac failure. These are associated with a fatality rate that ranges from 60% to 75%.[279] Several combinations of antibiotics have been used to improve survival. Kolasa et al.[284] noted that vancomycin plus gentamicin or rifampin was effective in eradicating methicillin-resistant *S. epidermidis* (MRSE) from valvular vegetations; treatment with vancomycin alone failed to do this. The results of treatment of infective endocarditis caused by MRSE were similar to those observed in animals.[285] The survival rate was 81% in patients treated with vancomycin and rifampin, with or without gentamicin. Fifty-one percent of individuals treated with a beta-lactam agent, alone or combined with rifampin and an aminoglycoside, lived. Individuals treated with vancomycin alone fared no better than those who received a beta-lactam. Resistance to vancomycin did not develop over the course of treatment. However, cultures obtained during surgery grew organisms resistant to rifampin; these probably developed during treatment. Resistance to gentamicin was present in 12 of 15 isolates; all were resistant to teicoplanin and amikacin.

Karchmer et al.[285] conducted a prospective randomized study of the treatment of prosthetic valves infected by multiply resistant streptococci. Two groups of patients were included. One was treated with vancomycin plus rifampin for 6 weeks; the other received these agents plus gentamicin for the first 2 weeks of therapy. Both groups achieved the same level of success. Thirty-seven percent of patients not treated with gentamicin developed resistance to rifampin. This did not occur in those given an aminoglycoside.

Treatment with rifampin plus vancomycin for 6 weeks has been recommended for patients with MRSE. Because the MIC of vancomycin is high, peak levels in serum should approach 30–35 μg/ml.[286] Gentamicin must be administered for the first 2 weeks to individuals infected by an organism sensitive to this agent. This augments the bactericidal activity of the other antimicrobial agents and decreases the risk of development of resistance to rifampin. When methicillin-sensitive CONS are involved, therapy with beta-lactam antibiotics plus rifampin and gentamicin is recommended.[91,279]

The increasing resistance of MRSE to aminoglycosides may make this therapy useless. Studies in animals have indicated that the fluorquinolones may be substituted for by an aminoglycoside.[287] Aquinolone is the drug of choice[283] when an isolate is resistant to gentamicin.

Native valve endocarditis caused by CONS is associated with a high incidence of complications (e.g., paravalvular abscesses); this is also true when prosthetic valves are involved. About 50% of these patients require valvular replacement.[288] Unlike infection of prosthetic valves, up to 70% of CONS that infect native valves are sensitive to penicillinase-resistant penicillins. All organisms acquired in the community are sensitive to penicillinase-resistant penicillins. The incidence of methicillin-sensitive S. epidermidis (MSSE) is highest in individuals with infection of native valves.

Because the incidence of complications is high in patients with infective endocarditis caused by MRSE, treatment with more than one antimicrobial agent is mandatory.[289] This must include 3–7 days of therapy with gentamicin.[288] It has been suggested that individuals with infected prosthetic valves be treated for 6 weeks.[290] From 27% to 46% of endocardial infections that involve native valves caused by CONS require cardiac surgery.[288,289,291] Table 13.3 summarizes the antibiotic therapy of endocarditis caused by CONS.

Gram-Negative Organisms

About 5% of native valves and 15% of prosthetic infections are caused by gram-negative organisms.[292,293] There has been a steady increase in the incidence of disease produced by these examples since the 1960s. The bacteria most often responsible for the development of infective endocarditis are the Enterobacteriaceae, including E. coli; Klebsiella species; S. marcesens; Pseudomonas species, including Ps. aeruginosa and Ps. cepacia; Salmonella species; the HACEK group (Haemophilus, Actinobacillus, Cardiobacterium, Eikenella, and Kingella species); Bacteriodes species; and Neisseria species.

The treatment of infective endocarditis caused by these organisms is associated with a fatality rate of 80%. Many patients with this disease are resistant to treatment because of the impaired activity of their host defenses. Among the causes of impairment are cirrhosis, intravenous drug abuse, and the presence of intracardiac foreign material (e.g., prosthetic

Table 13.3. Therapy of Coagulase-Negative Staphylococcal Endocarditis*†

Valve Type	Antibiotic	Dose in Adults	Comments
Native‡	Vancomycin	1 g IV every 12 hr for 6 weeks	All isolates must be assumed to be resistant to beta-lactam antibiotics unless proven otherwise (see text)
Prosthetic	Vancomycin	1 g IV every 12 hr for 6 weeks	As above
	plus rifampin	300 mg PO every 8 hr for 6 weeks	
	plus gentamicin	1.0 mg/kg IV every 8 hr or 1.5 mg/kg every 12 hr for 2 weeks	See text for gentamicin dosing intervals

*For patients with normal renal function.
†See text for alternative regimens.
‡May be combined with gentamicin for first 3–7 days of therapy (see text).

valves).[294] Both the paucity of controlled studies on the effectiveness of the antibiotics against them and the low incidence of valvular infection produced by gram-negative bacteria has inhibited efforts to improve the therapeutic outcome of this type of endocarditis. Many of the pathogens listed above require the use of antimicrobial agents with a low therapeutic:toxic ratio, such as the aminoglycosides.

The development of the third-generation cephalosporins, imipenem, and the broad-spectrum penicillins has increased the options for treatment. All of these agents were developed to improve the efficacy and decrease the toxicity of drugs like the aminoglycosides. However, they have created new problems, one of which is an increase in the incidence of disease produced by *Enterobacter* species in patients treated with the new cephalosporins. These organisms are now the third most common cause of gram-negative nosocomial infections. Only *E. coli* and *Ps. aeruginosa* are involved more often in nosocomial disease.[294–297] There is an increase not only in the prevalence of infection caused by *Enterobacter* species, but also in their resistance to the cephalosporins.[294–298]

Although in vitro studies may indicate that a strain of *Enterobacter* is sensitive to a cephalosporin, the organism may be resistant to this agent because it produces a cephalosporinase that neutralizes all members of this group of antibiotics.[298] It is not expressed constitutively but must be induced by exposure to a cephalosporin.[298,299] This process is rapid and confers resistance both to the cephalosporins and to many other beta-lactam antibiotics. Other gram-negative organisms, including *Serratia* species, *Proteus* species, and *Citrobacter freundii*, may produce this same enzyme. *Enterobacter* is the primary source of the cephalosporinases, partly because these organisms are the most common colonizers of the gastrointestinal tract.[300] The bowel has been found to be the source of infection in all patients and in health care workers.[301,302] *Pseudomonas* species produces an enzyme that is inducible on exposure to the new cephalosporins.[294] Although *E. coli* and *K. pneumoniae* do not possess an enzyme similar to the one described above, these organisms may alter their beta-lactamases and destroy the activity of third-generation cephalosporins and broad-spectrum penicillins. Disease caused by *E. coli* and *Klebsiella* species have had a significant impact in several institutions, including a chronic care facility.[303,304]

Inhibitors of the beta-lactamases, such as clavulinic acid and sulbactam, may be destroyed by inducible beta-lactamases.[305] This may reach the point at which the antibacterial activity of a combination of drugs, such as ticarcillin and clavulinic acid or ampicillin and sulbactam, is destroyed.

It is important to limit the use of the third-generation cephalosporins in order to decrease the risk of the development of potent cephalosporinases. Standard in vitro studies of sensitivity are not reliable for identifying inducible resistance of gram-negative organisms to the cephalosporins or the inhibitors of the beta-lactamases among strains of enterobacter, serratia and *Proteus sp*. Infective endocarditis caused by gram-negative organisms that may produce an inducible cephalosporinase (e.g., *Enterobacter* species) is best treated with a broad-spectrum penicillin (e.g., ticarcillin) and an aminoglycoside. This provides optimal therapy without stimulating the production of these enzymes. Treatment with a penicillin improves the therapeutic activity of the aminoglycosides.[306] This is due, in part, to the ability of the beta-lactams to produce a bactericidal effect when the level of the aminoglycoside in serum falls below the MBC of the drug used to treat the organism responsible for the disease. The use of "double beta" regimens—that is, two beta-lactam drugs—probably act as a strong stimulus for the induction of cephalosporinases.[294]

Aztreonam and the quinolones have been used to treat infective endocarditis.[307–309] Experience with these agents is limited. The development of resistance of various gram-negative organisms to these antimicrobial agents has been documented.[309] These drugs have been successful in suppressing active disease for long periods in patients with endocarditis caused by *Pseudomonas*.[310]

In general, gram-negative organisms, excluding *Pseudomonas* species, the fastidious HACEK group, and miscellaneous gram-negative bacteria, are Enterobacteriaceae.[311] Treatment of these infections is based on the results of studies of their in vitro sensitivity to various antimicrobial agents.[312] (Table 13.4). Ampicillin and cefazolin are effective in the treatment of disease caused by *E. coli* and *Proteus* species.[313] The addition of gentamicin to ampicillin increases the effectiveness of therapy.[306] However, when these organisms are highly sensitive to ampicillin, there is no need for an additional antibiotic. The addition of an aminoglycoside increases the risk of nephrotoxicity. Combined therapy is required for the management of disease caused by other gram-negative bacilli. It is probably best to avoid the

Table 13.4. Therapy of Infective Endocarditis Caused by Enterobacteriaceae and HACEK Organisms

Organism	Antibiotic Regimen*	Alternative Antibiotic Regimen*†
E. coli and P. mirabilis	Ampicilin‡ (12 g/day IV) for 4–6 weeks ± gentamicin§ (5 mg/kg/day) for 4–6 weeks	Cefazolin‡ (1 g IV every 8 hr for 4–6 weeks) or cefotaxime‡ (2 g IV every 6 hr) for 4–6 weeks or aztreonam§ (2 g IV every 6 hr) or 4–6 weeks or gentamicin (5 mg/kg/day) for 4–6 weeks
Klebsiella sp.	Cefotaxime‡ (2 g IV every 8 hr) for 4–6 weeks + gentamicin§ (5 mg/kg/day) for 4–6 weeks	Aztreonam§ (2 g IV every 6 hr) for 4–6 weeks + Gentamicin (5 mg/kg day) for 4–6 weeks
Enterobacter sp. Citrobacter sp. Providencia sp. S. marcescens	Ticarcillin (3 g IV every 4 hr) for 4–6 weeks + Gentamicin (5 mg/kg/day IV) for 4–6 weeks	Same as above for Klebsiella sp.
Ps. aeruginosa	Ticarcillin (3 g IV every 4 hr) for 6 weeks + Tobramycin (5 mg/kg/day IV) for 6 weeks	Ceftazadime‡ (2 g IV every 8 hr) or aztreonam§ (2 g IV every 6 hr) for 6 weeks + tobramycin (5 mg/kg IV per day) for 6 weeks
Salmonella sp.	Ampicillin (2 g IV every 4 hr) for 4–6 weeks	Cefotaxime‡ (2 g IV every 6 hr) for 4–6 weeks or chloramphenicol‖ (1 g IV every 6 hr) for 4–6 weeks or ciprofloxacin‖ (400 mg every 12 hr) for 4–6 weeks
HACEK group	Ampicillin (2 g every 4 hr) for 4–6 weeks + Gentamicin (5 mg/kg/day) for 4–6 weeks	Cefotaxime‡ (2 g every 8 hr IV) for 4–6 weeks + gentamicin (5 mg/kg/day) or chloramphenical‖ (1 g every 6 hr) for 4–6 weeks

*For normal renal function.
†See text for discussion of dosing regimens for the aminoglycosides.
‡Suitable for use in patients with minor allergic reactions to penicillin.
§For use in patients with severe allergic reactions to penicillin.
‖For use against resistant isolates.

sole use of aminoglycosides for the treatment of endocarditis caused by gram-negative bacteria. This is so because the difference between the therapeutic and toxic levels in serum of these antibiotics is so small.

The selection of an antibiotic to treat infection caused by *Citrobacter* species, indole-positive *Proteus, Enterobacter,* and *Pseudomonas* species must be based on the results of in vitro sensitivity tests (Table 13.4). In most instances, ticarcillin plus an aminoglycoside is required. This may produce a synergistic effect against many gram-negative organisms.[314] Disease caused by *Salmonella* species is usually treated with ampicillin or chloramphenicol. However, resistance to these drugs has been increasing. Third-generation cephalosporins and the quinolones appear to be promising in the management of infections due to *Salmonella* species.[315–318]

The broadest experience with the therapy of infective endocarditis caused by *Ps. aeruginosa* has involved studies of IVDA.[319] Paradoxically, the prognosis of nonaddicts is dismal. Reyes et al.[320] noted that the addition of carbenicillin to a large dose of gentamicin (8 mg/kg/day) decreased the fatality rate in patients with endocarditis caused by *Pseudomonas*. Lack of a synergistic effect predicted therapeutic failure.[320,321] Tobramycin is the drug of choice for the treatment of severe infection caused by *Ps. aeruginosa*. The MBC of agents active against this organism is two to four times lower than that of gentamicin. Peak levels of tobramycin in serum must be at least 12 µg/ml to achieve a maximum therapeutic effect.[322] Therapy must be continued for about 6 weeks. Although very large doses of tobramycin are administered (8 mg/kg/day), patients treated with this drug do not appear to be at higher risk of developing nephrotoxicity than those given a standard dose of the drug.[323]

There is no evidence that any of the broad-spectrum penicillins is more effective than ticarcillin. Third-generation cephalosporins must not be administered because they induce the development of cephalosporinases. There is little experience that supports the use of aztreonam and imipenem for the management of infective endocarditis caused by *Pseudomonas*. Ciprofloxacin administered orally or intravenously has been used to treat valvular infections caused by *Pseudomonas*.[310,324] The quinolones may be more effective against this organism than the penicillins and aminoglycosides.[325] Valvular infections of the left side of the heart caused by *Ps. cepacia* fail to respond to the regimens described above but do to trimethoprim-sulfamethoxazole.[326]

Many of the features of infective endocarditis produced by *Serratia* are similar to those caused by *Pseudomonas*.[327] Infections of native valves of the left side of the heart in IVDA are rarely cured by treatment with antibiotics. In vitro studies have indicated that gentamicin plus carbenicillin or chloramphenicol is the most effective approach to the treatment of endocardial disease caused by various isolates of *Serratia*. Two of 13 patients infected by this organism were cured by treatment with an aminoglycoside alone. In another study, 29 patients were given an aminoglycoside plus either trimethoprim-sulfamethoxazole chloramphenicol, or carbencillin; 18 were cured.[328] It has been reported that the therapy of infective endocarditis caused by resistant *Serratia* with ceftazadime or the quinolones is successful.[329] However treatment with third-generation cephalosporins alone against this and many other gram-negatives is not recommended. They are to be combined with an aminoglycoside.

HACEK Group

The HACEK group includes *Hemophilus* species, *A. actinomycetemcomitans*, *C. hominis*, *E. corrodens* and *K. kingii*. Of these, *H. parainfluenzae* and *H. aphrophilus* are most often involved in the pathogenesis of infective endocarditis.[330] These organisms are susceptible to penicillin or ampicillin; some strains may be resistant to these agents because they produce beta-lactamases. Determination of the antibiotic susceptibility of these bacteria is difficult because of their fastidious nutritional requirements.[331–333] Current recommendations for the treatment of valvular infections produced by members of the HACEK group include 12 g of ampicillin and 5 mg/kg of gentamicin per day (Table 13.4). There is no evidence that an aminoglycoside is necessary in all cases. For those infected by organisms resistant to ampicillin, the third-generation cephalosporins are an alternative choice; however, clinical experience with these agents is limited. If patients are highly allergic to the beta-lactams or if the organism responsible for the disease is resistant to the beta-lactams, chloramphenicol is the drug of choice.[334]

Brucellosis

Infective endocarditis is the most common cause of death in patients with brucellosis.[335] The diagnosis of this disease may be difficult because about 30% of patients have sterile cultures of blood. Serological studies are required in this situation. The tetracyclines and streptomycin have been effective in the therapy of this disease. However, a fatality rate of 80%[336,337] has led to therapy with a combination of bactericidal drugs. The administration of doxycycline (100 mg intravenously every 12 hr) plus rifampin (600–900 mg/day) cures most patients with this disease.[338,339] Some physicians continue to treat patients with streptomycin and rifampin.[335,340] Therapy must be continued for at least 8 weeks. Extended periods of treatment are required when intracardiac abscesses are identified during surgery.

Neisseria Species

The most common species of *Neisseria* involved in the pathogenesis of infective endocarditis is *N. gonorrhoeae*. Most strains of this organism are sensitive to penicillin (20 million units/day intravenously for 4 weeks).[341] However, strains resistant to this agent are increasing in frequency.[342] It is now recommended that initial therapy involve a third-generation cephalosporin until adequate sensitivity data are available.

Other Organisms Involved in the Pathogenesis of Endocarditis

Although rare, other species of gram-negative organisms are involved in the pathogenesis of infective endocarditis. There has been an increase in the frequency of endocardial disease caused by corynebacteria (diphtheroids, group JK) in patients with infection of prosthetic valves[343]; native valves are rarely infected. A major controversy has developed regarding the appropriateness of treatment with penicillin plus gentamicin when the organism is resistant to the former but sensitive to the latter (Table 13.5). When this is a problem, therapy with vancomycin alone [344–346] or with this drug plus gentamicin is employed. Treatment with vancomycin and gentamicin is recommended for patients with early-onset PVE caused by corynebacteria because the fatality rate is 73%; it is only 11% with late-onset PVE. Treatment must be continued for at least 6 weeks (Table 13.5).

Listeria monocytogenes

L. monocytogenes is sensitive in vitro to a number of antimicrobial agents, including penicillin, ampicillin, gentamicin, erythromycin, tetracycline, chloramphenicol, and trimethoprim-sulfamethoxazole.[347–350] Ampicillin plus gentamicin appears to be the regimen of choice for the treatment of infective endocarditis caused by this organism (Table 13.5). Gentamicin enhances the bactericidal activity of the penicillins. Treatment with trimethoprim-sulfamethoxazole has not been successful in penicillin-allergic patients. The use of this agent in such patients is not recommended because there is a higher incidence of allergic reactions. Native valve endocarditis (NVE) caused by *Listeria* requires treatment for 6–8 weeks. The fatality rate is similar in individuals with either PVE or NVE (40%) (Table 13.5).

Q Fever Endocarditis

The treatment of infective endocarditis caused by *Coxiella burnetii*, the agent of Q fever, is hampered by difficulty in establishing the diagnosis. The symptoms are chronic and nonspecific. Cultures of the blood are almost always sterile. Serological studies are required for the diagnosis.[351] The infection is usually present for about 1 year before it is identified. *C. burnetii* is resistant to many antibiotics. Tetracycline is the drug of choice because this agent is bacteriostatic and because the organism resides in a protected, intracellular environment. Treatment must be administered for at least 1 year. It has been suggested that therapy be continued until

Table 13.5. Therapy of Various Forms of Endocarditis*

Organism	Treatment Regimen	Reference
Corynebacterium sp.	Crystalline penicillin G (20 million units/day every 4 hr IV) for 6 weeks + Gentamicin (5 mg/kg/day)[†] for 6 weeks or Vancomycin[‡§] (1 IV every 12 hr) for 6 weeks	See text
L. monocytogenes	Ampicillin (12 g/day every 6 hr) for 6 weeks + Gentamicin (5 mg/kg/day)[†] for 6 weeks or Trimethoprim-sulfamethoxazole (10 mg/kg/day every 6 hr based on trimethoprim component) for 4-6 weeks	See text
C. burnetii	Doxycycline (100 mg PO every 12 hr) + Ciprofloxacin (500 mg every 12 hr) for at least 3 years	See text
B. fragilis	Metronidazole (500 mg IV every 6 hr) for 4–6 weeks	See text
Culture-negative endocarditis	Ampicillin (2 g IV every 4 hr) for 4 weeks + Gentamicin (5 mg/kg/day)[†] for the first 2 weeks if culture remains negative + Oxacillin (2 g every 4 hr) if the patient is an intravenous drug abuser or if MRSA is suspected or if prosthetic material is present, vancomycin[§] (one g IV every 12 hr) for 4 weeks	See text
Bacillus sp.	Vancomycin (1 g IV every 12 hr) for 4–6 weeks + Gentamicin (5 mg/kg/day)[†] for 4–6 weeks	359
Lactobacillus sp.	Crystalline penicillin G (20,000,000 units/day IV every 4 hr) for 4–6 weeks + Gentamicin (5 mg/kg/day IV)[†] for 4–6 weeks	360, 366
Chlamydia sp.	Doxycycline (100 mg IV every 12 hr) for 6 weeks + Rifampin (300 g IV every 12 hr) for 6 weeks then Doxycycline (100 g every 12 hr) for indefinite period	361, 362
Proprionobacterium acnes	Penicillin (20,000,000 units/day IV every 4 hr for 4–6 weeks + Gentamicin (5 mg/kg/day IV)[†]	363
E. rhusiopathiae	Crystalline penicillin G (20,000,000 units/day IV every 4 hr) for 4–6 weeks or Ciprofloxacin[‡] (400 mg IV every 12 hr) for 4–6 weeks	364, 365

*for patients with normal renal function.

[†] See text for gentamicin dosing.

[‡] For penicillin-resistant isolates.

[§] For patients allergic to penicillin.

serological titers return to normal. Some physicians have suggested that therapy be continued indefinitely. This conclusion has been based on anecdotal experiences with surgical specimens in which the organism was identified after 5 years of treatment with tetracycline.[352,353] Recent in vitro studies have supported the use of synergistic combinations of antibiotics. The widest experience with this disease has been acquired from clinical studies involving treatment with a quinolone and doxycycline.[354] A trial of therapy of infective endocarditis and Q fever indicated that the quinolones, rifampin, and trimethoprime-sulfamethoxazole failed to cure the disease after 2 years.[355] Treatment with doxycycline plus a quinolone for 3 years decreased the incidence of death significantly (Table 13.5).

Endocarditis Caused by Anaerobic Organisms

B. fragilis is the anaerobic organism most often involved in the pathogenesis of infective endocarditis. Metronidazole is the drug of choice for treatment because it is bactericidal for the bacteroides.[356] Clindamycin and chloramphenicol are bacteriostatic (Table 13.5).

Sterile Endocarditis

Patients with persistently sterile cultures of blood who have not been treated with antimicrobial agents, but in whom infective endocarditis is suspected but not proved, require treatment with antimicrobial agents active against enterococci and a variety of gram-negative organisms.[357,358] A regimen of 12 g of ampicillin plus 5 mg/kg of gentamicin per day is standard therapy in individuals with normal renal function.

Narcotic addicts and patients with sterile prosthetic valves require treatment with a penicillinase-resistant penicillin, oxacillin, or vancomycin to cover for the presence of MSSA and MRSA. Individuals whose blood is sterile prior to initiation of therapy, should be treated for no longer than 2 weeks with an aminoglycoside. Ninety-two percent of individuals become afebrile after 7 days of therapy. About 50% require a longer period of treatment before they defervesce. The antimicrobial therapy of other causes of infective endocarditis is presented in Table 13.5 and 13.6.[359–373]

Fungal Endocarditis

The incidence of infective endocarditis caused by fungi is increasing and is probably due to (1) the increased number of immunocompromised patients; (2) the higher prevalence of narcotic addiction; (3) the rising frequency of cardiac surgery; and (4) the increased use of broad-spectrum antibiotics. In the 1970s, 17.6% of patients with fungal endocarditis survived.[374–376] Presently, 22% survive when treated medically; 55.4% are

Table 13.6. Therapy of Endocarditis Caused by selected Gram-Negative Bacteria*†

Organism	Treatment	Reference
S. moniliformis	Crystalline penicillin G (3 million units IV every 4 hr)	366
Y. enterocolitica	Gentamicin (5 mg/kg/day IV)‡ for 4–6 weeks or chloramphenical (1 g IV every 6 hr) for 4–6 weeks	367, 369
P. multocida	Crystalline penicillin G (3 million units IV every 4 hr) for 4–6 weeks or ciprofloxacin (400 mg IV every 12 hr) for 4–6 weeks	370, 371
Acinetobacter sp.	Gentamicin (5 mg/kg/day IV)‡ for 4–6 weeks or chloramphenicol (1 g IV every 6 hr) for 4–6 weeks	372, 373

*For normal renal function.
†These regimens are suggestions. Exact dosages not well established.
‡See text for discussion of dosing regimens for the aminoglycosides.

cured by medical plus surgical therapy.[377] About 75% of the cases of infective endocarditis are caused by *Candida*.[378] The organisms most often recovered from IVDA are *C. albicans, C. parapsilosis,* and *Aspergillus* species. These species are becoming more frequent in association with cardiac surgery. Overall survival is better when less virulent fungi (*Torulopsis glabrata* and *Histoplasma*) are involved. These usually infect native valves. About 45% of patients with endocarditis caused by *Histoplasma* are cured when treated with amphotericin alone.[379]

Poor therapeutic results are associated with (1) continued difficulty in establishing the diagnosis before death; (2) significantly impaired host defenses; (3) relative paucity of effective antifungal agents; and (4) large, friable valvular vegetations that may embolize and penetrate the myocardium.[380]

Amphotericin is the drug of choice for the management of fungal endocarditis.[381–384] This agent penetrates masses of fibrin that contain *C. albicans*. It decreases the number of fungi but does not sterilize vegetations completely. Amphotericin is less effective in infection caused by *C. parapsilosis*. Fibrin protects these organisms when they are exposed to concentrations of amphotericin that kill *Candida* species in vitro. The dose of amphotericin and the duration of therapy have not been defined. However, it has been suggested that treatment with 2.5–3 g of amphotericin plus surgery is required to cure infective endocarditis caused by the fungi described above. Treatment with amphotericin plus 5-flurocytosine may improve the results of medical therapy. This combination of drugs has not consistently produced as constant or synergistic effect.

The roles of ketoconazole, itraconazole, and fluconazole for treatment of fungal endocarditis have not been defined.[385–387] Itraconazole has proved to be most effective in disease caused *Aspergillus*. Although fluconazole suppresses PVE caused by *C. parapsilosis*,[387] the fungistatic activity of this agent is inferior to that of amphotericin. Surgery is almost always required to cure fungal endocarditis that involves native or prosthetic valves.

References

1. Weinstein L: Infective endocarditis, in Braunwald E (ed): *Heart Disease: A Textbook of Cardiovascular Medicine,* ed 3. Philadelphia, WB Saunders, 1988, chap 34.
2. Watanakunakorn C: Clindamycin therapy for *Staph. aureus* endocarditis: Clinical relapse and development of resistance to clindamycin, lincomycin and erythromycin. *Am J Med* 1976;60:419.
3. Levinson M: Treatment of endocarditis due to viridans streptococci in experimental models, in Bisno A (ed): *Treatment of Infective Endocarditis.* New York, Grune and Stratton, 1981, chap 2.
4. Carizosa J, Kobsa WD, Kaye D: Antagonism between chloramphenicol and penicillin in streptococcal endocarditis in rabbits. *J Lab Clin Med* 1975;85:307.
5. Zak O, Sande MA: Correlation of in vitro antimicrobial activity of antibiotics with results of treatment in experimental animal models and human infection, in Sabath Bern LD (ed): *Action of Antibiotics in Patients.* Bern, Hans Huber, 1982, p 28.
6. Durack DT, Beeson PB: Experimental bacterial endocarditis. I. Colonization of a sterile vegetation. *Br J Exp Pathol* 1972;53:44.
7. Durack DT, Beeson PB: Experimental bacterial endocarditis. II. Survival of bacteria in endocardial vegetations. *Br J Exp Pathol* 1972;53:50.
8. Cremieux AC, Cardon C: Pharmacokinetics and pharmacodynamic requirements for antibiotic therapy of experimental endocarditis. *Antimicrob Agents Chemother* 1992;36:2069.
9. Friedman M: A study of the fibrin factor in relation to subacute endocarditis. *J Pharmacol Exp Ther* 1938;63:173.
10. Nathanson MH, Liebhold RA: Diffusion of sulfonamides and penicillin into fibrin. *Proc Soc Exp Biol Med* 1946;62:83.
11. Weinstein L, Daikos GK, Perin TS: Studies of relationship of tissue fluids and blood levels of penicillin. *J Lab Clin M* 1951;38:712.
12. Barza M, Brusch J, Bergeron MG, et al: Penetration of antibiotics into fibrin loci in vivo. III. Intermittent vs. continuous infusion and the effect of probenecid. *J Infect Dis* 1974;129:73.
13. Barza M, Weinstein L: Penetration of antibiotics into fibrin loci in vivo. I. Comparison of penetration of ampicillin into fibrin clots, abscesses and "interstitial fluid." *J Infect Dis* 1974;129:59.
14. Garrisson PK, Freedman LR: Experimental endocarditis. I. Staphylococcal endocarditis in rabbits resulting from placement of a polyethylene catheter in the right side of the heart. *Yale J Biol Med* 1970;42:394.
15. Contrepois AJ, Callois JM, Garaud JJ, et al: Kinetics and bactericidal effect of gentamicin and latamoxef (moxalactam) in experimental *Escherichia coli* endocarditis. *J Antimicrob Chemother* 1986;17:227.
16. Gengo FM, Schentag JJ: Rate of methicillin penetration into normal heart valves and experimental endocarditis lesions. *Antimicrob Agents Chemother* 1982;21:456.
17. McColm AA, Ryan DM: Penetration of β-lactam antibiotics into cardiac vegetations, aorta, and heart muscle in experimental *Staphylococcus aureus* endocarditis: Comparison of ceftazidime, cefuroxime and methicillin. *J Antimicrob Chemother* 1985;16:349.
18. Cremieux AC, Maziere B, Vallois JM, et al: Evaluation of antibiotic diffusion into cardiac vegetations by quantitative autoradiography. *J Infect Dis* 1989;159:938.
19. Cremieux AC, Maziere B, Vallois JM, et al: Ceftriaxone diffusion into cardiac fibrin vegetations: Qualitative and quantitative evaluation by autoradiography. *Fundam Clin Pharmacol* 1991;5:53.
20. Cremieux AC, Saleh-Mghir A, Vallois JM, et al: Pattern of diffusion of three quinolones

throughout infected cardiac vegetation studied by autoradiography. *In* Programs and Abstracts of the 31st Interscience Conference of Antimicrobial Agents and Chemotherapy, Chicago, 1991, p 158.

21. Bundtzen R, Garber A, Cohn D, et al: Postantibiotic suppression of bacterial growth. *Rev Infect Dis* 1981;3:28.

22. Drusano GL: Role of pharmacokinetics in the outcome of infection. *Antimicrob Agents Chemother* 1988;32:289.

23. Vogelman B, Gudmundsson S, Leggett J, et al: Correlation of antimicrobial pharmacokinetic parameters with therapeutic efficacy in an animal model. *J Infect Dis* 1988;158:831.

24. Durack DT, Beeson PB: Experimental bacterial endocarditis. II. Survival of bacteria in endocardial vegetations. *Br J Exp Pathol* 1972;53:50.

25. Frehel C, Hellio R, Cremieux AC, et al: Nutritionally variant streptococci develop ultrastructural abnormalities during experimental endocarditis. *J Microb Pathogen* 1988; 4:247.

26. Dall L, Bernes WG, Lane JW, et al: Enzymatic modification of glycocalyx in the treatment of experimental endocarditis due to viridans streptococci. *J Infect Dis* 1987;156:736.

27. Joly V, Pangon B, Vallois JM, et al: Value of antibiotic levels in serum and cardiac vegetations for predicting antibacterial effect of ceftriaxone in experimental *Escherichia coli* endocarditis. *Antimicrob Agents Chemother* 1987;31:1632.

28. Ingerman MJ, Pitsakis PG, Rosenberg AF, et al: The importance of pharmacodynamics in determining the dosing interval in therapy for experimental *Pseudomonas* endocarditis in the rat. *J Infect Dis* 1986;153:707.

29. Franciolli M, Bille J, Glauser MP, et al: β-Lactam resistance mechanisms of methicillin-resistant *Staphylococcus aureus. J Infect Dis* 1991;163:514.

30. Gengo F, Schentag J: Rate of methicillin penetration into normal heart valve and experimental endocarditis lesion. *Antimicrob Agents Chemother* 1982;21:456.

31. Weinstein L, Goldfield M, Chang TW: Infection occurring during chemotherapy: A study of their frequency, type and predisposing factors. *N Engl J Med* 1954;261:247.

32. Tan JS: Successful two-week treatment schedule for penicillin-susceptible *Streptococcus viridans* endocarditis. *Lancet* 1971;2:1340.

33. Carbon C, Cremieus AC, Fantin B: Pharmacokinetic and pharmacodynamic aspects of therapy of experimental endocarditis. *Infect Dis Clin NA* 1993;7:37.

34. Hambreger M, Kaplan S, Walker W: Subacute bacterial endocarditis caused by penicillin sensitive streptococci. *JAMA* 1961;17:554.

35. Philips B, Watson G: Oral treatment of subacute endocarditis in children. *Arch Dis Child* 1977;52:235.

36. Weinstein L, Schlesinger J: Treatment of infective endocarditis. *Prog Cardiovasc Dis* 1973;6:275.

37. Schlicter J, MacLean H, Milzo A: Effective penicillin therapy in subacute bacterial endocarditis and other classic infections. *Am J Med Sci* 1949;217:600.

38. Reller LB, Stratton CW: Serum dilution test for bactericidal activity. II. Standardization and correlation with antimicrobial assay and susceptibility tests. *J Infect Dis* 1977; 136:196.

39. Weinstein MP, Stratton CW, Ackley A, et al: Multicentre collaborative evaluation of a standardized serum bactericidal test as a prognostic indicator in infective endocarditis. *Am J Med* 1985;78:262.

40. Cooper R, Moll J: *Serratia* endocarditis: A follow-up report. *Arch Intern Med* 1980; 140:199.

41. Mellors JW, Coleman DL, Andriole VT: Value of the serum bactericidal test in management of patients with bacterial endocarditis. *Eur J Clin Microbiol* 1986;5:67.

42. Hackbarth CJ, Chambers HF, Sande MA: Serum bactericidal titer as a predictor of outcome in endocarditis. *Eur J Clin Microbiol* 1986;5:93.

43. Bisno AL, Dismukes WE, Durack DT: Antimicrobial treatment of infective endocarditis due to viridans streptococci and staphylococci. *JAMA* 1989;261:1471.

44. Vosti K: Serum bactericidal test: Past, present and future use in the management of

patients with infections, in Remington JS, Swartz MN (eds): *Current Clinical Topics in Infectious Diseases.* Boston, Blackwell Scientific, 1990, 43:10.

45. Wolfson JS, Swartz MN: Serum bactericidal activity as a monitor of antibiotic therapy. *N Engl J Med* 1985;312:968.

46. Steckleberg J, Melton L, Ilstrup D: Influence of referral bias on the apparent clinical spectrum of infective endocarditis. *Am J Med* 1990;88:582.

47. Tice AD: An office model of outpatients parenteral antibiotic therapy. *Rev Infect Dis* 1991;13(Suppl 2):S184.

48. Rubenstein E. Cost implications of home care in serious infections. *Hosp Formul* 1993; 28:46.

49. Nightingale C: Impact of nosocomial infections on hospital costs. *Hosp Formul* 1993; 28:51.

50. Foran RM, Butt JL, Wulf PH: Evaluating the cost impact of intravenous antibiotic dosing frequencies. *Ann Pharmacother* 1991;25:546.

51. Tanner DJ, Nazarian MQ: Cost containment associated with decreased parenteral antibiotic administration frequencies. *Am J Med* 1984;77:104.

52. Francioli P and the BE Collaborative Study Group: Ceftriaxone as a single daily dose for 4 weeks in the treatment of bacterial endocarditis (Abstr. 480). *Program and Abstracts of the International Congress for Infectious Diseases*, Rio de Janeiro, 1988.

53. Chambers HF, Mills J, Drake TA, et al: Failure of a once-daily regimen of cefonicid for treatment of endocarditis due to *Staphylococcus aureus. Rev Infect Dis* 1984; 6(Suppl 4):870.

54. Moore RD, Liebman PS, Smith CR: Clinical response to aminoglycoside therapy: Importance of the ratio of peak concentration to minimal inhibitory concentration. *J Infect Dis* 1987;155:93.

55. Balinsky W, Nesbitt S: Cost-effectiveness of outpatient parenteral antibiotics: A review of the literature. *Am J Med* 1989;87:301.

56. Williams DN, Gibson JA, Bosch D: Home intravenous antibiotic therapy using a programmable infusion pump. *Arch intern Med* 1989;149:1157.

57. Brown RB: Selection and training of patients for outpatient intravenous antibiotic therapy. *Rev Infect Dis* 1991;13(Suppl 2):S147.

58. Douglas A, Moore-Gillon J, Eykyn S: Fever during the treatment of infective endocarditis. *Lancet* 1986;1:1341.

59. Lederman MM, Sprague L, Wallis RS, et al: Duration of fever during treatment of infective endocarditis. *Medicine (Baltimore)* 1992;71:52.

60. Blumberg E, Robbins N, Adimora A, et al: Persistent fever in association with infective endocarditis. *Clin Infect Dis* 1992;15:983.

61. Lichtlen P: General principles of conservative treatment of infective endocarditis, in Horstkotte D, Bodnar E (eds): *Infective Endocarditis.* Aylesberg, Becks, England, ICR Publishers, 1991, p 85.

62. Wilson W, Gilbert D, Bisno A: Evaluation of new anti-infective drugs for the treatment of infective endocarditis. *Clin Infect Dis* 1992;15(Suppl 1):S89.

63. Wilson W, Giuliani E, Danielson G, et al: Management of complications of infective endocarditis. *Mayo Clin Proc* 1982;57:162.

64. Mansur A, Grinberg M, Lemoda-Luz P, et al: Complications of infective endocarditis: A reappraisal in the 1980's. *Arch Intern Med* 1992;152:2428.

65. von Reyn CF, Levy BS, Arbeit RF, et al: Infective endocarditis: An analysis based on strict case definitions. *Ann Intern Med* 1981;94(pt 1):505.

66. Calderwood SB, Swinski LA, Karchmer AW, et al: Prosthetic valve endocarditis: Analysis of factors affecting outcome of therapy. *J Thorac Cardiovasc Surg* 1986;92:776.

67. Pelletier LL Jr, Petersdorf RG: Infective endocarditis: A review of 125 cases from the University of Washington Hospitals, 1963–72. *Medicine* 1977;56;287.

68. Tornos MKP, Permanyer-Miralda G, Montserrat O: Long term complication of native valve infective endocarditis in non-addicts. *Ann Intern Med* 1992;117:567.

69. Rain RJI, Glover D, Littler WA, et al: The impact of a policy of collaborative management on mortality and morbidity from infective endocarditis. *Int J Cardiol* 1988;19:47.

70. Garvey GJ, Neu HC: Infective endocarditis—an evolving disease: A review of endocarditis at the Columbia-Presbyterian Medical Center, 1968–1973. *Medicine* 1978;57:105.

71. Brandenburg RO, Giuliani E, Wilson WR, et al: Infective endocarditis: A 25 year overview of diagnosis and therapy. *J Am Coll Cardiol* 1983;1:280.

72. Lerner PI, Weinstein L: Infective endocarditis in the antibiotic era. *N Engl J Med* 1966;247:199.

73. Karchmer AW, Moellering RC Jr, Maki DG, et al: Single antibiotic therapy for streptococcal endocarditis. *JAMA* 1979;241:1801.

74. Wilson WC, Thompson R, Wilkowski C: Short term therapy for streptococcal infective endocarditis: Combined intramuscular administration of penicillin and streptomycin. *JAMA* 1981;245:360.

75. Wilson W, Wilkoski C, Wright A: Treatment of streptomycin susceptible and streptomycin resistant enterococcal endocarditis. *Ann Intern Med* 1970;126:255.

76. Watanakunakorn C, Tan J, Phair J: Some salient features of *Staphylococcus aureus* endocarditis. *Am J Med* 1973;54:473.

77. Malacoff RF, Frank E, Andriole VT: Streptococcal endocarditis (nonenterococcal, nongroup A): Single vs combination therapy. *JAMA* 1979;241:1807.

78. Phair JP, Tan JS: Therapy of *Streptococcus viridans* endocarditis, in Laplan EL, Taranta AV (eds): *Infective Endocarditis—An American Heart Association Symposium.* Dallas, American Heart Association, 1977, p 55.

79. Almirante G, Tornos M, Gargul M, et al: Prognosis of enterococcal endocarditis. *Rev Infect Dis* 1991;13:1248.

80. Dajuni A, Bisno A, Chung T, et al: Prevention of bacterial endocarditis: Recommendations of the American Heart Association. *JAMA* 1990;264:2919.

81. Stinson EB: Surgical treatment of infective endocarditis. *Prog Cardiovasc Dis* 1979;22:145.

82. Pelletier LL, Petersdorf RG: Infective endocarditis: A review of 125 cases from the University of Washington Hospitals, 1963–72. *Medicine (Baltimore)* 1977;56:287.

83. Croft CH, Woodward W, Elliott A, et al: Analysis of surgical versus medical therapy in active complicated native valve infective endocarditis. *Am J Cardiol* 1983;589:88.

84. Levinson M, Kaye D, Mandell G, et al: Characteristics of patients with multiple episodes of bacterial endocarditis. *JAMA* 1980;211:1355.

85. Welton DE, Young JB, Gentry WO, et al: Recurrent infective endocarditis: Analysis of predisposing factors and clinical features. *Am J Med* 1979;66:932.

86. Baddour LM: Twelve year review of recurrent native valve endocarditis: A disease of the modern antibiotic era. *Rev Infect Dis* 1980;10:1163.

87. Shanson D: Antibiotic treatment of endocarditis due to penicillin-sensitive streptococci, in Horstkotte D, Bodnar E (eds): *Infective Endocarditis.* London, ICR Publishers, 1991, p 79.

88. Shanson DC: Short course treatment of streptococcal endocarditis. *J Antimicrob Chemother* 1981;8:427.

89. Report of a Working Party of the British Society for Antimicrobial Chemotherapy. Antibiotic treatment of streptococcal and staphylococcal endocarditis. *Lancet* 1985;2:815.

90. Karchmer AW: Staphycococcal endocarditis. Laboratory and clinical basis for antibiotic therapy. *Am J Med* 1985;78(6B):116.

91. Bisno A, Dismukes W, Durack D, et al: Antimicrobial treatment of infective endocarditis due to viridans streptococci, enterococci and staphylococci. *JAMA* 1989;261:1421.

92. Karchmer AW, Moellering RC Jr, Make DC, et al: Single-antibiotic therapy for streptococcal endocarditis. *JAMA* 1979;241:1801.

93. Roberts RB, Krieger AG, Schiller NL, et al: Viridans streptococcal endocarditis: The role of various species including pyridoxal-dependent streptococci. *Rev Infect Dis* 1979;1:955.

94. Wilson WR, Giuliani ER, Gerace JE: Treatment of penicillin-sensitive streptococcal infective endocarditis. *Mayo Clin Proc* 1982;57:95.

95. Farber BF, Eliopoulos GM, Ward JI, et al: Resistance to penicillin-streptomycin synergy among clinical isolates of viridans streptococci. *Antimicrob Agents Chemother* 1983;24:871.

96. Roberts R, Krieger A, Schiller Z, et al: Viridans streptococcal endocarditis: The role of various species, including pyridoxal-dependent streptococci. *Rev Infect Dis* 1979; 1:955.

97. Cooksey R, Swenson J: In vitro antimicrobial inhibition patterns of nutritionally variant streptococci. *Antimicrob Agents Chemother* 1979;16:514.

98. Roberts R, Wilson W, Bouvet A, et al: Nutritionally variant streptococcal (NVS) endocarditis. 22nd Interscience Conference on Antimicrobial Agents and Chemotherapy. In *Programs and Abstracts* 1982, 130.

99. Holloway Y, Dankert J: Penicillin tolerance in nutritionally variant streptococci. *Antimicrob Agents Chemother* 1982;22:1073.

100. Wilson WR: Antimicrobial therapy of streptococcal endocarditis. *J Antimicrob Chemother* 1987;20(Suppl A):147.

101. Pulliam L, Inokuchi S, Hadley WK, et al: Penicillin tolerance in experimental streptococcal endocarditis. *Lancet* 1979;2:957.

102. Rahal JJ, Mehers BR, Weinstein L: Treatment of bacterial endocarditis with cephalothin. *N Engl J Med* 1968;279:1305.

103. Cremieux AC, Maziere B, Vallois JM: Evaluation of antibiotic diffusion into cardiac vegetation by quantitative autoradiography. *J Infect Dis.* 1989;159:938.

104. Richards DM, Heel RC, Brogden RN: Ceftriaxone: A review of its antibacterial activity, pharmacological properties and therapeutic use. *Drugs* 1984;27:469.

105. Etienne J, Vendenesch F, Fauvel JP: Susceptibilities to ceftriaxone of streptococcal strains associated with infective endocarditis. *Chemotherapy* 1989;35:355.

106. Glauser MP, Francioli P, Meylan P: Antibiotic prophylaxis for patients with prosthetic valves. *Lancet* 1983;1:237.

107. Francioli PB, Glauser MP: Synergistic activity of ceftriaxone combined with netilmicin administered in one daily dose in the treatment of experimental streptococcal endocarditis. *Antimicrob Agents Chemother* 1993;37:438.

108. Stamboulain D, Bonvehi P, Arevalo C: Antibiotic management of outpatients with endocarditis due to penicillin-susceptible streptococci. *Rev Infect Dis* 1991;13(Suppl 2):S160.

109. Wolfe J, Johnson W: Penicillin-sensitive streptococcal endocarditis: In vitro and clinical observations on penicillin-streptomycin therapy. *Ann Intern Med* 1974;81:178.

110. Sande M, Irvin R: Penicillin aminoglycoside synergy: An experimental streptococcal viridans endocarditis continued. *J Infect Dis* 1974;129:572.

111. Stamboulian D, Francioli P, and SE Collaborative Study Group: Two-week treatment of streptococcal endocarditis with single daily dose of ceftriaxone plus netilmicin (abstract). *ENNMID Oslo* 1991;1600.

112. Farber BF, Eliopoulos GM, Ward JI, et al: Resistance to penicillin-streptomycin synergy among clinical isolates of viridans streptococi. *Antimicrob Agents Chemother* 1983; 24:871.

113. Farber BF, Yee Y: High level aminoglycoside resistance mediated by aminoglycoside-modifying enzymes among viridans streptococci: Implications for the therapy of endocarditis. *J Infect Dis* 1987;155:948.

114. Moellering R Jr, Krogstad D: Antibiotic resistance in enterococci, in Schlessinger D (ed): *Microbiology.* Washington, American Society for Microbiology, 1979, p 293.

115. Cates JE, Christie RV: Subacute bacterial endocarditis. *Q J Med* 1950;20:93.

116. Hoppes WL: Treatment of bacterial endocarditis caused by penicillin sensitive streptococci (editorial). *Arch Intern Med* 1977;137:1122.

117. Drake TA, Sande MA: Studies of the chemotherapy of endocarditis: Correlation of in vitro, animal model, and clinical studies. *Rev Infect Dis* 1983;5(Suppl 1):345.

118. Hamburger M, Stein L: *Streptococcus viridans* subacute bacterial endocarditis: Two weeks treatment schedule with penicillin. *JAMA* 1952;149:542.

119. Wilson WR, Geraci JE: Treatment of streptococcal infective endocarditis. *Am J Med* 1985;78(Suppl 6B):128.

120. Hunter TH, Patterson PV: Bacterial endocarditis. *Disease of the Month* 1956;November:1.

121. Tompsett R, Robbins WC, Bertson C: Short term penicillin and dihydrostreptomycin

therapy of streptococcal endocarditis: Results of the treatment of 35 patients. *Am J Med* 1958;24:57.

122. Wilson W, Geraci J, Wilkowski C, et al: Short-term intramuscular therapy with procaine penicillin plus streptomycin for infective endocarditis due to viridans streptococci. *Circulation* 1971;57:1158.

123. Ter Braak EW, de Vries PJ, Bouter KP: Once-daily dosing regimen for aminoglycoside plus β-lactam combination therapy of serious bacterial infections: Comparative trial with netilmicin plus ceftriaxone. *Am J Med* 1990;89:58.

124. Phair J, Tan J, Venezio F: Therapy of infective endocarditis due to penicillin susceptible streptococci: Duration of disease is a major determinant of outcome in treatment of infective endocarditis, in Bisno A (ed): *Treatment of Infective Endocarditis*. New York, Grune and Stratton, 1981.

125. Roberts R: Streptococcal endocarditis: The viridans and beta hemolytic streptococci, in Kaye D (ed): *Infective Endocarditis*, ed 2. New York, Raven Press, 1992, p 191.

126. Prins J, Buller H, Kuijper E, et al: Once versus thrice daily gentamicin in patients with serious infections. *Lancet* 1993;341:335.

127. Moellering R Jr: Treatment of endocarditis caused by resistant streptococci, in Horstkotte D, Bodnar E (eds): *Infective Endocarditis*. London, ICR Publishers, 1991, p 102.

128. Farber BF, Yee Y: High level aminoglycoside resistance mediated by aminoglycoside-modifying enzymes among viridans streptococci: Implications for the therapy for endocarditis. *J Infect Dis* 1987;155:948.

129. Schliefer KH, Kilpper-Balz R: Transfer of *Streptococcus faecalis* and *Streptococcus faecium* to the genus *Enterococcus nom. rev.* as *Enterococcus faecium comb. nov. int. J Syst Bacteriol* 1984;34:31.

130. Ruoff KL, Maza L, Murtagh MJ, et al: Species identities of enterococci isolated from clinical specimens. *J Clin Microbiol* 1990;28:435.

131. Murray B: Antibiotic resistance among enterococci: Current problems and management strategies, in Remington J, Swartz M (eds): *Current Clinical Topics in Infectious Diseases*. Cambridge, MA, Blackwell Scientific, 1991, p 94.

132. Report on the Rockefeller University Workshop. Multiple-antibiotic-resistant pathogenic bacteria. *NEJM* 1994;330(17):1247–1251.

133. Williamson R, Le Bourguenec C, Gutmann L, et al: One or two low affinity penicillin-binding proteins may be responsible for the range of susceptibility of *Enterococcus faecium* to benzylpenicillin. *J Gen Microbiol* 1985;131:1933.

134. Zighlboim-Daum S, Moellering RC Jr: Mechanisms and significance of antimicrobial resistance in enterococci, in Actor P, Daneo-Moore L, Higgins ML, et al (eds): *Antibiotic Inhibition of Bacterial Cell Surface Assembly and Function*. Washington, DC, American Society of Microbiology, 1988, p 505.

135. Toala PA, Solliday J, Crossley KB: Susceptibility of group D streptococcus (enterococcus) to 21 antibiotics in vitro, with special reference to species differences. *Am J Med Sci* 1984;258:416.

136. Eliopoulos GM, Moellering RC Jr: Antibiotic synergism and antimicrobial combinations in clinical infections. *Rev Infect Dis* 1982;4:282.

137. Fass RJ: In vitro activities of β-lactam and aminoglycoside antibiotics: A comparative study of 20 parenterally administered drugs. *Arch Intern Med* 1988;140:766.

138. Tofte RW, Solliday J, Crossley KB: Susceptibilities of enterococci to twelve antibiotics. *Antimicrob Agents Chemother* 1984;25:532.

139. Moellering RC Jr, Korzeniowski OM, Sande MA, et al: Species-specific resistance to antimicrobial synergism in *Streptococcus faecium* and *Streptococcus faecalis*. *J Infect Dis* 1979;140:203.

140. Moellering RC: Antimicrobial susceptibility of enterococci: In vitro studies of the action of antibiotics alone and in combination in treatment of infective endocarditis. Bisno A (ed): *Treatment of Infective Endocarditis*. New York, Grune and Stratton, 1981, p 81.

141. Bush LM, Calmon J, Cherney CL, et al: High-level penicillin resistance among isolates of

enterococci. Implications for treatment of enterococcal infections. *Ann Intern Med* 1989;110:515.

142. Gordon S: Enterococcal susceptibility patterns in the United States. *J Clin Microbiol* 1992;30:2373.

143. Spera R, Farber B: Multiply-resistant enterococcus faecium: The nosocomial pathogen of the 1990's. *JAMA* 1992;268:2563.

144. Krogstad DJ, Parquette AR: Defective killing of enterococci: A common property of antimicrobial agents acting on the cell wall. *Antimicrob Agents Chemother* 1980;17:965.

145. Moellering RC Jr, Wennerstern C, Weinberg AN: Studies on antibiotic synergism against enterococci. I. Bacteriologic studies. *J Lab Clin Med* 1971;77:821.

146. Hunter TH: Use of streptomycin in the treatment of bacterial endocarditis. *Am J Med* 1947;2:436.

147. Moellering RC Jr, Weinberg AN: Studies on antibiotic synergism against enterococci. II. Effect of various antibiotics on the uptake of ^{14}C-labeled streptomycin by enterococci. *J Clin Invest* 1971;50:2580.

148. Murray B: The life and times of the enterococcus. *Clin Microbiol Rev* 1992;3:46.

149. Watanakunakorn C, Bakie C: Sunergism of vancomycin-gentamicin and vancomycin-streptomycin against enterococci. *Antimicrob Agents Chemother* 1973;4:120.

150. Watanakunakorn C, Glotzbecker C: Comparative in vitro activity of nafcillin, oxacillin and methicillin in combination with gentamicin and tobramycin against enterococci. *Antimicrob Agents Chemother* 1977;11:88.

151. Glew RH, Moellering RC Jr, Wennerstern C: Comparative synergistic activity of nafcillin, oxacillin and methicillin in combination with gentamicin against enterococci. *Antimicrob Agents Chemother* 1975;7:828.

152. Marier RL, Joyce N, Andriole VY: Synergism of oxacillin and gentamicin against enterococci. *Antimicrob Agents Chemother* 1975;8:571.

153. Glew RH, Moellering RC Jr: Effect of protein binding on the activity of penicillin in combination with gentamicin against enterococci. *Antimicrob Agents Chemother* 1979; 15:87.

154. Weinstein AJ, Moellering RC Jr: Studies of cephalothin: Aminoglycoside synergism against enterococci. *Antimicrob Agents Chemother* 1975;7:522.

155. Murillo J, Standiford H, Holley A, et al: Prophylaxis against enterococcal endocarditis: Comparison of the aminoglycoside components of parenteral antimicrobial regimens. *Antimicrob Agents Chemother* 1986;18:448.

156. Iannini PB, Ehret J, Eickhoff TC: Effect of ampicillin-amikacin and ampicillin-rifampin on enterococci. *Antimicrob Agents Chemother* 1976;9·448.

157. Clewell DB: Conjugative transposons and the dissemination of antibiotic resistance in streptococci. *Ann Rev Microbiol* 1986;40:635.

158. Calderwood SA, Wennersten C, Moellering RC Jr, et al: Resistance to six aminoglycoside aminocyclitol antibiotics among enterococci: Prevalence, evolution and relationship to synergism with penicillin. *Antimicrob Agents Chemother* 1977;12:401.

159. Eliopoulos GM, Farber BF, Murray BE, et al: Ribosomal resistance of clinical enterococci isolates to streptomycin. *Antimicrob Agents Chemother* 1984;25:398.

160. Horodniceanu T, Bouquelert L, El-Solh N, et al: Righ level, plasmid-borne resistance to gentamicin in *Streptococcus faecalis* subsp. zymogens. *Antimicrob Agents Chemother* 1979;16:686.

161. Mederski-Samoraj BD, Murray BE: High-level resistance to gentamicin in clinical isolates of enterococci. *J Infect Dis* 1983;147:751.

162. Preventing the spread of vancomycin resistance—report from the Hospital Infection Control Practices Advisory Committee, *Federal Register* 1994, May 17;59(94):25758–25763.

163. Zervos MJ, Kauffman CA, Therasse PM, et al: Epidemiology of nosocomial infection caused by gentamicin-resistant *S. faecalis. Ann Intern Med* 1987;106:687.

164. Kathpalia S, Lolans V, Levandowski R, et al: Resistance to all aminoglycoside antibiotics in enterococcal endocarditis. *Clin Res* 1984;32:327A.

165. Nachamkin I, Axelrod P, Talbot GH, et al: Multiple high level aminoglycoside resistant

enterococci isolated from patients in a university hospital (Abstr. 120). *Abstracts of the Eighty-sixth Annual Meeting of the American Society for Microbiology.* Washington, DC, American Society for Microbiology, 1986.

166. Murray BE, Mederski-Samorap BD: Transferable beta-lactamase: A new mechanism for in vitro penicillin resistance in *Staphylococcus faecalis. J Clin Invest* 1983;72:1168.

167. Zscheck KK, Hull R, Murray BE: Restriction mapping and hybridization studies of a β-lactamase-encoding fragment from *Streptococcus (Enterococcus) faecalis. Antimicrob Agents Chemother* 1988;2:768.

168. Hindes RG, Willey SH, Eliopoulos GM, et al: Treatment of experimental endocarditis due to a beta-lactamase-producing high-level gentamicin-resistant *Enterococcus faecalis. Antimicrob Agents Chemother* 1989;33:1019.

169. Berger-Bachi B: Genetics of methicillin resistance to *Staphylococcus aureus. J Antimicrob Chemother* 1989;23:671.

170. Uttley AHC, Collins CH, Naidoo J, et al: Vancomycin-resistant enterococci. *Lancet* 1988;57:8.

171. Lutticken R, Kunstmann G: Vancomycin-resistant Streptococcaceae from clinical material. *Zbl Bakt Hyg* 1988;A267:379.

172. Johnson D, Barnes J, McLeod E: Subacute bacterial endocarditis caused by *Streptococcus faecalis* and successfully treated with ampicillin. *Med J Aust* 1965;2:1026.

173. Louris D: Discussion of a paper activity of broad spectrum endocarditis. *Ann NY Acad Sci* 1967;145:471.

174. Wilson WR: Antimicrobial therapy of streptococcal endocarditis. *J Antimicrob Chemother* 1987;20(Suppl A):147.

175. Matsumoto JY, Wilson WR, Wright AJ, et al: Synergy of penicillin and decreasing concentration of aminoglycosides against enterococci from patients with infective endocarditis. *Antimicrob Agents Chemother* 1980;18:944.

176. Ingerman M, Pitsakis PG, Rosenberg A, et al: β-Lactamase production in experimental endocarditis due to aminoglycoside-resistant *Streptococcus faecalis. J Infect Dis* 1987;155:1226.

177. Thauvin C, Eliroulos GM, Willey S, et al: Continuous infusion ampicillin therapy of enterococcal endocarditis in rats. *Antimicrob Agents Chemother* 1987;31:139.

178. Fernandez-Guerrero M, Rouse MS, Henry NK, et al: In vitro and in vivo activity of ciprofloxacin against enterococci isolated from patients with infective endocarditis. *Antimicrob Agents Chemother* 1987;31:430.

179. Markowitz S, Wells L, Williams D, et al: Antimicrobial susceptibility and molecular epidemiology of β-lactamase producing aminoglycoside resistant isolates of *Enterococcus faecalis. Antimicrob Agents Chemother* 1992;1075:35.

180. Crider SR, Colby SD: Susceptibility of enterococci to trimethoprim and trimethoprim-sulfamethoxazole. *Antimicrob Agents Chemother* 1985;27:71.

181. Hamilton-Miller JMY: Reversal of activity of trimethoprim against gram-positive cocci by thymidine, thymine and "folates." *J Antimicrob Agents Chemother* 1987;31:800.

182. Lavoie S, Wong E, Coudron P, et al: Comparison of Ampicillin-Sulbactam with Vancomycin for Treatment of Experimental Endocarditis Due to β-Lactamase-Producing, Highly Gentamicin-Resistant Isolate of *Enterococcus faecalis. Antimicrob Agents Chemother* 1992;37:1447.

183. Caron F, Lemeland J, Humbert G, et al: Triple Combination Penicillin-Vancomycin Gentamicin for Experimental Endocarditis Caused by Highly Penicillin- and Glyco-peptide-Resistant Isolate of enterococcus faecium. *J Infect Dis* 1993; 168:681.

184. Bisno AL, Dismukes WE, Durack DT, et al: Antimicrobial therapy of infective endocarditis due to streptococci, enterococci and staphylococci. *JAMA* 1989;261:1471.

185. Matsumoto JY, Wilson WR, Wright AJ, et al: Synergy of penicillin and decreasing concentrations of aminoglycosides against enterococci from patients with infective endocarditis. *Antimicrob Agents Chemother* 1980;18:944.

186. Spiegel CA, Huycke M: Endocarditis due to streptomycin-susceptible *Enterococcus faecalis* with high-level gentamicin resistance. *Arch Intern Med* 1989;148:1873.

187. Libertin CR, McKinley KM: Gentamicin-resistant enterococcal endocarditis: The need

for routine screening for high-level resistance to aminoglycosides. *South Med J* 1990; 83:458.

188. Wilson W, Geraci J: Antimicrobial therapy for penicillin-sensitive streptococcal infective endocarditis: Two week regimen in treatment of infective endocarditis. Bisno A (ed): *Treatment of Infective Endocarditis.* New York, Grune and Stratton, 1981, p 61.

189. Friedberg C, Rosen K, Beinstock P: Vancomycin therapy for enterococcal and streptococcal viridans endocarditis. *Arch Intern Med* 1968;122:134.

190. Farber B, Moellering RC Jr: Retrospective study of the toxicity of preparations of vancomycin from 1974–1981. *Antimicrob Agents Chemother* 1983;23:138.

191. Moellering RC Jr, Krogstad D, Greenblatt D: Vancomycin therapy in patients with impaired renal function by nomogram for dosage. *Ann Intern Med* 1981;93:343.

192. Mylotte J, McDermott C, Spooner J: Prospective study of episodes of *Staphylococcus aureus* bacteremia. *Rev Infect Dis* 1987;9:891.

193. Watanakunakorn C, Tan J, Phair J: Some salients featuring *Staphylococcus aureus* endocarditis. *Am J Med* 1973;54:473.

194. Reisberg B: Infective endocarditis in the narcotic addict. *Prog Cardiovasc Dis* 1979;22: 193.

195. Wilson W, Danielson G, Guiliani E, et al: Prosthetic valve endocarditis. *Mayo Clin Proc* 1982;52:155.

196. Mayer KH, Schoenbaum SC: Evaluation and management of prosthetic valve endocarditis. *Prog Cardiovasc Dis* 1982;25:43.

197. Karchmer AW, Archer GL, Dismukes WE: *Staphylococcus epidermidis* causing prosthetic valve endocarditis: Microbiologic and clinical observations as guides to therapy. *Ann Intern Med* 1983;447:455.

198. Arber N, Militianu A, Ben-Yehwdo A, et al: Native valve *Staphylococcus epidermidis* endocarditis: Report of seven cases and review of the literature. *Am J Med* 1991; 90:758.

199. Reisberg B: Infective endocarditis in the narcotic addict. *Prog Cardiovasc Dis* 1979;22: 193.

200. Chambers HF, Korzeniowski O, Sande MA, et al: *Staphylococcus aureus* endocarditis: Clinical manifestations in addicts and nonaddicts. *Medicine* 1983;62:170.

201. Sande M, Korzeniowski O: the antimicrobial therapy of staphylococcal endocarditis in treatment of infective endocarditis. Bisno A (ed): *Treatment of Infective Endocarditis.* New York, Grune and Stratton, 1981, p 113.

202. Sabath LD, Postic B, Finland M: Methicillin treatment of severe staphylococcal disease. *N Engl J Med* 1962;267:1049.

203. Eickoff TA, Kislak JW, Finland M: Clinical evaluation of nafcillin in patients with severe staphylococcal disease. *N Engl J Med* 1965;272:699.

204. Egert J, Carrizosa J, Kaye D: Comparison of methicillin, nafcillin, and oxacillin in therapy of *Staphylococcus aureus* endocarditis in rabbits. *J Lab Clin Med* 1977;89:1262.

205. Dismukes WE: Oxacillin-induced hepatic dysfunction. *JAMA* 1973;226:861.

206. Masur H, Murray HW, Roberts RB: Nafcillin therapy for *Staphylococcus aureus* endocarditis. *Antimicrob Agents Chemother* 1978;14:457.

207. Kind A, Typasi T, Kirby W, et al: Mechanism responsible for plasma levels of nafcillin lower than those of oxacillin. *Arch Intern Med* 1970;125:685.

208. Brusch JL, Barza M, Brown RB, et al: Comparative pharmacokinetics of thirteen antibiotics in dogs. *Infection* 1976;4(Suppl 2):S82.

209. Korzeniowski O, Sande MA, The National Collaborative Endocarditis Study Group: Combination antimicrobial therapy for *Staphylococcus aureus* endocarditis in patients addicted to parenteral drugs and in nonaddicts. A prospective study. *Ann Intern Med* 1982;97:496.

210. Chapman S, Steigbigel R: Staphylococcal β-lactamase and efficiency of β-lactam antibiotics: In vitro and in vivo evaluation. *J Infect Dis* 1983;147:1078.

211. Chambers H: Antibiotic treatment of staphylococcal endocarditis. In *Infective Endocarditis,* Horstkotte D, Bodnar E (eds): London, ICR Publishers, 1991, p 110.

212. Carrizosa J, Lobasa WD, Snepar R, et al: Cefazolin versus cephalothin in β-lactamase-

producing *Stahylococcus aureus* endocarditis in a rabbit experimental model. *J Antimicrob Chemother* 1982;9:387.

213. Bryant RE, Alford RH: Unsuccessful treatment of staphylococcal endocarditis with cefazolin. *JAMA* 1977;237:569.

214. Kaye D, Hewitt W, Remington JS, et al: Cefaxolin and *Staphylococcus aureus* endocarditis. *JAMA* 1977;237:2601.

215. Regamey C, Libke RD, Engelking ER, et al: Inactivation of cefazolin, cephloridine and cephalothin by methicillin-sensitive and methicillin-resistant strains of *Staphylococcus aureus*. *J Infect Dis* 1975;131:291.

216. Carrizosa J, Santoro J, Kaye D: Treatment of experimental *Staphylococcus aureus* endocarditis: Comparison of cephalothin, cefazolin and methicillin. *Antimicrob Agents Chemother* 1978;13:74.

217. Goldman PL, Petersdorf RG: Importance by β-lactamase inactivation in treatment of experimental endocarditis caused by *Staphylococcus aureus*. *J Infect Dis* 1980;141:331.

218. Kaye D: Treatment of staphylococcal endocarditis, in Sande M, Kaye D, Root R (eds): *Endocarditis*. New York, Churchill Livingstone, 1984, p 135.

219. Moellering RC, Krogstad DJ, Greenblatt DJ. Vancomycin therapy in patients with impaired renal function: A normogram for dosing. *Ann Intern Med* 1981;94:343.

220. Sorrell TC, Collingnon PJ: A prospective study of adverse reactions associated with vancomycin therapy. *J Antimicrob Chemother* 1985;16:235.

221. Gopal V, Bisno AL, Silverblatt FJ: Failure of vancomycin treatments in *Staphylococcus aureus* endocarditis: In vivo and in vitro observations. *JAMA* 1976;236:1604.

222. Geiseler PJ, Rice TW, McCulley DJ, et al: Failure of medical therapy in tricuspid endocarditis due to *Staphylococcus aureus*. *Chemotherapy* 1984;30:408.

223. Small PM, Chambers HF: Vancomycin for *Staphylococcus aureus* endocarditis in intravenous drug abusers. *Antimicrob Agents Chemother* 1990;34:1227.

224. Harstein AL, Mulligan ME, Morthland VH, et al: Recurrent *Staphylococcus aureus* bacteremia. *J Clin Microbiol* 1991;30:670.

228. Celain P, Krause KH, Vaudaux P, et al: Early termination of a prospective randomized trial comparing teicoplanin and flucloxacillin for treating severe staphylococcal infections. *J Infect Dis* 1987;155:187.

226. GalankisN, Giamarellou H, Vlachogiannis, et al: Poor efficacy of teicoplanin in treatment of deep-seated staphylococcal infections. *Eur J Clin Microbiol Infect Dis* 1988;7:130.

227. Gilbert DN, Wood CA, Kimbrough RC, et al: Failure of treatment of teicoplanin at 6 milligrams/kilogram/day in patients with *Staphylococcus aureus* intravascular infection. *Antimicrob Agents Chemother* 1991;35:79.

228. Ryback MJ, Bailey EM, Lamp KC, et al: Pharmkacokinetics and bactericidal rates of daptomycin and vancomycin in intravenous drug abusers being treated for gram-positive endocarditis and bacteremia. *Antimicrob Agents Chemother* 1992;36:1109.

229. Ryback MJ, Lerner SA, Levine DP, et al: Teicoplanin pharmacokinetics in intravenous drug abusers being treated for bacterial endocarditis. *Antimicrob Agents Chemother* 1991;35:696.

230. Kaatz G, Sen S, Dorman N, et al: Emergency teicoplanin resistance during therapy of *Staphylococcus aureus* endocarditis. *J Infect Dis* 1990;162:103.

231. Miller M, Wexler M, Steigbigel N: Single and combination antibiotic therapy of *Staphylococcus aureus* experimental endocarditis: Emergence of gentamicin-resistant mutants. *Antimicrob Agents Chemother* 1978;14:336.

232. Watanakunakorn C, Tisons JC: Synergism between vancomycin and gentamicin or tobramycin for methicillin-susceptible and methicillin-resistant *Staphylococcus aureus* strains. *Antimicrob Agents Chemother* 1982;22:903.

233. Sande MA, Courtney KB: Nafcillin-gentamicin synergism in experimental staphylococcal endocarditis. *J Lab Clin Med* 1976;88:118.

234. Licht JH: Penicillinase-resistant penicillin/gentamicin synergism. *Arch Intern Med* 1979;139:1094.

235. Abrams B, Sklaver A, Hoffman T, et al: Single or combination therapy of staphylococcal endocarditis in intravenous drug abusers. *Ann Intern Med* 1979;90:789.

236. Watanakunakorn C, Baird IM: Prognostic factors in *Staphylococcus aureus* endocarditis and results of therapy with penicillin and gentamicin. *Am J Med Sci* 1977;273:133.

237. Korzeniowski O, Sande MA, the National Collaborative Endocarditis Study Group. Combination microbial therapy for *Staphylococcus aureus* endocarditis in patients addicted to parenteral drugs and non-addicts: A prospective study. *Ann Interns Med* 1982;97:496.

238. Chambers HF, Miller T, Newman MD: Right-sided *Staphylococcus aureus* endocarditis in intravenous drug abusers—two-week combination therapy. *Ann Intern Med* 1988;109:619.

239. Mandell GL, Vest TK: Killing of intraleukocitic *Staphylococcus aureus* by rifampin: In vitro and in vivo studies. *J Infect Dis* 1972;125:486.

240. Lobo MC, Mandell GL: Treatment of experimental staphylococcal infection with rifampin. *Antimicrob Agents Chemother* 1972;2:195.

241. Sande JA, Johnson ML: Antimicrobial therapy of experimental endocarditis caused by *Staphylococcus aureus. J Infect Dis* 1975;131:367.

242. Zinner SH, Lagast H, Klastersky J: Anti-staphylococcal acitivity of rifampin with other antibiotics. *J Infect Dis* 1981;144:365.

243. Zak O, Scheld WM, Sande MA: Rifampin in experimental endocarditis due to *Staphylococcus aureus* in rabbits. *Rev Infect Dis* 1983;5(Suppl 1):S481.

244. Massanari RM, Donta ST: The efficacy of rifampin as adjunctive therapy in selected cases of staphylococcal endocarditis. *Chest* 1978;73:371.

245. Van der Auwera P, Meunier-Carpenter F, Klastersky J: Clinical study of combination therapy with oxacillin and rifampin for staphylococcal infections. *Rev Infect Dis* 1983;5(Suppl):S515.

246. Fernandez-Guerrero M, Rouse M, Henry M, Wilson Walter: Ciprofloxacin therapy of Experimental endocarditis caused by methicillin-susceptible or methicillin-resistant *Staphylococcus aureus. Antimicrob Agents Chemother* 1988;32:747.

247. Chambers H, Huckbarth C, Drake T, et al: Endocarditis due to methicillin-resistant *Staphylococcus aureus* in rabbits: Expression of resistance IV β-lactam antibiotics in vivo administration. *J/D* 1904;449:897.

248. Harnett N, Brown S, Krishnan C: Emergence of quinolone resistance among clinical isolates of methicillin-resistant *Staphylococcus aureus* in Ontario, Canada. *Antimicrob Agents Chemother* 1991;35:1911.

249. Trucksis N, Hooper D, Wolfsan J: Emerging resistance to fluroquinolones in staphylocci. *Alert Ann Int Med* 1991;114:429.

250. Tamer MA, Bray JD: Trimethoprim-sulfamethoxazole treatment of multiantibiotic-resistant staphylococcal endocarditis and meningitis. *Clin Pediatr* 1986;21:125–126.

251. Markowitz N, Quinn E, Saravolatz L: Trimethoprim-sulfamethoxazole compared with vancomycin for the treatment of *Staphylococcus aureus* infection. *Ann Int Med* 1992;117:390.

252. Scheld W, Sande M: Endocarditis and intravascular infections. *Infectious diseases* (4th ed). Mandell G, Bennett J, Dolin R (eds). New York, Churchill Livingstone, 1995.

253. Handwerger S, Tomasz A: Antibiotic tolerance among clinical isolates of bacteria. *Rev Infect Dis* 7:368–86, 1985.

254. Mayhall CG, Medoff G, Marr TT: Variation in the susceptibility of strains of *Staphylococcus aureus* to oxacillin, cephalothin, and gentamicin. *Antimicrob Agents Chemother* 1976;10:707.

255. Rajashekaraiah K, Rice T, Rao V, et al: Clinical significance of tolerant strains of *Staphylococcus aureus* in patients with endocarditis. *Ann Intern Med* 1980;93:796.

256. Woolfrey B, Lally R, Ederer M: Evaluating oxacillin tolerance in *Staphylococcus aureus* by a novel method. *Antimicrob Agents Chemother* 1985;28:381.

257. Watanakunakorn C: Antibiotic-tolerant *Staphylococcus aureus. Antimicrob Agents Chemother* 1978;4:561.

258. Sheagren J: *Staphylococcus aureus*, the persistent pathogen (second of two parts). *N Engl J Med* 1984;310:1437.

259. Karchmer A: Staphylococcal endocarditis: Laboratory and clinical basis for antibiotic therapy. *Am J Med* 1985;78(Suppl 6b):116.

260. Hackbarth CJ, Chambers HF: Methicillin-resistant staphylococci: Detection methods and treatment of infections. *Antimicrob Agents Chemother* 1989;995:999.

261. Chambers H, Sande M: Teicoplanin versus nafcillin in the treatment of experimental endocarditis caused by methicillin-susceptible or resistant *Staphylococcus aureus*. *Antimicrob Agents Chemother* 1990;34:2081.

262. Gilbert DN, Wood CA, Kimbrough RC, et al: Failure of treatment with teicoplanin at 6 milligramks/kilogram/day in patients with *Staphylococcus aureus* intravascular infection. *Antimicrob Agents Chemother* 1991;35:79.

263. Karchmer A: Staphylococcal endocarditis, in Kaye D (ed): *Infective Endocarditis*, ed 2. New York, Raven Press, 1992, p 225.

264. Levine D, Fromm B, Reddy B: Slow response to vancomycin or vancomycin plus rifampin in methicillin-resistant *Staphylococcus aureus* endocarditis. *Ann Intern Med* 1991; 115:674.

265. Kaatz G, Barriere S, Schaberg D, et al: Ciprofloxacin versus vancomycin in the therapy of experimental methicillin-resistant *Staphylococcus aureus* endocarditis. *Antimicrob Agents Chemother* 1987;31:527.

266. Markowitz N, Saramolatz L, Pohlod D, et al: Comparative efficacy and toxicity of trimethoprim-sulfamethoxazole versus vancomycin in the therapy of serious *S. aureus* infections (638). *Abstracts of the 25th Interscience Conference on Antimicrobial Agents and Chemotherapy, American Society for Microbiology, Las Vegas, October 1983.*

267. Hirano L, Bayer A: β-lactam-β-lactamase inhibitor combinations are active in experimental endocarditis caused by β-lactamase-producing oxacillin-resistant staphylococci. *Antimicrob Agents Chemother* 1991;35:605.

268. Kloss W: Coagulase-negative staphylococci. *Clin Microbiol Newsletter* 1982;4:75.

269. Kloss W: Natural populations of the genus *Staphylococcus*. *Ann Rev Microbiol* 1982;34: 559.

270. Karchmer AW, Archer GL, Dismukes WE: *Staphylococcus epidermidis* causing prosthetic valve endocarditis: Microbiologic and clinical observations as guides to therapy. *Ann Intern Med* 1983;98:447.

271. Heimberger TS, Duma RJ: Infections of prosthetic heart valves and cardiac pacemakers. *Infect Dis Clin North Am* 1989;3(2):221.

272. Patrick C: Coagulase-negative staphylococci: Pathogens with increasing clinical significance. *J Pediatr* 1990;116:497.

273. Archer GL: Antimicrobial susceptibility and detection of resistance among *Staphylococcus epidermidis* isolates recovered from patient with infections of indwelling foreign devices. *Antimicrob Agents Chemother* 1978;14:353.

274. Christensen G, Bisno A, Paris J: Nosocomial septicemia due to multiple antibiotic-resistant *Staphylococcus epidermidis*. *Ann Intern Med* 1982;9:61.

275. Archer GL: Antibiotic resistance in coagulase-negative staphylococci, in Mardh P-A, Schliefer KH (eds): *Coagulase-Negative Staphylococci*. Stockholm, Almquist and Wiskell, 1986, p 93.

276. Chambers HF, Coagulase-negative staphylococcal resistant to beta-lactam antibiotics in vivo produces penicillin-binding protein 2a. *Antimicrob Agents Chemother* 1987;31:1919.

277. Archer GL, Basquez GJ, Johnson JL: Antibiotic prophylaxis of experimental endocarditis due to methicillin-resistant *Staphylococcus epidermidis*. *J Infect Dis* 1980;142:725.

278. Berry AJ, Johnson JL, Archer GL: Imipenem therapy of experimental *Staphylococcus epidermidis* endocarditis. *Antimicrob Agents Chemother* 1986;29:748.

279. Karchmer A, Archer G, Dismukes W: *Staphylococcus epidermidis* prosthetic valve endocarditis: Microbiological and clinical observations as guides to therapy. *Ann Intern Med* 1983;98:447.

280. Varaldo PE, Debbia E, Schito GC: In vitro activity of teichomycin and vancomycin alone and in combination with rifampin. *Antimicrob Agents Chemother* 1983;23:402.

281. Gemmell CG: Virulence characteristics of *Staphylococcus epidermidis*. *Med Microbiol* 1985;22:287.

282. Schwalbe RS, Stapleton JT, Gilligan PH: Emergence of vancomycin resistance in coagulase-negative staphylococci. *N Engl J Med* 1987;316(3):927.

283. Wilson APR, O'Hare MD, Felmingham D, et al: Teicoplanin-resistant coagulase-negative staphylococcus. *Lancet* 1986;2:973.

284. Kolasa WD, Kaye KL, Shapiro T, et al: Therapy for experimental endocarditis due to *Staphylococcus epidermidis*. *Rev Infect Dis* 1983;5:5533.

285. Karchmer AW, Archer GL, the Endocarditis Study Group: Methicillin-resistant *Staphylococcus epidermidis* prosthetic valve endocarditis: A therapeutic trial in *Programs and Abstracts of the Twenty-fourth Interscience Conference of Antimicrobial Agents and Chemotherapy, Washington, DC, for Microbiology, 1984*.

286. Whitener C, Caputo G, Weitekamp M, et al: Endocarditis due to coagulase-negative staphylococci: Microbiologic, epidemiologic and clinical considerations in infective endocarditis, eds. Wilson W, Steckelbert J, in *ICNA* 1993, p 7.

287. Rouse MS, Wilcox RM, Henry NK, et al: Ciprofloxacin therapy of experimental endocarditis caused by methicillin-resistant *Staphylococcus epidermidis*. *Antimicrob Agents Chemother* 1990;34:273.

288. Etienne J, Eykyn SJ: Increase in native valve endocarditis caused by coagulase-negative staphylococci: An Anglo-French clinical and microbiological study. *Br Heart J* 1990;64:381.

289. Caputo GM, Archer GL, Calderwood SB, et al: Native valve endocarditis due to coagulase-negative staphylococci: Clinical and microbiologic features. *Am J Med* 1987;83:625.

290. Tuazon CU, Miller H: Clinical and microbiological aspects of serious infections caused by *Staphylococcus epidermidis*. *Scand J Infect Dis* 1983;15:347.

291. Arber N, Militianu A, Ben-Yehude A, et al: Native valve *Staphylococcus epidermidis* endocarditis: Report of seven cases and review of the literature. *Am J Med* 1991;90:758.

292. Cohen PS, Maguire JH,Weinstein L: Infective endocarditis caused by gram-negative bacteria: A review of the literature, 1945–1977. *Prog Cardiovasc Dis* 1980;22:205.

293. Geraci JE, Wilson WR: Endocarditis due to gram-negative bacteria. Report of 56 cases. *Mayo Clin Proc* 1982;57:145.

294. Sanders C: New β-lactams: New problems for the internist. Editorial. *Ann Intern Med* 1991;115:650.

295. Chow JW, Fine MJ, Shlaes DM, et al: *Enterobacter* bacteremia: Clinical features and emergence of antibiotic resistance during therapy. *Ann Intern Med* 1991;115:585.

296. Quinn J, DiVencenzo C, Foster J: Emergence of resistance to ceftozadime during therapy for *enterobacter cloacae* infections. *J Infect Dis* 1982;115:942.

297. Heasser M, Patterson J, Kuritzor A, et al: Emergence of resistance to beta-lactams in *Enterobacter cloacae* during treatment for neonatal meningitis with cefotaxime. *Pediatr Infect Dis* 1990;29:509.

298. Sanders WE Jr, Sanders CC: Inducible β-lactamases: Clinical and epidemiologic implications for use of newer cephalosporins. *Rev Infect Dis* 1988;10:830.

299. Sanders CC: Chromosomal cephalosporinases responsible for multiple resistance to newer beta-lactam antibiotics. *Annu Rev Microbiol* 1987;41:573.

300. Tancrede CH, Andremont AO, Leonard FC: Epidemiology of enterobacteria resistant to cefotaxime in hospital. *J Antimicrob Chemother* 1984;14(Suppl B):53.

301. Bryan CS, John FJ Jr, Pal MS, et al: Gentamicin vs. cefotaxime for therapy of neonatal sepsis. Relationship to drug resistance. *Am J Dis Child* 1985;139:1086.

302. Modi N, Damjamovic V, Cooke RW: Outbreak of cephalosporin resistant *Enterobacter cloacae* infection in a neonatal intensive care unit. *Arch Dis Child* 1987;62:148.

303. Rice LB, Willey SH, Papanicolaou GA, et al: Outbreak of ceftazidime resistance caused by extended-spectrum β-lactamases at a Massachusetts chronic-care facility. *Antimicrob Agents Chemother* 1990;34:2193.

304. Cooksey R, Swenson J, Clark N, et al: Patterns and mechanisms of β-lactam resistance among isolates of *Escherichia coli* from hospitals in the United States. *Antimicrob Agents Chemother* 1990;34:739.

305. Sanders CC, Iaconis JP, Bodey GP, et al: Resistance to ticarcillin-potassium clavulanate among clinical isolates of the family Enterobacteriaceae: Role of PSE-1 β-lactamase and

high levels of TEM-1 and SHV-1 and problems with false susceptibility in disk diffusion tests. *Antimicrob Agents Chemother* 1988;32:1365.

306. Levison ME, Kobasa WD: Mezlocillin and ticarcillin alone and combined with gentamicin in the treatment of experimental *Entrobacter aerogenes* endocarditis. *Antimicrob Agents Chemother* 1984;25:683.

307. Kobasa WD, Kaye D: Aztreonam, cefoperazone and gentamicin in the treatment of experimental *Enterobacter aerogenes* endocarditis in rabbits. *Antimicrob Agents Chemother* 1983;24:321.

308. Dickinson G, Rodriguez K, Arcey S, et al: Efficacy of imipenem/cilastin in endocarditis. *Am J Med* 1985;78(Suppl 6A):117.

309. Bayer AS, Hirano L, Yih J: Development of beta-lactam resistance and increased quinolone MIC's during therapy of experimental *Pseudomonas* endocarditis. *Antimicrob Agents Chemother* 1988;32:231.

310. Daikos GL, Kathpalia SB, Lolans VT, et al: Long term oral ciprofloxacin experience in the treatment of incurable infective endocarditis. *Am J Med* 1988;84:786.

311. King K, Harkness J: Infective endocaarditis in the 1980's. *Med J Aust* 1989;144:588.

312. Wilson W, Geraci J: Antibiotic treatment of infective endocarditis. *Annu Rev Med* 1983;34:413.

313. Weinstein L, Schlesinger J: Treatment of infective endocarditis—1973. *Prog Cardiovasc Dis* 1973;16:275.

314. Giamerellou H: Aminoglycoside plus β-lactams against gram-negative organisms: Evaluation of in vitro synergy and chemical interactions. *Am J Med* 1986;80(Suppl B):126.

315. Carruthers MM: Endocarditis due to enteric bacilli other than Salmonellae: Case reports and literature review. *Am J Med Sci* 1977;273:203.

316. Cohen JI, Bartlett JA, Corey GR: Extra-intestinal manifestations of *Salmonella* infections. *Medicine* 1987;66:349.

317. Rodriguez C, Olcoz MT, Izquierdo G, et al: Endocarditis due to ampicillin-resistant nontyphoid *Salmonella:* Cure with a third generation cephalosporin. *Rev Infect Dis* 1990;12:817.

318. Fernandez GC, Chapman AJ, Bolli R, et al: Gonococcal endocarditis: A case series demonstrating modern presentation of an old disease. *Am Heart J* 1984;108:1326.

319. Currathers M, Kanokvechayost R: *Pseudomonas aeruginosa:* Report of a case with a review of the literature. *Am J Med* 1973;55:811.

320. Reyes MP, Brown WJ, Lerner AM: Treatment of patients with *Pseudomonas* endocarditis with high dose aminoglycoside and carbenicillin therapy. *Medicine* 1978;57:57.

321. Reyes MP, El-Khatib MR, Frown WJ, et al: Synergy between carbenicillin and an aminoglycoside (gentamicin or tobramycin) against *Pseudomonas aeruginosa* isolated from patients with endocarditis and sensitivity of isolates to normal human serum. *J Infect Dis* 1979;140:192.

322. Reyes M, Lerner A: Current problems in the treatment of infective endocarditis due to *Pseudomonas aeruginosa. Rev Infect Dis* 1983;5:314.

323. Rybak M, Bolke S, Levine D, et al: Clinical use and toxicity of high-dose tobramycin in patients with pseudomonal endocarditis. *J Antimicrob Chemother* 1989;17:115.

324. Fass RJ, Plouffe JF, Russell JA: Intravenous/oral ciprofloxacin vs. ceftazidime in the treatment of serious infections. *Am J Med* 1989;87(Suppl 5A):164S.

325. Traub W, Spohr M, Bauer D: *Pseudomonas aeruginosa:* In vitro susceptibility to antimicrobial defibrinated human blood. *Chemotherapy* 1988;34:284.

326. Street AC, Durack DT: Experience with trimethoprim-sulfamethoxazole in treatment of infective endocarditis. *Rev Infect Dis* 1988;10:915.

327. Cooper R, Mills J: *Serratia* endocarditis: A follow-up report. *Arch Intern Med* 1980;140:199.

328. Cooper R, Mills J: *Serratia* endocarditis. *Arch Intern Med* 1980;140:199.

329. Berkowitz FR, Colsen P, Raw K: *Serratia marcescens* endocarditis treated with ceftazidime. *S Afr Med J* 1983;64:105.

320. Lynn DJ, Kane JG, Parker RH: *Haemophilus parainfluenzae* and influenzae endocarditis: A review of forty cases. *Medicine* 1977;56:115.
331. Reller LB, Baines RD, Brandt D, Lichtenstein KA, Johnson ZT: Activity of ceftriaxone against HACEK bacteria and efficacy in treatment of *Hemophilus* spp. endocarditis in *Program and Abstracts of the 27th Interscience Conference on Antimicrobial Agents in Chemotherapy, Oct. 7, 1987, New York.*
332. Bryan JP, Pankey GA: *Haemophilus paraphrophilus* endocarditis. *South Med J* 1986;79: 480.
333. Chann C, Jones S, McCatchan R, et al: *Haemophilus parainfluenzae* infective endocarditis. *Medicine* 1977;56:99.
334. Greenspan J, Noble J, Tenenbaum M: Care of *Haemophilus parainfluenzae* endocarditis with chloramphenicol. *Arch Intern Med* 1981;141:1222.
335. Flugelman M, Galvin E, Gen-chetrit E, et al: Brucellosis in patients with heart disease: When should endocarditis be diagnosed? *Cardiology* 1990;77:313.
336. Jacobs F, Abramowicz P, Voreerstraetan P, et al: *Brucella* endocarditis: The role of combined medical and surgical treatment. *Rev Infect Dis* 1990;12:740.
337. Valliattu J, Shuhaiber H, Kiwan Y, et al: *Brucella* endocarditis. *J Cardiovasc Surg* 1989;30:782.
338. Ariza J, Gudiol F, Pallarej R, et al: Treatment of human brucellosis with doxycycline plus rifampin or doxycycline plus streptomycin. *Ann Intern Med* 1992;117:25.
339. Pratt D, Tenney J, Bjork C, et al: Successful treatment of *Brucella melitensis* endocarditis. *Am J Med* 1980;69:857.
340. Joint FAO/WHO Expert Committee on Brucellosis: Geneva, World Health Organization, 1986.
341. Weisner P, Handsfield H, Holmes K: Low antibiotic resistance of gonococci causing disseminated infection. *N Engl J Med* 1973;288:1221.
342. Bush L, Boscia J: Disseminated multiple antibiotic resistant gonococcal infection: Needed changes in antimicrobial therapy. *Ann Intern Med* 1987;197:692.
343. Murray BE, Karchmer AW, Moellering RC Jr: Diphtheroid prosthetic valve endocarditis. *Am J Med* 1980;69:838.
344. Harchmer A: Prosthetic valve endocarditis, in Magilligan L, Quinn A (eds): *Endocarditis: Medical and Surgical Management.* New York, Marcel Dekker, 1989, p 241.
345. Cauda R, Tamburrini E, Ventura G, et al: Effective vancomycin therapy for *Corynebacterium pseudodiphtheriticum* endocarditis. *South Med J* 1987;80(12):1598.
346. Gerry JL, Greenough WB III: Diphtheroid endocarditis. Report of nine cases and review of the litcrature. *John Hopkins Med J* 1976;139:61.
347. Carvajal A, Fredericksen W: Fatal endocarditis due to *Listeria* monocytogenes. *Rev Infect Dis* 1988;10:616.
348. Gallagher PG, Watanakunakorn D: *Listeria monocytogenes* endocarditis: A review of the literature 1950–1986. *Scand J Infect Dis* 1988;20:359.
349. Moellering R, Medoff C, Leech T, et al: Antibiotic synergism against *Listeria monocytogenes. Antimicrob Agents Chemother* 1972;1:30.
350. Treatment of *Listeria monocytogenes* infection with trimethoprim-sulfamethoxazole: Case report and review of literature. *Rev Infect Dis* 1986;8:427.
351. Raoult D, Etienne J, Massip P, et al: Q fever endocarditis in the south of France. *J Infect Dis* 1987;155(3):570.
352. Varma MPS, Adgey AAJ, Connolly JH: Chronic Q fever endocarditis. *Br Heart J* 1980;43:695.
353. Turck W, Howitt G, Turnberz H, et al: Chronic Q fever. *Am J Med* 1976;45:197.
354. Yeaman M, Mitscher A, Baca O: In vitro susceptibility of *Coxiella burnetii* to antibiotics, including several types of quinolones. *Antimicrob Agents Chemother* 1987;31:1079.
355. Levy P, Drancourt M, Etienne J, et al: Comparison of different antibiotic regimens for therapy of 32 cases of Q fever endocarditis. *Antimicrob Agents Chemother* 1991;35:533.
356. Jackson R, Dopp A: *Bacteroides fragilis* endocarditis. *South Med J* 1988;81:781.
357. Tunbel A, Kaye D: Endocarditis with negative blood culture. *N Engl J Med* 1992;325: 1215.

358. Pesanti E, Smith I: Infective endocarditis with negative blood culture: An analysis of 52 cases. *Am J Med* 1979;66:43.

359. Sliman R, Rehm S, Shlaes DM: Serious infections caused by *Bacillus* species. *Medicine* 1987;66(s):218.

360. Sussman JI Baron EJ, Goldberg SM, et al: Clinical manifestations and therapy of *Lactobacillus* endocarditis: Report of a case and review of the literature. *Rev Infect Dis* 1986;8(5):771.

361. Jariwalla AG, Daview BH, White J: Infective endocarditis complicating psittacosis: Response to rifampicin. *Br Med J* 1980;280:155.

362. Marrie TJ, Harczy M, Mann OE, et al: Culture-negative endocarditis probably due to *Chlamydia pneumoniae*. *J Infect Dis* 1990;161:127.

363. O'Neill P, Hone R, Blake S: Prosthetic valve endocarditis caused by *Propionibacterium acnes*. *Br Med J* 1988;296(6634):1444.

364. Grieco MH, Sheldon C: *Erysipelothrix rhusiopathiae*. *Ann NY Acad Sci* 1970;174:523.

365. MacGowen AP, Reeves DS, Wright C, et al: Tricuspid valve infective endocarditis and pulmonary sepsis due to *Erysipelothrix rhusiopathiae* successfully treated with high doses of ciprofloxacin but complicated by gynecomastia. *J Infect Dis* 1991;22(1):100.

366. Edwards R, Finch R: Characterization and antibiotic susceptibilities of *Streptobacillis moniliformis*. *J Med Microbiol* 1986;21:39.

367. Appelbaum J, Wilding G, Morse L: *Yersinia enterocolitica* endocarditis. *Arch Intern Med* 1983;193:2150.

368. Larsen J: The spectrum of clinical manifestations of infections with *Yersinia enterocolitica* and their pathogenesis. *Contrib Microbiol Immunol* 1979;5:257.

369. Urbano-Marquez A, Estruch R, Agusti A, et al: Infectious endocarditis due to *Yersinia enterocolitica*. *J Infect Dis* 1983;148:1899.

370. Weber D, Wolfson J, Swartz M: *Pasturella multocida* infections: Report of 34 cases and review of the literature. *Medicine* 1989;63:133.

371. Goldstein E, Citron D, Richwald G: Lack of in vitro efficacy of oral forms of certain cephalosporins, erythromycin and oxacillin against *Pasteurella multocida*. *Antimicrob Agents Chemother* 1988;32:213.

372. Altman H, Sacks F: Bronchopneumonia and endocarditis caused by *Acinetobacter anitratum cherella vaginicola*. *NY State J Med* 1979;79:1434.

373. Ramphal R, Kluge R: *Acinetobacter calcoaceticus* variety *anitratus:* An increasing nosocomial problem. *Am J Med Sci* 1979;277:57.

374. Wilson WR, Danielson GK, Giuliani ER, et al: Prosthetic valve endocarditis. *Mayo Clin Proc* 1982;57:155.

375. McLeod R, Remington JS: Fungal endocarditis, in Rahimtoola SH (ed): *Infective Endocarditis*. New York, Grune and Stratton, 1978, p 211.

376. Atkinson J, Connor P, Robinowitz M, et al: Cardiac fungal infections. Review of autopsy findings in 60 patients. *Hum Pathol* 1984;15:935.

377. Leaf H, Simberkoff M: *Fungal Endocarditis in Infective Endocarditis*. London, ICR Publishers, 1991.

378. Rubenstein E, Noriega C, Simberkoff M, et al: Fungal endocarditis: Analysis of 24 cases and review of the literature. *Medicine* 1975;54:331.

379. Kanawaty DS, Stalker JB, Munt PW: Nonsurgical treatment of *Histoplasma* endocarditis involving a bioprosthetic valve. *Chest* 1991;1:253.

380. Smith BM, Hoeprich PD, Huston AC, et al: Activity of two polyene and two imidazole antimicrobics on *Candida albicans* in human fibrin clots. *J Lab Clin Med* 1983;102:126.

381. Rubinstein E, Noreiga E, Simberkoff MS, et al: Tissue penetration of amphotericin B in *Candida* endocarditis. *Chest* 1974;66:376.

382. Turnier E, Kay JH, Bernstein S, et al: Surgical treatment of *Candida* endocarditis. *Chest* 1975;67:262.

383. Sande MA, Bowman CR, Calderone RA: Experimental *Candida albicans* endocarditis: Characterization of the disease and response to therapy. *Infect Immun* 1977;17:140.

384. Maisch PA, Calderone RA: Adherence of *Candida albicans* to a fibrin-platelet matrix formed in vitro. *Infect Immun* 1980;27:650.

385. Longman LP, Martin MV: A comparison of the efficacy of itraconazole, amphotericin B and 5-fluorocytosine in the treatment of *Aspergillus fumigatus* endocarditis in the rabbit. *J Antimicrob Chemother* 1987.

386. Ernst JD, Rusnak M, Sande MA: Combination antifungal chemotherapy for experimental disseminated candidiasis: Lack of correlation between in vitro and in vivo observations with amphotericin B and rifampin. *Rev Infect Dis* 1983;5:S626.

387. Witt M, Bayer A: Comparison of fluconazole and amphotericin B for prevention and treatment of experimental *Candida* endocarditis. *Antimicrob Agents Chemother* 1991;35: 2481.

14

Surgical Management

Advances in cardiac surgery have played an important role in the successful management of infective endocarditis. A number of surgical techniques, including the placement of prosthetic valves, have been developed to repair the damage produced by these infections. In addition, their use has resulted in an entirely new set of challenges in the management of endocardial infection.

About 15–25% of patients with infective endocarditis are presently treated surgically. This proportion is the same for individuals confined in tertiary institutions and in community hospitals.[1,2] Data published in the 1970s indicated that infection of native valves was cured by medical treatment alone in 75–85% of patients.[3,4]

Because there has been an increase in endocardial disease caused by *S. aureus*, enterococci, gram-negative organisms, and fungi, therapeutic success has not improved overall. Fifty percent of some valvular infections presently fail to respond to intensive medical therapy or surgery.[5–9] The enlarging spectrum of pathogens has been responsible for an increase in the intra- and extracardiac complications of infective endocarditis. Both the aggressiveness of the invading organisms and concurrent decrease in the defense mechanisms of the host have been responsible for this situation.

Since the time valvular replacement was first performed, there has been ongoing debate over the role of cardiac surgery in treating infective endocarditis. Indications for this mode of treatment have been defined over the past 10 years[10–12]. They include (1) the presence of congestive cardiac failure; (2) persistent bacteremia; (3) valvular dysfunction; (4) intracardiac abscesses; and (5) fungal endocarditis. Lesser criteria are (1) systemic embolization; (2) valvular vegetations detected by echocardiography; and (3) difficulty in treating disease caused by gram-negative bacilli and fungi. Several scaling systems have been developed to characterize cases of infective endocarditis in which the outcome might be improved by surgery[13,14] (Table 14.1). A score of 5 or higher indicates that surgical intervention is warranted. We emphasize that the decision should be based on the clinical features of the disease, and not solely on scoring guidelines. Most signifi-

Table 14.1 Indications for Surgical Intervention in Acute NVE

Finding	Prognostic Score
Congestive cardiac failure	
Manifest refractory to therapy, and/or progressive	5
Manifest, medically compensated	3
Concealed	1
Fungal endocarditis (except that caused by *Histoplasma capsulatum*)	5
Persistent sepsis (>72 hr) despite antimicrobical therapy	5
Nonstreptococcal infective endocarditis (IE)	1
Single episode of thromboembolism	3
Recurrent septic thromboembolism	5
Vegetations detected by echocardiography	1
IE restricted to right-sided valves	−2*
Rupture of aneurysms of the sinus of Valsalva	5
AV block, conduction disturbances, abscesses	5
Kissing infection of the anterior mitral leaflet in IE of the aortic valve	4
Isolated IE of the aortic valve or of more than one valve	2
Isolated IE of the mitral valve	1

*According to the experience of the Duesseldorf Heart Center, the prognosis is improved with an operation in patients demonstrating more than 5 points, according to the following score (adapted Ref. 13). Because of the overall favorable prognosis of isolated, conservatively treatable IE of the right-sided valves, this finding is scored −2.

Source: Adapted from Horstkotte D, Schulte H, Bircks W: Factors influencing prognosis and indication for surgical intervention in acute native valve endocarditis, in Horstkotte D, Bodner E (eds): *Infective Endocarditis.* London, ICR Publishers, 1991, p 187a.

cant are the level of experience of surgeons and appropriate postoperative management in the hospital.[15]

Michael et al.[16] defined the need for surgery and its timing early or late in the course of infective endocarditis. Most patients were free of complications when the study was initiated. Three stages were identified as the disease progressed: *Stage 1*—This involves treatment with an effective antimicrobial agent for 4 weeks. Surgery is required in individuals who develop severe aortic regurgitation that starts after medical therapy is completed. *Stage 2*—Individuals who suffer severe complications such as congestive cardiac failure or persistent bacteremia not reversed by appropriate treatment must have surgery immediately. *Stage 3*—Individuals who have cardiac failure but who respond rapidly to medical management must have surgery earlier than later in the course of their disease.

Congestive cardiac failure is the primary indication for surgical intervention in patients with infective endocarditis.[17–20] Ninety-one percent of those who die have had moderate to severe congestive failure.[4] Griffin et al.[21] were among the earliest investigators to recognize the significance of congestive cardiac failure in individuals with infective endocarditis. They noted that surgery decreased the fatality rate of the disease. This has been confirmed by others.[20–26] Croft et al.[26] reported that medical plus surgical therapy led to survival in 91% of patients compared to only 4% of those treated medically. Infection of the mitral valve by *S. viridans* was treatable medically even when mild congestive cardiac failure was present. Horstkotte et al.[15] confirmed this finding.

Severe progressive congestive cardiac failure demands surgical removal of the malfunctioning valve. Aortic insufficiency is less responsive to medical therapy than cardiac decompensation caused by an incompetent mitral valve. Signs of heart failure in the presence of aortic dysfunction indicate the need for immediate surgical consultation.[27,28] The presence of true clinical congestive cardiac failure, not just echocardiographically detected valvular insufficiency, is prognostically very significant.[29] However, the absence of valvular insufficiency early in the course of the infection does not guarantee a favorable clinical outcome.

The congestive failure of infective endocarditis is usually related to perforation of valvular cusps.[30] Obstruction of the orifice by a large vegetation rarely leads to cardiac decompensation.[31] However, when this occurs, it is due to interference with the functioning of the mitral valve by a fibrin clot.

Persistent Infective Endocarditis

Infective endocarditis uncontrolled by antimicrobial therapy is an indication for surgery. This is almost always the case in patients with fungal endocardial disease. Early replacement of the valve and treatment with antifungal agents is optimal therapy.[32,33] However, the fatality rate remains high, probably related to an increase in the incidence of embolization, metastatic infections (70% of cases), and paravalvular and myocardial abscesses.[34-36] When surgery is performed prior to the development or early on in the course of these complications, the outcome may be better than average. Removal or debridement of the involved valve is often adequate to eradicate infection in patients with fungal endocarditis involving the tricuspid valves. Some evidence suggests that the removal of emboli from areas in which they are deposited improves survival.[37]

Several studies have pointed out that the persistence of bacteremia after 7 days of antimicrobial therapy is associated with a poor clinical outcome.[38] Early valvular surgery decreases the fatality rate from 34–90% to 9–13%.[13,26,39,40] By removing large valvular vegetations that are poorly penetrated by antibiotics, surgery eradicates the sources of emboli and permits the repair of damaged leaflets.[41,42] Bacterial infection of the tricuspid valve may be treated successfully by valvulectomy or excision of one or two leaflets.[43,44] Earlier studies recommended total replacement of an infected tricuspid valve[45]; this is usually not required. A simple valvulectomy, without replacement, decreases the risk of reinfection of prosthetic valves in intravenous drug abusers (IVDA).

Replacement of a native valve in patients with fungal or bacterial endocarditis involving the left side of the heart raises concern that the implanted valve may become infected. Experience has indicated that placement of a

prosthetic valve during treatment of infective endocarditis does not constitute a significant infectious risk.[11,13,25,46–48] Reinfection after valve replacement occurs in 20–40% of IVDA[49,50] but in only 5% of nonaddicts.[46–48]
There is no increase in the risk of paravalvular infection invading prosthetic valves inserted in infected individuals than in those inserted in individuals with noninfectious disorders. It is important to note that before
surgery is performed in individuals with persistent bacteremia or fungemia, other sources of bacteremia, especially splenic abscesses, must be
ruled out.[51]

Valvular Vegetations

A major area of controversy in the management of infective endocarditis is
the ability of valvular vegetations to produce single or recurrent emboli.
The incidence of detectable arterial embolization is about 43%; 27% of
emboli lodge in the carotid circulation.[52,53] Early studies with TTE failed to
prove a clear association between the deposition of emboli and the presence
of valvular thrombi and embolization.[54,55] By using TEE, Mugge et al.[56]
noted a close association between the deposition of emboli and the presence
of thrombi in native aortic valves larger than 10 mm in diameter. Vegetations in other areas were not associated with embolic phenomena. Other
studies indicated that there is no relation between the presence of valvular
thrombi, the complications of cardiac failure, and death.[56,57] An association
between cardiac failure and the presence of vegetations larger than 10 mm
has been reported by Bayer et al.[58]

Studies by Steckelberg et al.[59] have indicated that the incidence of embolization peaks in the first 2 weeks of treatment with an antimicrobial agent.
There appears to be no relation between the size of a thrombus and the risk
of embolization. According to these investigators, the danger of embolism is
most significant in patients with infective endocarditis caused by S. viridans.
However, other studies have indicated that disease produced by S. aureus is
associated with the highest incidence of embolization.[60]

An investigation of the development of vegetations over 74 weeks by
Rohmamn et al.[61] indicated that an increase or a lack of decrease in the size
of a vegetation greater than 8 mm in diameter predicted an extended
period of healing of the valvular infection. This was associated with a
higher incidence of embolization, congestive cardiac failure, perivalvular
abscesses, and death. Disease caused by S. viridans was associated with rapid
resolution of the thrombus. The reverse was the case when emboli were
caused by S. aureus. Consideration of surgery is mandatory when embolization occurs in the absence of healing or during an increase in the size of the
thrombus. Even when embolization recurs, antimicrobial therapy is continued unless the vegetation is growing larger. A decision to undertake surgery requires a comprehensive review of the clinical situation. Based on
current date, we favor downgrading of the significance of embolization
when evaluating the need for valvular surgery.

Myocardial Abscess

Heart block is usually produced by the spread of infection from the valvular bend to the conducting system. Dinubile[62] established the following criteria for urgent surgery when cardiac block developed in the course of infective endocarditis: (1) the onset or progression of heart block; (2) the presence of infection of the aortic valve; (3) persistence of block for at least 1 week of treatment with antimicrobial agents; and (4) elimination of other causes of abnormal conduction (e.g., digitalis toxicity). However, only about 15% of patients with a burrowing valvular ring abscess exhibit new electrocardiographic disturbances.[63] About 14% of patients with endocardial infections that involve native valves develop some type of defect in conduction. The persistence of unexplained fever during treatment may be the only evidence of an intracardiac abscess.[64] TTE detects about 30% of suppurative complications; TEE identifies 87%.[65] Myocardial abscess must be at least 1 cm in diameter to be detected by TTE. A very high proportion of false positives in PVE are due to technical problems.

An asymptomatic abscess detected by echocardiography does not require surgical treatment unless complications develop.[66] Among these are (1) a new or progressive delay in conduction; (2) persistent bacteremia; and (3) rupture of the abscess into the pericardial sac, leading to the development of acute pericarditis. Inflammation of the aortic valvular ring may progress to an aneurysm of the sinus of Valsalva that can further injure the valve or produce fistulas between the root of the aorta and either ventricle. These aneurysms are more easily detected than those of the coronary arteries or myocardial abcesses.

Relapse of Infection

A relapse of infection is defined as the return of the symptoms and signs consistent with active infective endocarditis and the presence of bacteremia within 3 months after an apparent cure. The first relapse is treated in the same manner as the initial episode if complications are absent.[67] Exceptions to this rule are secondary diseases caused by drug-resistant organisms such as gram-negative bacteria or rickettsiae. Surgery is indicated when this occurs. A second relapse, during or after completion of treatment, mandates surgical replacement of the involved valve and therapy with antibiotics to which the organism is susceptible.

Infection may recur more than 6 months after successful treatment. When the original valve is involved, the therapy is identical to that applied during the first episode of infection.

Metastatic Complications

Mycotic aneurysms develop in 2–15% of patients with infective endocarditis.[68] The incidence did not decrease after antimicrobial therapy became available. These lesions appear late in the course of endocardial infection. The most comon mechanism in the pathogenesis of aneurysms is the deposition of infected emboli in the vasa vasorum of the blood vessels. Their common "final resting place" is at the branchpoints of the vascular tree.[68] *S. viridans* produces mycotic aneurysms more frequently that does *S. aureus* but those caused by the staphylococcus rupture more often. The cerebral arteries, abdominal coronary and pulmonary arteries, abdominal aorta, and ligated ductus arteriosus are involved most often.[69–74] The arteries of the legs, small bowel, valvular leaflets, and annulus of the mitral valve are other sites at which aneurysms may develop.[75,76] These have been identified in 23% of patients.[77,78] The clinical course of aneurysms does not always parallel that of infective endocarditis. An aneurysm may require surgery even when the infected valve is responding to medical treatment.[79]

Aneurysms are often silent until they start to leak; 66% are mycotic.[80] A study by Bohmfalk et al.[81] indicated that 80% of patients with ruptured aneurysms died compared to only 30% of those with intact lesions. Sixty-five percent of aneurysms ruptured spontaneously.

Wilson et al.[75] described a somewhat more encouraging clinical result. They identified an aneurysm in eight patients, all of whom had severe headaches and visual field defects. Four had mycotic aneurysms and three were thought to have had an intracranial hemorrhage. CT scans identified the secondary signs of mycotic aneurysms, such as inflammation caused by small leaks. Angiography was noted to be the definitive approach to establishing the presence of a cerebral aneurysm. A CT scan was recommended in patients with a headache and neurological symptoms, especially homonymous hemianopsia, in order to rule out the presence of a mycotic aneurysm. Arteriography is called for when this is not identified by the scan but clinical suspicion remains high.[75]

It has been recommended that all cerebral aneurysms be excised because there is a high incidence of fatal rupture.[82] However, 30% of these aneurysms may heal when treated medically.[80,83] Surgical removal or "clipping" is indicated when the lesion begins to leak. The management of asymptomatic aneurysms remains controversial.

Surgery may be considered when an aneurysm is present in the periphery of the cerebral circulation.[84] When it is located close to the midline, there is an increased risk of surgically induced neurological dysfunction. In this case, the aneurysm would be followed by angiography at 2-week intervals. Surgery is mandatory when an aneurysm increases in size while being observed.[84–87] A similar approach is recommended for multiple intracranial aneurysms.

Asymptomatic aneurysms detected early in the course of infective endocarditis may initially increase in size but may eventually become thrombosed.[84] This observation must be considered when inaccessible aneurysms enlarge but remain clinically silent. In the absence of leaks, surgery is indicated only when continued growth is documented despite several weeks of antimicrobial therapy.

Mycotic aneurysms of peripheral vessels require resection and ligation.[80]

In most instances, the placement of a bypass graft is unnecessary if the collateral circulation is adequate. When this is not the case, a venous graft is required. Prosthetic devices must be avoided, if possible, in order to minimize the risk of infection.[88–90] This is true for mycotic aneurysms of the abdominal aorta and its branches.[87] Embolization of these arteries may be attempted when resection is impossible.[91]

Large cerebral abscesses require drainage. Multiple abscesses less than 1 cm in diameter usually resolve when treated with antibiotics.[92] Drainage is required before cardiac surgery is undertaken because the abscess may be the source of bacteremia and secondary infection of a newly placed cardiac valve.

The presence of a splenic abscess must be ruled out before replacement of an infected cardiac valve in patients with bacteremia. Aspiration may be performed prior to surgery when nuclear or CT scans are positive. Splenectomy is indicated when the aspirate contains polymorphonuclear cells and/ or organisms. However, when it is sterile and a scan identifies only a scar, splenectomy may be withheld.[93]

Because of difficulty in eradicating organisms from prosthetic devices, surgery plays a more important role in the treatment of PVE than in native valve endocarditis (NVE).[94] However, operative intervention is not always required for cure.[83,95,96] Factors that predict a favorable outcome in patients not treated surgically are (1) infection caused by organisms susceptible to penicillin or other antimicrobial agents; (2) late infection of a prosthetic valve; (3) infection of the mitral valve; and (4) initiation of treatment early in the course of infection of a bioprosthetic valve.[97–100] Late-onset disease is usually caused by organisms similar to those responsible for NVE. The incidence of complications is much higher in individuals with early-onset PVE (80%) than in those with late disease.[97–102] This may be related to the tendency of infections to burrow into adjacent myocardium early in the course of the disease. About 65% of patients with PVE eventually require cardiac surgery.[91] Regardless of the nature of the infecting organism, mitral valvular disease produces less spread of infection into the adjacent myocardium than into an infected aortic valve. Infection of bioprosthetic valves involves the valvular leaflets but not the surrounding ring.

Complications are the most important determinant of the outcome of PVE (Table 14.2). The indications for surgery are determined mainly by the severity of the clinical manifestations, not by whether disease onset is early or late. The indications for surgery in PVE are essentially identical to those for NVE (Table 14.1) plus the presence of a small paravalvular dehiscence in early PVE. The absolute indications for surgery include (1) moderate to severe congestive cardiac failure; (2) persistent sepsis; (3) fungal PVE; (4) an unstable prosthetic valve; and (5) the onset of cardiac block and infection of the valvular bed. Relative indications are (1) infection by organisms other than streptococci; (2) early onset of PVE; (3) embolization; (4) congestive cardiac failure; (5) paravalvular leak; (6) relapse of infection; and (7) culture-negative endocarditis[103] (Table 14.3). During the first 12–24 months after implantation, bioprosthetic valves are less likely to become

Table 14.2. Cardiac and Noncardiac Complications of Acute Infective Endocarditis in 103 Consecutive Patients After Mitral (MVR), Aortic (AVR), and Mitral-Aortic Valve Replacement (DVR).

	MVR (n = 35)	AVR (n = 56)	DVR (n = 12)	
Persistent sepsis (>72 hr)	8	10	3	21 (20.4%)
Periprosthetic dehiscence	21	47	11	79 (76.7%)
Interference of vegetation and valve occluder	3	4	3	10 (9.7%)
Cardiac failure	13	27	8	48 (46.6%)
Myocarditis/pericarditis	4	8	2	14 (13.6%)
Intracardiac fistulas/abscesses	4	6	3	13 (12.6%)
Conduction disturbances	8	11	6	25 (24.3%)
Ventricular arrhythmias	1	3	1	5 (4.9%)
Septic thromboembolism	9	12	7	28 (27.2%)
Hematuria/proteinuria	18	30	7	55 (53.4%)
Acute renal failure	5	9	3	17 (16.5%)
Mycotic aneurysms	2	2	0	4 (3.9%)
Diffuse vasculitis	3	4	3	10 (9.7%)
Nonembolic involvement of the central nervous system	8	11	4	23 (22.3%)

Source: Adapted from Horstkotte D: Prosthetic valve endocarditis, in Horstkotte D, Bodnar E (eds): *Infective Endocarditis.* London, ICR Publishers, 1991, p 241.

infected than mechanical ones.[104,105] There appears to be no difference in the risk of infection when either type of prosthetic valve replaces an acute infected valve (Figure 14.1) Because of their longevity, mechanical prostheses are presently preferred.

Anticoagulation

Thill and Myer[106] reported their experience with penicillin and dicumarol in the treatment of subacute bacterial endocarditis in 1947. They speculated that anticoagulation might potentiate antibacterial activity by decreasing the size of an infected vegetation. Earlier studies in animals had supported this concept.[107] Unfortunately, the patients who received the anti-coagulant frequently experienced cerebral bleeding. Anticoagulation in individuals with infective endocarditis remains controversial. It is our opinion that this practice be avoided. An exception is infection of prosthetic valves, for which continuous anticoagulation is required.[108]

Wilson et al.[109] studied the role of coumadin in the therapy of infected mechanical prosthetic valves. They noted that 30% of the patients not treated with an anticoagulant experienced significant neurological compli-

Table 14.3. Indications for Surgical Intervention in Prosthetic Valve Endocarditis

Finding	Prognostic Score
Congestive cardiac failure	
Manifest, refractory to therapy, and/or progressive	5
Manifest, medically compensated	4
Concealed	2
Fungal endocarditis (except that caused by *Histoplasma capsulatum*)	5
Persistent sepsis (>72 hr) despite antimicrobical therapy	5
Nonstreptococcal PVE	2
Single episode of thromboembolism	3
Recurrent septic thromboembolism	5
Vegetations detected by echocardiography	1
PVE restricted to right-sided valves	0
Rupture of aneurysms of the sinus of Valsalva	5
AV block, conduction disturbances, abscesses	5
Small perivalvular dehiscence	2
Significant perivalvular dehiscence, tilting movement of prosthetic valve	5
Early prosthetic valve endocarditis (<60 days of surgery)	2
Kissing infection of the anterior mitral leaflet in infective endocarditis (IE) of the aortic valve	4
Isolated IE of the aortic valve or of more than one valve	2
Isolated IE of the mitral valve	1

Source: Adapted from Horstkotte D: Prosthetic valve endocarditis, in Horstkotte D, Bodnar E (eds): *Infective Endocarditis.* London, ICR Publishers, 1991, p 248.

cations. A study at the Massachusetts General Hospital confirmed this experience.[97] However, another report indicated that untoward cerebral events were more common in individuals receiving coumadin[110]. It is our opinion that when a cerebrovascular event occurs in patients with PVE, treatment with coumadin should be discontinued for 48–72 hr and reinstituted when the bleeding has ceased. If anticoagulation is resumed, heparin is the drug of choice because its activity is rapidly reversed when complications develop. The need for continued coagulation must be decided on an individual basis. When thrombosis develops in areas other than the cardiac valves, such as the legs, appropriate anticoagulation is indicated. The insertion of an umbrella in the vena cava to interrupt migration of a clot must be given serious consideration in these situations.

Treatment

The earlier medical treatment is begun, the better the clinical outcome. This is so whether surgery is or is not required. Lerner and Weinstein[111] pointed out that 90% of patients with subacute infective endocarditis were cured when treatment was initiated 2 weeks after the appearance of symp-

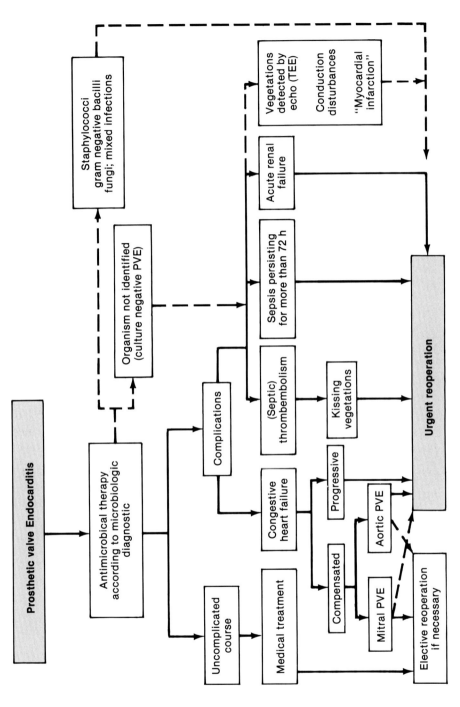

Fig. 14.1. Algorithm of the need for urgent surgery in a patient with PVE. (Adapted from Horstkotte D: Prosthetic valve

toms. This rate was reduced to 74% when the disease was present for 8 weeks. The two classical complications of infective endocarditis, cardiac failure and myocardial abscess, were responsible for the decrease in the response to treatment.

Myocardial infarction may occur during treatment in about 3% of patients and is responsible for sudden death in about 1%.[112,113] Infarctions in patients with infective endocarditis are caused by emboli that break off from valvular vegetations and obstruct the coronary circulation. Candidates for surgery must be evaluated for the presence of atherosclerotic disease because myocardial infarction plays an important role in the development of postoperative congestive cardiac failure.[114]

Renal failure that develops during or after clinical recovery is a serious complication.[1] It is responsible for about 10% of deaths in patients with infective endocarditis treated medically, with or without surgery. Severe renal failure may be significantly improved by antimicrobial therapy.

Surgical management has improved the outcome of infective endocarditis. Prior to this, 5% of patients died after the endocardial disease was cured.[115] Fifty percent of those with aortic insufficiency when they left the hospital succumbed to their disease within 5 years. Others died within 2 years after discharge of congestive cardiac failure. Richardson et al.[116] noted that the fatality rate in patients treated with antimicrobial agents alone was 44%; it was only 14% in those managed surgically. Surgical therapy reduced this figure in individuals with mild to moderate congestive cardiac failure from 66% in those treated medically to 25% in those who underwent valvular surgery.[116] Karchmer and Stinson reported similar results.[117] The fatality rate was highest in individuals who underwent surgery within 6 weeks of the initiation of antimicrobial therapy. About 5% of those operated on required additional procedures.[118] Surgery performed in the presence of uncontrolled sepsis led to a significant incidence of death.[119]

The risk of a fatal outcome was directly related to the pathological findings identified during surgery. The death rate in patients with disease limited to the valvular leaflets was similar to that in those treated medically. Twenty-seven percent of individuals with an infected annulus or valvular abscesses died.[120] This was especially the case when the aortic valve was involved. Fifty-five percent of these individuals had severe injury of the valvular ring, annulus, and paravalvular tissues to an extent that made placement of a prosthetic valve impossible. A variety of techniques was used to produce tight-fitting valves. However, the use of these valves was associated with 23% operative mortality; 8% of patients required reoperation.[120]

Surgery in patients with infection of a mitral valve is beneficial due to the decrease in the incidence of paravalvular complications. The risk of death increases to 21% when both the aortic and mitral valves are replaced.

Persistent or recurrent infection produced by the same organisms present before valvular replacement ranges from 0% to 4% postoperatively.[117,121] Paravalvular leaks develop in 7–14% postoperatively[117,122]; most require surgical repair. A positive Gram stain or culture obtained during surgery indicates an increased risk of postoperative paravalvular leaks.

It must be emphasized that (1) the incidence of death following replacement of a valve is highest in patients with active infection; (2) the presence and severity of congestive cardiac failure at the time of surgery are major determinants of survival; (3) patients with infective endocarditis fare as well as those receiving replacement valves for noninfectious disorders; (4) an implanted valve is not at risk of infection when effective antimicrobial therapy is initiated; and (5) "buff up" of a patient prior to replacement of a valve is not indicated and may be dangerous because the required surgery is delayed.

Infection of Pacemakers

Six percent of permanent pacemakers are infected by a variety of organisms; this may be associated with bacteremia.[123] The average fatality rate is about 2% but is increases to 35% when infective endocarditis is present.[124,125] The risk factors include (1) the development of chronic dermatitis or a hematoma in areas where a pacemaker has been placed; (2) therapy with corticosteriods and/or anticoagulants; and (3) the presence of diabetes mellitus. Seventy-five percent of infections are caused by staphylococci, including *S. aureus* and *S. epidermidis*.

Infection of pacemakers includes (1) involvement of the pocket in the skin in which the pacemaker generator has been placed; (2) infection of the area proximal to the leads of the pacemaker; and (3) infection of distal areas contiguous with the endocardium. The diagnosis is established by (1) the presence of an abscess or inflammation of the overlying skin; (2) erosion of the skin at the site of the pacemaker generator; and (3) fever and/or positive culture of the blood in the absence of an identifiable focus of infection. Bacteremia, usually caused by *S. aureus*, develops in about 23% of patients. The presence of bacteremia, especially when it appears early in the course of the disease, does not indicate the presence of endocardial infection.

The management of infected pacemakers is controversial. This is so because the need to remove the leads of the apparatus to achieve cure has not been established. Local drainage, together with appropriate antimicrobial therapy, is adequate.[126] There is evidence that failure to remove the wires of a pacemaker is responsible for a high incidence of relapse. The system must be removed when infective endocarditis is present. This must not be undertaken lightly because it usually requires open cardiac surgery.[127] Suppressive antimicrobial therapy is indicated when this is not feasible.[128]

References

1. McAnulty J, Rahimtoola S: Surgery for infective endocarditis. *JAMA* 1979;242:77.
2. Wantanakunakorn C, Burbert T: Infective endocarditis at a large community teaching hospital 1980–1990: A review of 210 episodes. *Medicine* 1993;72:90.

3. Kaye D: Changes in the spectrum, diagnosis and management of bacterial and fungal endocarditis. *Med Clin North Am* 1973;57:941.

4. Pelletier LL, Petersdorf RG: Infective endocarditis: A review of 125 cases from the University of Washington Hospitals, 1963–1972. *Medicine (Baltimore)* 1977;56:287.

5. Bayliss R, Clarke C, Oakley CM: The microbiology and pathogenesis of infective endocarditis. *Br Heart J* 1983;50:513.

6. Geraci J, Wilson W: Endocarditis due to gram-negative bacteria. Report of 56 cases. *Mayo Clin Proc* 1982;57:145.

7. Reyes M, Lerner A: Current problems in the treatment of infective endocarditis due to *Pseudomonas aeruginosa:* A report of 10 cases and a review of the literature. *Medicine* 1989;65:180.

8. Walsh TJ, Hutchins GM, Bulkley BH, et al: Fungal infections of the heart: Analysis of 51 autopsy cases. *Am J Cardiol* 1980;45:357.

9. Carvagal A, Frederisksen W: Fatal endocarditis due to *Listeria monocytogenes. Rev Infect Dis* 1988;10:616.

10. Dinubile M: Surgery in active endocarditis. *Ann Intern Med* 1980;96:650.

11. D'Agostino R, Miller D, Stinson E: Valve replacement in patients with native valve endocarditis: What really determines operative outcome. *Ann Thorac Surg* 1985; 40:429.

12. Karp RB: Role of surgery in infective endocarditis. *Cardiovasc Clin* 1987;17(3):141.

13. Cobbs C, Gnann J: Indications for surgery, in Sande M, Kaye D, Root R, (eds): *Endocarditis.* New York, Churchill Livingstone, 1984, chap 11.

14. Alsip SG, Blackstone EH, Kirklin JW: Indications for cardiac surgery in patients with active infective endocarditis. *Am J Med* 1985;78(Suppl 6B):138.

15. Horstkotte D, Bircks W, Loogen F: Infective endocarditis of native and prosthetic valves—the case for prompt surgical intervention? A retrospective analysis of factors affecting survival. *Z Kardiol* 1986;75(Suppl 2):168.

16. Michel P, Vitoux B, Hage A: Early or delayed surgery in acute native valve endocarditis, in Horstkotte D, Bodnar E. (eds): *Infective Endocarditis.* London, ICR Publishers, 1991, p 22.

17. Mills J, Utlay J, Abbott J: Heart failure in infective endocarditis: Predisposing factors, course and treatment. *Chest* 1974;66:151.

18. Cukingnan RA, Carey JS, Witting JH, et al: Early valve replacement in active infective endocarditis. *J Thorac Cardiovasc Surg* 1983;85:163.

19. Argulu A, Asfaw I: Management of infective endocarditis: 17 years experience. *Ann Thorac Surg* 1987;43:144.

20. Dreyfus G, Serraf A, Jebara VA: Valve repair in acute endocarditis. *Ann Thorac Surg* 1987:43:144.

21. Griffin FM, Jones G, Cobbs CG: Aortic insufficiency in bacterial endocarditis. *Ann Intern Med* 1972;76;23.

22. Mills J, Utley J, Abbott J: Heart failure in infective endocarditis: Predisposing factors, course and treatment. *Chest* 1974;66:151.

23. Wilson WR, Danielson GK, Giuliani ER: Cardiac valve replacement in congestive heart failure due to infective endocarditis. *Mayo Clin Proc* 1979;54:223.

24. Young JB, Welton DE, Raizner AE: Surgery in active infectious endocarditis. *Circulation* 1979;60(Suppl I):77.

25. Richardson JD, Karp RB, Kirklin JW, et al: Treatment of infective endocarditis: A ten year comparative analysis. *Circulation* 1978;58:589.

26. Croft CH, Woodward W, Elliott A: Analysis of surgical versus medical therapy in active complicated native valve infective endocarditis. *Am J Cardiol* 1983;51:1650.

27. Lakier JB: Congestive heart failure, in Magilligan D, Quinn E (eds): *Endocarditis—Medical and Surgical Management.* New York, Marcel Dekker, 1986, p 139.

28. Mann T, McLaurin L, Grossman W, et al: Assessing the haemodynamic severity of acute aortic regurgitation due to infective endocarditis. *N Engl J Med* 1975;293:108.

29. Karalis D, Blumberg E, Vilaro J: Prognostic significance of valvular regurgitation in patients with infective endocarditis. *Am J Med* 1991;90:193.

30. Buchbinder NA, Roberts WC: Left sided valvular active endocarditis—a study of 45 necropsy patients. *Am J Med* 1972;53:20.

31. Karchmer AW, Stinson EB: The role of surgery in infective endocarditis, in Remmington JS, Swartz MS (eds): *Current Clinical Topics in Infectious Diseases*, vol 1. New York, McGraw-Hill, p. 124.

32. Turnier E, Kay J, Bernstein S: Surgical treatment of candida endocarditis. *Chest* 1975; 67:262.

33. Utley J Jr, Mills J, Roe B: The role of valve replacement in the treatment of fungal endocarditis. *J Thorac Cardiovasc Surg* 1975;69:255.

34. McLeod R, Remington JS: Fungal endocarditis, in Rahimtoola SH (ed): *Infective Endocarditis*. New York, Grune and Stratton, 1978, p 211.

35. Kammer RB, Utz JP: *Aspergillus* species endocarditis: The new face of a not so rare disease. *Am J Med* 1974;56:506.

36. Blair TP, Waugh RA, Pollack M, et al: *Histoplasma capsulatium* endocarditis. *Am Heart J* 1980;99:783.

37. Woods CH, Wood RP, Shaw HW Jr: *Aspergillus* endocarditis in patients without prior cardiovascular surgery: Report of a case in a liver transplant recipient and review. *Rev Infect Dis* 1989;11:263.

38. Yee ES, Khonsari S: Right-sided infective endocarditis: Valvuloplasty, valvulectomy, or replacement. *J Cardiovasc Surg* 1989;30:744.

39. Boyd AD, Spencer SC, Isom OW: Infective endocarditis: Analysis of 54 surgically treated patients. *J Thorac Cardiovasc Surg* 1977;73:23.

40. Ormiston JA, Neutze JM, Agnew TM: Infective endocarditis: A lethal disease. *Aust NZ Med* 1981;11:620.

41. Stimmel B, Dack S: Infective endocarditis in narcotic addicts, in Rahimtoola SH (ed): *Infective Endocarditis*. New York, Grune and Stratton, 1977, p 195.

42. Stimmel B, Donoso E, Dack S: Comparison of infective endocarditis in drug addicts and nondrug users. *Am J Cardiol* 1973;32:924.

43. Yee ES, Khonsari S: Right-sided infective endocarditis: Valvuloplasty, valvectomy or replacement. *J Cardiovasc Surg* 1989;30:744.

44. Arbulu A, Holmes R, Asfaw I: Surgical treatment of intractable right-sided infective endocarditis in drug addicts: 25 years experience. *J Heart Valve Dis* 1993;2:129.

45. Arneborn P, Bjork VO, Rodriquez I, et al: Two-stage replacement of tricuspid valve in active endocarditis. *Br Heart J* 1977;39:1276.

46. Magilligan DJ Jr: Active infective endocarditis of a native valve, in Magilligan DJ Jr, Quinn EL (eds): *Endocarditis—Medical and Surgical Management*. New York, Marcel Dekker, 1986, p 207.

47. Defraigne JO, Dalem AM, Demoulin JC, et al: Surgical management of left heart endocarditis. *Acta Chi Belg* 1989;89:247.

48. David TE, Bos J, Christakin CT: Heart valve operations in patients with active infective endocarditis. *Ann Thorac Surg* 1990;49:701.

49. Welton DE, Young JB, Gentry WO, et al: Recurrent infective endocarditis. *Am J Med* 1979;66:932.

50. Freedman LR: Endocarditis updated. *Dis of the Month* 1979;26:1.

51. Magilligan DJ Jr: Splenic abscess, in Magilligan DJ Jr, Quinn E (eds): *Endocarditis—Medical and Surgical Management*. New York, Marcel Dekker, 1986, p 197.

52. Weinstein L, Schlesinger JJ: Pathoanatomic, pathophysiologic and clinical correlations in endocarditis: *N Engl J Med* 1974;291:839.

53. Weinstein L, Schlesinger JJ: Pathonanatomic, pathophysiologic and clinical correlations in endocarditis. *N Engl J Med* 1974;291:1122.

54. Thompson KR, Nanda NC, Gramiak R: Reliability of echocardiography in the diagnosis of infectious endocarditis. *Radiology* 1977;125:473.

55. Wann LS, Hallam CC, Dillon JC, et al: Comparison of M-mode and cross-sectional echocardiography in infective endocarditis. *Circulation* 1979;60:728.

56. Mugge A, Daniel WG, Frank G, et al: Echocardiography in infective endocarditis: Reas-

sessment of prognostic implications of vegetation size determined by the transthoracic and transesophageal approach. *J Am Coll Cardiol* 1989;14:631.

57. Lutas EM, Roberts RB, Devereux RB, et al: Relation between the presence of echocardiographic vegetation and the complication rate in infective endocarditis. *Am Heart J* 1986;112:107.

58. Bayer AN, Blomquist IK, Bello E: Tricuspid valve endocarditis due to *Staphylococcus aureus*. Correlation of two-dimensional echocardiography with clinical outcomes. *Chest* 1988;93:247.

59. Steckelberg JN, Murphy JG, Ballard D: Emboli in infective endocarditis—the prognostic valve of echocardiography. *Ann Intern Med* 1991;114:635.

60. Stafford WJ, Petch J, Radford DJ: Vegetations in infective endocarditis: Clinical relevance and diagnosis by cross-sectional echocardiography. *Br Heart J* 1985;53:310.

61. Rohmann J, Ebel R, Darius H: Prediction of rapid versus prolonged healing of infective endocarditis by monitoring vegetation size. *J Am Soc Echocardiogr* 1991;4:465.

62. Dinubile M: Heart block during bacterial endocarditis: A review of the literature and guidelines for surgical intervention. *Am J Med Sci* 1989;287:30.

63. Douglas A, Moore-Gillen J, Ekyns S: Fever during treatment of infective endocarditis. *Lancet* 1989;1:1341.

64. Weisse AB, Khan MY: The relationship between new cardiac conduction defects and extensions of valve infection in native valve endocarditis. *Clin Cardiol* 1990;13:337.

65. Daniel WG, Mugge A, Martin RP, et al: Improvement in the diagnosis of abscesses associated with endocarditis by transesophageal echocardiography. *N Engl J Med* 1991;324:795.

66. Ryon DS, Pastor BH, Meyerson RM: Abscess of the myocardium. *Am J Med Sci* 1966;251:698.

67. Wilson W, Giuliani E, Danielson G, et al: Management of complications of infective endocarditis. *Mayo Clin Proc* 1982;57:162.

68. Roach MR, Drake CG: Ruptured cerebral aneurysms caused by microorganisms. *N. Engl J Med* 1963;273:246.

69. Kerr A: Bacterial endocarditis revisited. *Mon Con Cardiovasc Dis* 1991;33:831.

70. Kaufman S, Lynfield J, Hennigar G: Mycotic aneurysm of the intrapulmonary arteries in intravenous drug addicts; report of three cases and review of the literature. *Circulation* 1967;35:90.

71. Navarro C, Dickinson P, Kondlapool P, et al: Mycotic aneurysms in pulmonary arteries in intravenous drug addicts; report of three cases and review of the literature. *Am J Med* 1984;76:1124.

72. Escudier B, Becquenin J, Alexandre J: Aneurysmes jambiers compliquant les endocardits bacteriennes: Deux observations. *Presse Med* 1983;12:1595.

73. Wilson J, Ellis D, Lexclen M: Mycotic aneurysm of the small bowel presenting as gastrointestinal hemorrhage. *Med J Aust* 1989;191:119.

74. Ania F, Celona G, Filippone V: Echocardiographic detection of mitral valve aneurysm in patient with infective endocarditis. *Br Heart J* 1983;49:90.

75. Wilson WR, Lie JT, Houser OW, et al: The management of patients with mycotic aneurysm. *Curr Clin Top Infect Dis* 1981;2:151.

76. Stengel A, Wolferth CC: Mycotic (bacterial) aneurysms of intravascular origin. *Arch Intern Med* 1983;31:527.

77. Johansen K, Devin J: Mycotic aortic aneurysms: A reappraisal. *Arch Surg* 1983;118:583.

78. Robinson MJ, Ruedy J: Sequelae of bacterial endocarditis. *Am J Med* 1962;32:922.

79. Morgan WT, Bland EF: Bacterial endocarditis in the antibiotic era with special reference to the later complications. *Circulation* 1959;19:753.

80. Pruitt A, Rubin R, Karchmer A, et al: Neurologic complications of bacterial endocarditis. *Medicine* 1978,57:329.

81. Bohmfalk GL, Story JL, Wissinger JP, et al: Bacterial intracranial aneurysm. *J Neurol Surg* 1978;48:369.

82. Ziment I, Johnson BL Jr: Angiography in the management of intracranial mycotic aneurysms. *Arch Intern Med* 1968:122:349.

83. Gingham WF: Treatment of mycotic intracranial aneurysms. *J Neurosurg* 1977;46:428.
84. Cobbs G, Livingston E: Special problems in the management of infective endocarditis, in Bismo A (ed): *Treatment of Infective Endocarditis.* New York, Grune and Stratton, 1981, p 141.
85. Wilson WR, Giuliani ER, Danielson GK, et al: Management of complications of infective endocarditis. *Mayo Clin Proc* 1982;57:152.
86. Cantu RC, LeMay M, Wilkinson HA: The importance of repeated angiography in the treatment of mycotic-embolic intracranial aneurysms. *J Neurosurg* 1966;25:189.
87. Mundth ED, Darling RC, Alvarado RH, et al: Surgical management of mycotic aneurysms and the complications of infection in vascular reconstructive surgery. *Am J Surg* 1969;117:460.
88. Patel S, Johnston K: Classification and management of mycotic aneurysms. *Surg Gynecol Obstet* 1979;144:691.
89. Anderson BC, Butcher HR Jr, Ballinger WF: Mycotic aneurysms. *Arch Surg* 1974; 109:712.
90. Lawrence G: Surgical management of infected aneurysms. *Am J Surg* 1962;104:355.
91. Porter L, Houston M, Kadir S: Mycotic aneurysms of the hepatic artery: Treatment with arterial embolization. *Am J Med* 1979;67:697.
92. Ziment I: Nervous system complications in bacterial endocarditis. *Am J Med* 1969;47:593.
93. Magilligan D: Cardiac surgery in infective endocarditis, in Horstkotte D, Bodnar E (eds): *Infective Endocarditis.* London, ICR Publishers, 1991, p 210.
94. Watanakunakorn C: Prosthetic valve endocarditis: A review. *Prog Cardiovasc Dis* 1979; 22:181.
95. Robinson M, Greenberg J, Korn M, et al: Infective endocarditis at autopsy 1965–1969. *Am J Med* 1972;52:492.
96. Karchmer AW, Archer GL, Dismukes WE: *Staphylococcus epidermidis* causing prosthetic valve endocarditis: Microbiologic and clinical observations as guide to therapy. *Ann Intern Med* 1983;98:447.
97. Karchmer AW, Dismukes WE, Buckley MJ, et al: Late prosthetic valve endocarditis: Clinical features influencing therapy. *Am J Med* 1978;64:199.
98. Madison J, Wang K, Gobel F, et al: Prosthetic aortic valvular endocarditis. *Circulation* 1975;51:940.
99. Rossiter SJ, Stinson EB, Oyer PR, et al: Prosthetic valve endocarditis: Comparison of heterograft tissue valves and mechanical valves. *J Thorac Cardiovasc Surg* 1978;76:795.
100. Ferrans VJ, Boyce SW, Billingham ME: Infection of glutaraldehyde-preserved porcine valve heterografts. *Am J Cardiol* 1979;43:1123.
101. Calderwood S, Swinski L, Karchmer A: Prosthetic valve endocarditis: Analysis of factors affecting outcome of therapy. *J Thorac Cardiovasc Surg* 1986;92:776.
102. Slaughter L, Morris J, Starr A: Prosthetic valvular endocarditis: A 12 year review. *Circulation* 1976;417:1319.
103. Cowgill L, Addonigio L, Hopeman A, et al: Prosthetic valve endocarditis, in *Curr Probl Cardiol* 1986;11:620.
104. O'Brien MR, Stafford EG, Gardner MAH, et al: A comparison of aortic valve replacement with viable cryopreserved and fresh allograft valves, with a note on chromosomal studies. *J Thorac Cardiovasc Surg* 1987;4:812.
105. Ivert TSA, Dismukes WE, Cobbs GG, et al: Prosthetic valve endocarditis. *Circulation* 1984;69:223.
106. Thill C, Meyer O: Experience with penicillin and dicumanol in the treatment of subacute bacterial endocarditis. *Ann J Med Sci* 1947;213:500.
107. Freedman L, Valoni J: Experimental infective endocarditis. *Prog Cardiovasc Dis* 1979; 22:169.
108. Weinstein L: Infectious endocarditis, in Braunwald E (ed): *Heart Disease: Textbook of Cardiovascular Medicine,* ed 3. Philadelphia, WB Saunders, 1980, p 116.
109. Wilson W, GEraci J, Danielson G: Anticoagulant therapy and central nervous system complications in patients with prosthetic valve endocarditis. *Circulation* 1978:57:1004.

110. Carpenter J, McAllister C, U.S. Army Collaborative Group: Anticoagulation in prosthetic valve endocarditis. *South Med J* 1983;76:1372.

111. Lerner P, Weinstein L: Infective endocarditis in the antibiotic era. *N Engl J Med* 1966;274;387.

112. Buchbinder NA, Roberts WC: Left-sided valvular active infective endocarditis: A study of forty-five necropsy patients. *Am J Med* 1972;53:20.

113. Menzies C: Coronary embolism with infarction in bacterial endocarditis. *Br Heart J* 1961;23:464.

114. Jackson J, Allison F: Bacterial endocarditis. *South Med J* 1961;54;1331.

115. Kaye D: Cure rate and long term prognosis, in *Endocarditis*. Baltimore, University Park Press, 1976, p 201.

116. Richardson J, Karp R, Kirklin J, et al: Treatment of infective endocarditis: A ten year comparative analysis. *Circulation* 1978;58:589.

117. Karchmer A, Stinson E: The role of surgery in infective endocarditis, in Remington J, Swartz M (eds): *Current Clinical Topics in Infectious Disease*. New York, McGraw-Hill, 1980, p 129.

118. Croft C, Woodward W, Elliot A: Analysis of surgical vs. medical therapy in active complicated native valve infective endocarditis. *Am J Cardiol* 1983;51:1650.

119. Borst H, Hetzer R, Deyerling W: Surgery for active endocarditis. *Thorac Cardiovasc Surg* 1982;30:345.

120. Frank G, Lowes L, Burmester B: The prognostic value of intraoperative findings in infective endocarditis, in Horstkotte D, Bodner E (eds): *Infective Endocarditis*. London, ICR Publishers, p 198.

121. Nelson R, Harley D, French W, et al: Favorable ten year experience with valve procedures for active infective endocarditis. *J Thorac Cardiovasc Surg* 1989;87:493.

122. D'Agostino R, Miller C, Stinson E: Valve replacement in patients with native valve endocarditis: What really determines operative outcome? *Ann Thorac Surg* 1985;40:429.

123. Harjula A, Jarvinen A, Virtanen KS: Pacemaker infections—Treatment with total or partial pacemaker system removal. *Thorac Cardiovasc Surg* 1985;33:218.

124. Hakki AH: Permanent cardiac pacing: Complications and management, in Kakki AH (ed): *Ideal Cardiac Pacing*. Philadelphia, WB Saunders, 1984, p 160.

125. Helmberger T, Duma R: Infections of prosthetic heart valves and cardiac pacemakers, in Westenfelder G (ed): *Infections of Prosthetic Devices*. Infect Dis Clin N.A. Philadelphia, WB Saunders, 1989, p 321.

126. Arger N, Prav E, Cooperman Y: Pacemaker endocarditis: Report of 44 cases and review of the literature. *Medicine* 1994;73:299.

127. Rutter JH, Degener JE, Von Mechelen R: Late purulent pacemaker pocket infections caused by *Staphylococcus epidermidis*. *PACE* 1985;8:903.

128. Wade J, Cobbs C: Infections in cardiac pacemakers, in Remmington J, Swartz M (eds): vol 9. New York, McGraw-Hill, 1988, p 44.

15

Prophylaxis

Despite the availability of effective therapy, the incidence of infective endo-carditis has not decreased.[1,2] In fact, the number of cases has actually in-creased, due largely to changes in the profile of underlying valvular dis-eases. Rheumatic heart disease is now much less common. Calcific aortic stenosis, PVE, and the intravenous injection of drugs have replaced rheu-matic fever as major predisposing factors. In addition, there have been changes in the organisms involved in the pathogenesis of infective endocar-ditis. Enterococci, gram-negative organisms, fungi, and MRSA are now the most often isolated pathogens. These changes challenge the physician to cure the valvular infection expeditiously in order to minimize the risk of permanent cardiac damage and to avoid the necessity of performing car-diac surgery to correct the hemodynamic consequences of endocarditis (e.g., intractable congestive cardiac failure).[3]

It has been common practice for physicians to prescribe antimicrobial agents to prevent the development of endocarditis prior to initiating a procedure that might lead to a bacteremia that would seed a previously damaged valve. From 15% to 25% of cases of endocarditis are associated with these invasive procedures. Only about 50% of patients who develop endocarditis have a previously diagnosed cardiac disorder that would initi-ate the use of a preventive antibiotic.[8] Therefore, in total, about 10% of cases of endocarditis can be thwarted by the current regimens of an-timicrobial prophylaxis.[4–9]

A disproportionate effort has focused on iatrogenic disease and not on the most common sources of transient bacteremia, such as poor oral hy-geine. S. viridans is involved in 50% of patients with endocarditis. The mouth serves as the usual habitat of this organism.[8,10] About 10% of adults have significant periodontal disease, a most favorable environment for the proliferation of S. viridans and other bacteria.[11,12] About 25 years ago, Thom and Howe[13] and later Holbrook et al.,[14] documented significant dental pathology in about 50% of patients at risk of developing valvular infection. In 1962, Hook and Kaye[15] emphasized the importance of aggres-sive care of the mouth in order to prevent the transient bacteremia associated with brushing the teeth or chewing food. Since then, the American Heart Association and other organizations have emphasized the need to maintain excellent oral hygiene in patients at risk of developing infective endocarditis.[16-23] Despite this recommendation, nonpharmacological approaches to the prevention of endocardial infection have not been widely accepted. Recommendations for the prevention of bacteremia produced by the oral microflora include: (1) meticulous dental care; (2) regular brushing of the teeth; (3) flossing with waxed floss; (4) avoidance of irrigation devices (e.g., Water Pik); (5) avoidance of dental trauma; (6) rinsing of the mouth with an antiseptic; and (7) no dental work within 2 to 3 weeks after a cardiac procedure.[24] The application of chlorexidine to the gingiva 3–5 min prior to extraction of a tooth has been found to decrease the incidence of bacteremia. Povidone iodine may be equally effective.[23,24] It must be emphasized that the risk of bacteremia associated with chewing gum or food or brushing the teeth is directly related to the health of the periodontal tissues.[25]

Other nonpharmacological means of reducing transient bacteremia originating in sites other than the oral cavity are (1) avoidance of enemas; (2) no unnecessary invasive procedures; (3) avoidance of manipulation of various skin lesions; (4) investigation of any unexplained febrile illness; (5) medical evaluation prior to treatment with antibiotics; and (6) maintenance of bowel regularity.

A number of prophylactic regimens have been suggested since the initial recommendations for the prevention of rheumatic fever in 1955.[26,27] It is clear that none of these were based on statistically valid data obtained from clinical studies. Continued updates have been issued over the past 16 years.[28-32] During the same period, the Europeans developed a program for prophylaxis.[33-35] *The Medical Letter,* published in the United States, proposed still another approach to the prevention of infection.[36]

The current recommendations proposed by the American Hospital Association (AHA) constitute the most recent guidelines for prophylaxis.[23] They have been designed to be more flexible in order to improve their implementation. These guidelines published in 1990 by the AHA agree closely with those proposed by the Endocarditis Working Party of the British Society for Antibiotic Therapy and *The Medical Letter.*[35,36] The AHA guidelines are based on the results of in vivo studies of animal models and clinical experience with antibiotic prophylaxis.

The previous directives published by the AHA in 1977[30] were based, for the most part, on experimental data obtained from animal systems.[37-39] Adherence to them has been poor.[40-47] The rate of compliance had been estimated to be about 15–20%. They eventually failed for two major reasons. First, the dosage of drugs administered was too low. Dentists failed to use the recommended loading doses and very rarely administered the antibiotics parenterally. In addition, the timing of prophylaxis was often inappropriate.

These guidelines were simplified in 1984, leading to a marked increase in compliance (from 44% to 79%) by both dentists and physicians.[48-54] However, there were still defeciencies in the dose and timing of delivery of the antibiotic. Parenteral regimens were rarely used because of the difficulty of delivery in a dentist's office.

The present rate of compliance by physicians and dentists with the current AHA guidelines is not clear. This issue deserves close study.

Mechanisms of Antimicrobial Prophylaxis

Bayer[55] has identified three major steps in the development of infective endocarditis that are susceptible to the action of antibiotics: (1) killing of organisms in the bloodstream before they can adhere to a thrombus; (2) prevention of adherence to the vegetation of those pathogens that escaped destruction within the circulatory system; and (3) elimination of those organisms that have managed to attach to a thrombus before they can multiply.

The results of studies of animal models indicate that the prophylactic effect of an antibiotic depends on more than its ability to eradicate the invading organism. Even a subbactericidal level of an antibiotic may suppress the development of infective endocarditis.[56,57] Evidence derived from patients has indicated that the administration of an antibiotic eliminates the risk of bacteremia following invasive procedures.[58,59]

Successful prophylaxis involves (1) identification of patients at risk of developing endocarditis; (2) an understanding of procedures that require chemoprophylaxis; and (3) selection of an appropriate prophylactic regimen.[60]

The situations in which prophylaxis is required are listed in Table 15.1. Two factors are critical for the deposition of a thrombus on the leaflets of native or bioprosthetic valves, the struts of a mechanical valve, and the endocardium. First is the deposition of a collar of fibrin surrounding the orifice of the lower-pressure side when blood flows from an area of high pressure to one of low presure.[61] This is the Bernoulli effect. Second is the development of a fibrin thrombus on an area of abnormal endothelium due to an increase in its thrombogenicity. One or both of these complications may be present in patients with infective endocarditis.

Patients with prosthetic valves most clearly demonstrate these two major requisites for the deposition of fibrin. Antibiotic prophylaxis is critical in this situation because successful treatment of PVE often requires open heart surgery.[62] The incidence of infective endocarditis in patients with prosthetic valves is about 1 in 200 patients-years compared to 1 in 100,000 patient-years among individuals with native valves.[63] PVE usually occurs during the first year of placement of a cardiac prosthesis.[64–66]

A native valve that has been the site of a successfully treated endocardial infection is at high risk of recurrent disease.[67] Many reports of repeated episodes of the disease have been documented in patients with clear-cut, persistent risk factors such as addiction to intravenous injection of "recreational" drugs. More than 50% of individuals who suffer repeated episodes of infective endocarditis have no predisposition other than a previously

Table 15.1. Cardiac Conditions*

ENDOCARDITIS PROPHYLAXIS RECOMMENDED

Prosthetic cardiac valves, including bioprosthetic and homograft valves

Previous bacterial endocarditis, even in the absence of heart disease

Most congenital cardiac malformations

Rheumatic and other acquired valvular dysfunction, even after valvular surgery

Hypertrophic cardiomyopathy

Mitral valve prolapse with valvular regurgitiation

ENDOCARDITIS PROPHYLAXIS NOT RECOMMENDED

Isolated secundum atrial septal defect

Surgical repair without residua beyond 6 mo of secundum atrial septal defect,
   ventricular septal defect, or patent ductus arteriosus

Previous coronary artery bypass graft surgery

Mitral valve prolapse without valvular regurgitation[†]

Physiologic, functional, or innocent heart murmurs

Previous Kawasaki disease without valvular dysfunction

Previous rheumatic fever without valvular dysfunction

Cardiac pacemakers and implanted defibrillators

---

   *This table lists selected conditions but is not meant to be all-inclusive.

   [†]Individuals who have a mitral valve prolapse associated with thickening and/or redundancy of the valve leaflets may be at increased risk for bacterial endocarditis, particularly
men who are 45 years of age or older.

   Source: Ref. 22.

infected valve. Patients with congenital heart disease require antibiotic prophylaxis when they undergo invasive procedures.[68] Exceptions to this rule
are patients with isolated ostium secundum defects, or with closure of an
atrial septal defect either in the distant past or 6 weeks after ligature of a
patent ductus. Patients with a small ostium secundum defect do not require
antibiotic prophylaxis due to the absence of a pressure gradient between
the two atrial chambers. The risk of infective endocarditis involving valves
that are damaged by rheumatic fever is very similar to that of patients with
prosthetic valves.[69]

   Five percent of individuals with idiopathic hypertrophic subaortic stenosis are at risk of developing endocardial infections at some time in life.[70]

   Antibiotic prophylaxis in patients with mitral valve prolapse (MVP) is
presently controverial.[71–74] A recent study has pointed out that MVP might
be the cause of endocarditis in 29% of patients[73] At least 5% of the population have this variation of the mitral valve. When IVDA are excluded,
patients with MVP have an incidence of endocarditis five to eight times
higher than that of the general population for this type of valve. Although
this is a significant increase, it is much lower than the rate for patients with
rheumatic valvular disease.

   It is clear that not all patients with MVP are at risk of developing infective
endocarditis. The presence of a murmur is strongly associated with the
development of valvular infection.[73,74] A click on auscultation is an insig-

nificant finding in characterizing those individuals at risk of developing infection of a prolapsed valve. The incidence of endocardial infection in patients with MVP is higher in elderly men.[71] Echocardiographic studies have disclosed that thick, redundant valvular leaflets are associated with an increased incidence of infection.[74–81] About 3% of patients with these echocardiographic abnormalities will eventually develop infective endocarditis. The AHA has recommended that those patients with valvular regurgitation be given prophylaxis. The absence of a murmur does not rule out the presence of important redundancy.[81] Which patients with MVP should receive prophylaxis has not been settled.

Many elderly individuals who develop infective endocarditis have a history and physical findings inconsistent with the classical manifestations of valvular infection.[82] However, many of them describe a "murmur" present many years before the onset of endocardial infection. These murmurs are often related to the presence of calcific or degenerative disorders associated with aging of the aortic or mitral valve or both.[83] The need for chemoprophylaxis in individuals with these valvular disorders has not been addressed by the AHA except for the category "other acquired valvular dysfunction." Because endocardial infection of native valves in patients who are not IVDA has become a disease of old age, we recommend that antimicrobial prophylaxis be instituted in the elderly with degenerative changes even when these do not pose a hemodynamic threat. It must be emphasized that the fatality rate of valvular infection is higher in the aged.[84]

A very important cardiac disorder for which prophylaxis may be required is dysfunction of the papillary muscle leading to atrioventricular regurgitation. This may be due to either dilated cardiomyopathy or ischemic cardiac disease.[85,86]

Indications for Antimicrobial Prophylaxis

Transient bacteremia plays a critical role in the development of infective endocarditis. Not all invasive procedures that lead to bacteremia require antimicrobial prophylaxis in patients susceptible to endocardial infection. However, prophylaxis is indicated when there is clinical evidence that a procedure may pose a risk for the development of endocarditis. Any maneuver that poses a risk for bacteremia caused by *E. coli* in a patient with rheumatic valvular disease does not require prophylaxis because endocarditis with the organism is uncommon. An intervention that leads to the development of bacteremia with *S. viridans*, an organism that readily infects valvular endothelium, requires antimicrobial therapy in the susceptible patient. There are other variables determining the risk of infection.[87] Most of the procedures that require prophylaxis are listed in Table 15.2. Procedures that require rigid instruments, especially those used for a biopsy, are associated with a high incidence of bacteremia.[88–104] The use of a flexible instrument is associated with a decreased risk of bacteremia (Table 15.3).

Table 15.2. Surgical or Dental Procedures*

ENDOCARDITIS PROPHYLAXIS RECOMMENDED

Dental procedures known to induce gingival or mucosal bleeding, including professional cleaning

Tonsillectomy and/or adenoidectomy

Surgical operations that involve intestinal or respiratory mucosa

Bronchoscopy with a rigid bronchoscope

Sclerotherapy for esophageal varices

Esophageal dilatation

Gallbladder surgery

Cystoscopy

Urethral dilatation

Urethral catheterization if urinary tract infection is present[†]

Urinary tract surgery if urinary tract infection is present[†]

Prostatic surgery

Incision and drainage of infected tissue[†]

Vaginal hysterectomy

Vaginal delivery in the presence of infection[†]

ENDOCARDITIS PROPHYLAXIS NOT RECOMMENDED[‡]

Dental procedures not likely to induce gingival bleeding, such as simple adjustment of orthodontic appilances or fillings above the gum line

Injection of local intraoral anesthetic (except intraligamentary injections)

Shedding of primary teeth

Tympanostomy tube insertion

Endotracheal intubation

Bronchoscopy with a flexible branchoscope, with or without biopsy

Cardiac catheterization

Endoscopy with or without gastrointestinal biospsy

Cesarean section

In the absence of infection for urethral catheterization, dilatation and curettage, uncomplicated vaginal delivery, therapeutic abortion, sterilization procedures, or insertion or removal of intrauterine devices.

---

*This table lists selected procedures but is not meant to be all-inclusive.

[†] In addition to prophylactic regimen for genitourinary procedures, antibiotic therapy should be directed against the most likely bacterial pathogen.

[‡] In patients who have prosthetic heart valves, a previous history of endocarditis, or surgically constructed systemic-pulmonary shunts or conduits, physicians may choose to administer prophylactic antibiotics even for low-risk procedures that involve the lower respiratory, genitourinary, or gastrointestinal tracts.

Source: Ref. 22.

Table 15.3. Rate of Bacteremia Associated with Various Procedures

Procedure	Reference	Percent of Positive Blood Cultures	Organisms
Tonsillectomy	88	38	Streptococci
Bronchoscopy (rigid)	89	15	Streptococci or S. epidermidis
Bronchoscopy (flexible)	90	0	
Endoscopy	91	12	S. epidermidis, streptococci, and diphtheroids
Colonoscopy	92	6	E. coli and bacteroids
Barium enema	93	11.4	Enterococci; aerobic and anaerobic gram negative rods
Prostatectomy	94		
Sterile urine		13	Coliforms and
Infected urine		84	enterococci
Transurethal resection of the prostate	95	31	Coliforms and S. aureus
Cystoscopy		17	Coliforms and anaerobic, gram-negative rods
Catheterization of urethra		8.0	Enterococci and other streptococci
Childbirth	96	5	Anaerobic streptococci
Traumatic dental procedures	97, 95	60 (children) 70–80 (adults)	S. viridans
Liver biopsy	98	3–13 (in setting of cholangitis)	Coliforms and enterococci
Sclerotherapy of esophageal varices	99	5–50	S. viridans, gram-negative rods, S. aureus
Esophageal dilatation	100	45	S. aureus, S. viridans
Suction abortion	101	85	S. viridans and anaerobes
Transesophageal echocardiography	102, 103	7	Streptococci

The duration of a bacteremia plays an important role in the development of infective endocarditis. Dental procedures are the leading source of bacteremia caused by *S. viridans* and follow dental brushing or flossing of the teeth.[87] Bacteremia present for 15–30 min is required for the initiation of infection of a previously injured cardiac valve.[85] Only 15% of patients who undergo various manipulations develop a bacteremia that persists for this length of time.[105] Dental manipulations that cause bleeding (e.g., multiple extractions) and other invasive procedures that injure infected gingiva are more likely to lead to the development of bacteremia that persists for more than 30 min. Edentulous individuals may develop infective endocarditis due to *S. viridans*[106] This is usually related to the presence of poorly fitting dentures. Such patients should be advised to have periodic examinations of their gums and teeth at regular intervals. The dental problems described above may indicate the presence of an oropharyngeal lesion betrayed by the development of bacteremia. Endoscopy of the gastrointestinal tract may cause bacteremia in a small number of patients (Table 15.3). The American Society of Gastroenterology has recommended that patients with prosthetic valves or with a previous history of endocarditis receive prophylaxis.[107]

These recommendations are not inclusive. Clinical judgment is required because data supporting the use of antimicrobial prophylaxis are often not available.

AHA guidelines focus on patients with a moderate or high risk of developing endocarditis when they undergo procedures associated with a high incidence of bacteremia. Several procedures for which chemoprophylaxis was once recommended, no longer require preventive measures. Among these are fiberoptic bronchoscopy and other endoscopic studies. There has been a significant change in the AHA classification of the risk associated with prophylaxis in patients with MVP. Only patients with thick or damaged valvular leaflets associated with regurgitation, are considered to be candidates for chemoprophylaxis.

Choice of Antibiotic for Prophylaxis

Amoxicillin, administered orally, is the drug of choice for the prophylaxis of infective endocarditis in patients not sensitized to penicillin. Individuals unable to be treated orally should be given ampicillin intravenously. High-risk patients undergoing gastrointestinal or genitourinary procedures are best managed by intravenous administered ampicillin and gentamicin. This combination is followed by oral amoxicillin (Table 15.4). Patients at low risk of developing infective endocarditis are best managed by oral therapy with amoxicillin alone.

The recommendations proposed by the AHA differ from those formulated by the Endocarditis Working Party of the British Society for Antimicrobial Chemotherapy[108] and *The Medical Letter*.[109] Both of these groups have stated that a dose of amoxicillin administered 6 hr after the initial one is unnecessary. The British physicians declared that there is no role for parenterally administered antimicrobial agents in patients undergoing routine dental procedures even when prosthetic valves are present.

The targets of antimicrobial prophylaxis are *S. viridans* and enterococci. Amoxicillin has replaced Pen VK as the agent of choice because it is absorbed more efficiently by the gastrointestinal tract and has a longer half-life. It also provides highly effective protection during procedures involving the genitourinary and gastrointestinal tracts due to its activity against enterococci. How long this antibiotic will remain active against the

Table 15.4. Recommended Standard Prophylactic Regimen for Dental, Oral, or Upper Respiratory Tract Procedures in Patients Who Are at Risk*

Drug	Dosing Regiment†
	STANDARD REGIMEN
Amoxicillin	3.0 g orally 1 h before procedure; than 1.5 g 6 h after initial dose
	Amoxicillin/Penicillin-Allergic Patients
Erythromycin	Erythromycin ethylsuccinate, 800 mg, or erythromycin stearate, 1.0 g,
or	orally 2 h before procedure; then half the dose 6 h after initial dose
clindamycin	300 mg orally 1 h before procedure and 150 mg 6 h after initial dose

*Includes those with prosthetic heart valves and other high-risk patients.
†Initial pediatric doses are as follows: amoxicillin, 50 mg/km; erythromycin ethylsuccinate or erythromycin stearate, 20 mg/kg; and clindamycin, 10 mg/kg. Follow-up doses should be one-half the initial dose. Total pediatric dose should not exceed total adult dose. The following weight ranges may also be used for the initial pediatric dose of amoxicillin; <15 kg, 750 mg; 15 to 30 kg, 1500 mg; and >30 kg, 3000 mg (full adult dose).
Source: Ref. 22.

enterococci is unknown because these organisms are rapidly becoming resistant to ampicillin, amoxicillin, and gentamicin.[4]

Erythromycin and clindamycin are alternative agents for the prophylaxis in patients allergic to penicillin who require dental or respiratory procedures (Table 15.5). However, despite the better tolerance of the gastrointestinal tract to clindamycin, treatment with this antibiotic should be avoided, if possible, because it may produce pseudomembranous colitis. Clindamycin may be more acceptable to patients who require intravenous therapy because it produces significantly less phlebitis than does erythromycin. The new macrolide, clarithromycin, may be substituted for the older one because it produces fewer gastrointestinal disturbances.

There is considerable disagreement concerning the guidelines for prophylaxis in patients with prosthetic valves. We feel that, whenever possible, the antibiotics used as prophylaxis in this situation should be administered intravenously because of the dire consequences of an infective prosthetic valve. The prophylaxis of disease caused by enterococci requires the use of two antimicrobial agents in patients undergoing gastrointestinal and genitourinary procedures (Table 15.6). An aggressive approach to the prophylaxis of PVE is mandatory.

Drugs other than amoxicillin should be employed in patients receiving penicillin for the prophylaxis of rheumatic fever and in those who have been given penicillin within a few weeks of the procedure. Strains of *S. viridans* resistant to penicillin have been recovered from patients previously treated with this antibiotic.[110,111]

Streptococcal endocarditis has been caused by the penicillin-resistant organisms.[112] Patients treated with benzathine penicillin prophylactically for the prevention of rheumatic fever appear to develop fewer changes in the sensitivity of the organisms present in the oral microflora.[113] When penicillin has been administered recently, surgery should not be undertaken for

Table 15.5 Alternate Prophylactic Regimens for Dental, Oral, or Upper Respiratory Tract Procedures in Patients Who Are at Risk

Drug	Dosing Regimen*
PATIENTS UNABLE TO TAKE ORAL MEDICATIONS	
Ampicillin	Intravenous or intramuscular administration of ampicillin, 2.0 g, 30 min before procedure; then intravenous or intramuscular administration of ampicillin, 1.0 g, or oral adminstration of amoxicillin, 1.5 g, 6 h after initial dose
AMPICILLIN/AMOXICILLIN/PENICILLIN-ALLERGIC PATIENTS UNABLE TO TAKE ORAL MEDICATIONS	
Clindamycin	Intravenous administration of 300 mg 30 min before procedure and an intravenous or oral administration of 150 mg 6 h after initial dose
PATIENTS CONSIDERED HIGH RISK AND NOT CANDIDATES FOR STANDARD REGIMEN	
Ampicillin, gentamicin, and amoxicillin	Intravenous or intramuscular administration of ampicillin, 2.0 g, plus gentamicin, 1.5 mg/kg (not to exceed 80mg), 30 min before procedure; followed by amoxicillin, 1.5 g, orally 6 h after initial dose; alternatively, the parenteral regimen may be repeated 8 h after initial dose
AMPICILLIN/AMOXICILLIN/PENICILLIN-ALLERGIC PATIENTS CONSIDERED HIGH RISK	
Vancomycin	Intravenous administration of 1.0 g over 1 h, starting 1 h before procedure; no repeated dose necessary

*Initial pediatric doses are as follows: ampicillin, 50 mg/kg; clindamycin, 10 mg/kg; gentamicin, 2.0 mg/kg; and vancomycin, 20 mg/kg. Follow-up doses should be one half the initial dose. Total pediatric dose should not exceed total adult dose. No initial dose is recommended in this table for amoxicillin (25 mg/kg is the follow-up dose).
Source: Ref. 22.

2–4 weeks. If dental manipulation is required sooner, treatment with erythromycin is indicated.

A study by Clemens and Ransoho[75] estimated that some patients with MVP given penicillin intravenously for the prophylaxis of oral surgery were at risk of developing fatal anaphylactic reactions. Two to three cases of endocarditis were prevented for each fatal reaction to the drug administered. A similar study by Bor and Himmelstein[114] concluded that if prophylaxis was required, erythromycin was the drug of choice because anaphylactic reactions to penicillin were less common. Antimicrobial prophylaxis was first employed in patients undergoing cardiac surgery in the late 1960s[115] Because of the risk of MRSA, vancomycin rather than a cephalosporin became the drug of choice.[116]

Several cases of failure of antimicrobial prophylaxis have been reported.[111] Many of them occurred in the early days when few antibiotics were available.[111] Fifty-two cases of prophylaxis failure were published by

Table 15.6. Regimens for Genitourinaray/Gastrointestinal Procedures

Drug	Dosage Regimen*
	STANDARD REGIMEN
Ampicillin, gentamicin, and amoxicillin	Intravenous or intramuscular administration of ampicillin, 2.0 g, plus gentamicin, 1.5 mg/kg (not to exceed 80 mg), 30 min before procedure; followed by amoxicillin, 1.5 g, orally 6 h after initial dose; alternatively, the parenteral regimen may be repeated once 8 h after initial dose
	AMPICILLIN/AMOXICILLIN/PENICILLIN-ALLERGIC PATIENT REGIMEN
Vancomycin and gentamicin	Intravenous administration of vancomycin, 1.0 g, over 1 h plus intravenous or intramuscular administration of gentamicin, 1.5 mg/kg (not to exceed 80 mg), 1 h before procedure; may be repeated once 8 h after initial dose
	ALTERNATE LOW-RISK PATIENT REGIMEN
Amoxicillin	3.0 orally 1 h before procedure; then 1.5 g 6 h after initial dose

*Initial pediatric doses are as follows: ampicillin, 50 mg/kg; amoxicillin, 50 mg/kg; gentamicin, 2.0 mg/kg; and vancomycin, 20 mg/kg. Follow-up doses should be half the initial dose. Total pediatric dose should not exceed total adult dose.
Source: Ref. 22.

the AHA in 1983.[74] The results of this study indicated that most failures occurred in the course of various dental manipulations. O the resultant valvular infections that occurred, 75% were caused by *S. viridans*. Only 12% of the patients who developed endocarditis received state of the art prophylaxis. All strains of *S. viridans* recovered were sensitive to the antibiotic used; three patients were treated with penicillin and two received erythromycin. Although erythromycin was administered in only 15% of cases, two failures occurred. These may have been related to poor absorption of the antibiotic.[117] In addition, poor compliance may be related to the gastrointestinal intolerance of erythromycin. MVP was the most common underlying cardiac pathology in these patients.[117,118]

Failure of prophylaxis is probably related to an incomplete understanding of the risk posed by various procedures. Inadequate knowledge of the prevention of endocarditis by both children and parents has been well documented in the pediatric age group.[119–121] A report on one clinical series noted that 78% of patients recalled having received instructions about prophylaxis but only 20% of these individuals retained any specific knowledge concerning the prevention and recognition of infective endocarditis.[122]

For ethical and legal reasons, controlled studies in humans cannot be carried out. However, two controlled studies in animals have demonstrated that prophylaxis is effective in preventing infective endocarditis.[123,124]

In our opinion, there has been a large improvement in the recently published AHA guidelines on antibiotic prophylaxis. However, recommendations for the prophylaxis of patients with MVP are uncertain. It is very important to appreciate the role of calcified valves in the pathogenesis of infective endocarditis among the elderly. Lastly, we believe that prophlyaxis in patients with prosthetic valves should be given parenterally.

References

1. Danchim N, Voiriot P, Briancon S: Mitral valve prolapse as a risk factor for infective endocarditis. *Lancet* 1989;1:743.
2. Skehan JD, Murray M, Mills PG: Infective endocarditis: Incidence and mortality in the North East Thames Region. *Br Heart J* 1988;59:62.
3. Gray IR: Infective endocarditis. Editorial. *Br Heart J* 1987;57:211.
4. Geva E, Frank M: Infective endocarditis in children with congenital heart disease: The changing spectrum, 1965–86. *Eur Heart J* 1988;9:1244.
5. Shulman ST: Prevention of infective endocarditis: The view from the United States. *J Antimicrob Chemother* 1987;20(Suppl A):111.
6. Kaye D, Abrutyn E: Prevention of bacterial endocarditis. Editorial. *Ann Intern Med* 1991;114:803.
7. Guntheroth W: How important are dental procedures as a cause of infective endocarditis? *Am J Cardiol* 1989;54:797.
8. Weinstein L, Rubin R: Infective endocarditis—1973. *Prog Cardiovasc Dis* 1973;16:239.
9. Daracks V: Prevention of infective endocarditis. *N Engl J Med* 1995;332:38.
10. Bayliss R, Clarke C, Oakley C, et al: The teeth and infective endocarditis. *Br Heart J* 1983;50:506.
11. Morris KG: Infective endocarditis: A preventable disease? *Br Med J* 1985;290:1532.
12. Shanson DC: Antibiotic prophylaxis of infective endocarditis in the United Kingdom and Europe. *J Antimicrob Chemother* 1987;20(Suppl A):119.
13. Thom AR, Howe GL: The dental status of cardiac patients. *Br Heart J* 1972;34:1302.
14. Holbrook WP, Willey RF, Shaw TRD: Dental health in patients susceptible to infective endocarditis. *Br Med J* 1981;283:371.
15. Hook EW, Kaye D: Prophylaxis of bacterial endocarditis. *J Chronic Dis* 1962;15:635.
16. American Heart Association: Committee report on prevention of bacterial endocarditis. *Circulation* 1965;46:3.
17. American Heart Association: Committee report on prevention of bacterial endocarditis. *Circulation* 1972;46:3.
18. American Heart Association: Committee report on prevention of bacterial endocarditis. *Circulation* 1977;56:139A.
19. American Heart Association: Committee report on prevention of bacterial endocarditis. *Circulation* 1984;70:1123A.
20. Working party of the British Society for Antimicrobial Chemotherapy: Report on the antibiotic prophylaxis of infective endocarditis. *Lancet* 1982;2:1323.
21. Schweizerische Arbeitsgruppe fur Endokarditis-prophylaxe: Prophylaxe der bakteriellen Endokarditis. *Schweiz Med Wochenschr* 1984;114:1246.
22. Working Party of the European Society of Cardiology: Report on prophylaxis of infective endocarditis for dental procedures. *Eur Heart J* 1985;6:826.
23. Dajani AS, Bisno AL, Chung KJ: Prevention of bacterial endocarditis. Recommendations by the American Heart Association. *JAMA* 1990;264:2919.
24. Tzukert AA, Leviner E, Sela M: Prevention of infective endocarditis: Not by antibiotics alone. *Oral Surg Oral Med Oral Pathol* 1986;62:385.
25. Everett E, Hirschmann J: Transient bacteremia and endocarditis prophylaxis: A review. *Medicine* 1977;56:61.

26. Jones TD, Baumgartner L, Bellows MT: Prevention of rheumatic fever and bacterial endocarditis through control of streptococcal infections. *Circulation* 1955;11:317.

27. Oakley CM: Controversies in the prophylaxis of infective endocarditis: A cardiological view. *J. Antimicrob Chemother* 1987;20(Suppl A):105.

28. Wannamaker LW, Denny FW, Diehl A: Prevention of bacterial endocarditis. *Circulation* 1965;31:953.

29. Taranta A, Ayoub EM, Gordis L: Prevention of bacterial endocarditis. *Circulation* 1972;46:S3.

30. Kaplan EL, Anthony BR, Bisno AL: Prevention of bacterial endocarditis. *Circulation* 1977;56:139A.

31. Shulman ST, Amren DP, Bisno AL: Prevention of bacterial endocarditis. A statement for health professionals by the committee on rheumatic fever and infective endocarditis of the Council on Cardiovascular Disease in the Young. *Circulation* 1984;70:1118.

32. Chadwick EG, Shulman ST: Prevention of infective endocarditis. *Concepts Cardiovasc Dis* 1986;55:1.

33. Simmons NA, Cawson RA, Clarke C: Antibiotic prophylaxis of infective endocarditis. Recommendations from the Working Party of the British Society for Antimicrobial Chemotherapy. *Lancet* 1982;2:1323.

34. Delaye J, Etienne J, Delahaye F: Prophylaxis of bacterial endocarditis in 1987: From theory to practice. *Presse Med* 1988;17:185.

35. Endocarditis Working Party of the British Society for Antimicrobial Chemotherapy: Antibiotic prophylaxis of infective endocarditis. *Lancet* 1990;335:88.

36. Prevention of bacterial endocarditis. *Med Lett* 1986;28(issue 707):22.

37. Durack DT, Petersdorf RG: Chemotherapy of experimental streptococcal endocarditis. Comparison of commonly recommended prophylactic regimens. *J Clin Invest* 1973;52:592.

38. Pelletier LL Jr, Durack DT, Petersdorf RG: Chemotherapy of experimental streptococcal endocarditis. Further observations on prophylaxis. *J. Clin Invest* 1975;56:319.

39. Durack DT, Starkebaum MS, Petersdorf RG: Chemotherapy of experimental streptococcal endocarditis. VI. Prevention of enterococcal endocarditis. *J Lab Clin Med* 1977;90:171.

40. Durack DT: Current practice in prevention of bacterial endocarditis. *Br Heart J* 1975;37:478.

41. Brooks S: Survey of compliance with American Heart Association Guidelines for prevention of bacterial endocarditis. *J Am Dent Assoc* 1980;101:41.

42. Hashway T, Stone LJ: Antibiotic prophylaxis of subacute bacterial endocarditis for adult patients by dentists in Dade County, Florida. *Circulation* 1982;66:1110.

43. Holbrook WP, Willey RF, Shaw TRD: Prophylaxis of infective endocarditis. Problems in practice. *Br Dent J* 1983;154:36.

44. Sadowsky D, Kumzel D: Clinical compliance and the prevention of bacterial endocarditis. *J Am Dent Assoc* 1984;109:425.

45. Gould IM: Chemoprophylaxis for bacterial endocarditis—a survey of current practice in London. *J Antimicrob Chemother* 1984;14:379.

46. Gaidry D, Kudlick EM, Hutton JG, et al: A survey to evaluate the management of orthodontic patients with a history of rheumatic fever or congenital heart disease. *Am J Orthod* 1985;87:338.

47. Brooks RG, Notario G, McCabe RE: Hospital survey of antimicrobial prophylaxis to prevent endocarditis in patients with prosthetic heart valves. *Am J Med* 1988;84:817.

48. Woodman AJ: Prescribing for the prevention of infective endocarditis: A study into the use of prophylactic antibiotics in the Armed Forces Dental Services. *J R Nav Med Serv* 1984;70:149.

49. Scully CM, Levers BGH, Griffiths MJ, et al: Antimicrobial prophylaxis of infective endocarditis: Effect of BSAC recommendations on compliance in general practice. *J Antimicrob Chemother* 1987;19:521.

50. Levers BGH, Scully C: Antimicrobial prophylaxis of endocarditis: Compliance of dental practitioners with British recommendations. *J Dent Res* 1986;(special issue)65:789.

51. Holbrook WP, Higgins B, Shak TRD: Recent changes in antibiotic prophylactic measures taken by dentists against infective endocarditis. *J Antimicrob Chemother* 1987;20:439.

52. Jaspers MT, Little JW, Hartwick WL: Effectiveness of a dental school program in the prevention of infective endocarditis and other related infections. *J Dent Educ* 1984; 48:159.

53. Karpf A, Bertel O, Braun H: Luckenhafte Endokarditisprophylaxe trotz intensiver Patienteninformation bei valvularer Herzkrankheit. *Schweiz Med Wockenschr* 1988(Suppl 23):10.

54. Sadowsky D, Kunzel C: Recommendations for prevention of bacterial endocarditis: Compliance by dental general practitioners. *Circulation* 1988;77:1316.

55. Bayer AS: New concepts in the pathogenesis and modalities of the chemoprophylaxis of native valve endocarditis. *Chest* 1989;96:893.

56. Malinverni R, Overholser CD, Bille J, et al: Antibiotic prophylaxis of experimental endocarditis after dental extractions. *Circulation* 1988;77:182.

57. Glauser MP, Bernard JP, Moreillon P: Successful single-dose amoxicillin prophylaxis against experimental streptococcal endocarditis: Evidence for two mechanisms of protection. *J Infect Dis* 1983;147:568.

58. Francioli P, Glauser MP: Successful prophylaxis of experimental streptococcal endocarditis with single doses of sublethal concentrations of penicillin. *J Antimicrob Chemother* 1985;15:297.

59. Baltch AL, Pressman HL, Schaffer C: Bacteremia in patients undergoing oral procedures. Study following parenteral antimicrobial prophylaxis as recommended by the American Heart Association. *Arch Intern Med* 1988;148:1084.

60. Weinstein L: Infective endocarditis, in Braunwald E (ed): *Heart Disease: A Textbook of Cardiovascular Medicine*, ed 3. Philadelphia, WB Saunders, 1988, p 1127.

61. Rodbard S: Blood velocity and endocarditis. *Circulation* 1963;27:18.

62. Arnett E, Roberts W: Valve ring abscesses in active infective endocarditis: Frequency, location and clues to clinical diagnosis from the study of 95 autopsy patients. *Circulation* 1976;54:140.

63. Horstkotte D, Friedriche W, Pippert H, et al: Benefit of prophylaxis for infectious endocarditis in patients with prosthetic heart valves [in German with an English abstract]. *Z Kardiol* 1986;75:8.

64. Colanglu A, Brockman S: Selection of prosthetic heart valves, in Frankl W, Brest A (eds): *Valvular Heart Disease. Comprehensive Evaluation and Management*. Philadelphia, FA Davis, 1989, p 399.

65. Rossiter SJ, Stinson EB, Oyer PE: Prosthetic valve endocarditis. Comparison of heterograft tissue valves and mechanical valves. *J Thorac Cardiovasc Surg* 1978;76:795.

66. Calderwood SB, Swinski LA, Karchmer AW: Prosthetic valve endocarditis: Analysis of factors affecting outcome of therapy. *J Thorac Cardiovasc Surg* 1986;92:776.

67. Baddour LM: Twelve year review of recurrent native-valve infective endocarditis: A disease of the mordern antibiotic era. *Rev Infect Dis* 1988;10:1163.

68. Durack DT: Prophylaxis for infective endocarditis, in Mandel GL, Douglas RG Jr, Bennett JE (eds): *Principles and Practice of Infectious Diseases*, ed 3. New York, Churchill Livingstone, 1990, p 716.

69. Doyle EF, Spagnuolo M, Taranta A: The risk of bacterial endocarditis during rheumatic prophylaxis *JAMA* 1967;201:807.

70. Chagnac A, Rudnike C, Loebel H: Infectious endocarditis in idiopathic hypertrophic subaortic stenosis: Report of three cases and review of the literature. *Chest* 1982;81:346.

71. McKinsey DS, Ratts TE, Bisno AL: Underlying cardiac lesions in adults with infective endocarditis: The changing spectrum. *Am J Med* 1987;82:681.

72. Nolan C, Kane J, Grunow W: Infective endocarditis and mitral valve prolapse: A comparison with other types of endocarditis. *Arch Intern Med* 1981;131:477.

73. MacMahon S, Hickey A, Wilcken D: Risk of infective endocarditis in mitral valve prolapse with and without precordial systolic murmurs. *Am J Cardiol* 1989;58:105.

74. Durack D, Bisno A, Kaplan A: Apparent failure of endocarditis prophylaxis: Analysis of 52 cases submitted to a national registry. *JAMA* 1983;250:2318.

75. Clemens JD, Ransohoff DR: A quantitative assessment of pre-dental antibiotic prophylaxis for patients with mitral valve prolapse. *J Chronic Dis* 1984;37:531.

76. Clemens JD, Horwitz RI, Jaffe CC: A controlled evaluation of the risk of bacterial endocarditis in persons with mitral valve prolapse. *N Engl J Med* 1982;307:776.

77. Hickey AJ, MacMahon SW, Wilcken DE: Mitral valve prolapse and bacterial endocarditis: When is antibiotic prophylaxis necessary? *Am Heart J* 1985;109:431.

78. MacMahon SW, Roberts JK, Kramer-Fox R: Mitral valve prolapse and infective endocarditis. *Am Heart J* 1987;113:1291.

79. Baddour LM, Bisno AL: Mitral valve prolapse: Multifactorial etiologies and variable prognoses. *Am Heart J* 1986;112:1359.

80. Nishimura RA, McGoon MD, Shub C: Echocardiographically-documented mitral valve prolapse: Long-term follow-up of 237 patients. *N Engl J Med* 1985;313:1305.

81. Marks AR, Choong CY, Chir MBB: Idenification of high-risk and low-risk subgroups of patients with mitral valve prolapse. *N Engl J Med* 1989;320:1031.

82. Garvey GJ, Nru NC: Infective endocarditis: An evolving disease. *Medicine* 1978;57:105.

83. Sipes JN, Thompson RL, Hook EW: Prophylaxis of infective endocarditis: A re-evaluation. *Annu Rev Med* 1977;28:371.

84. Terpenning MS, Buggy BP, Kauffman CA: Infective endocarditis: Clinical features in young and elderly patients. *Am J Med* 1987;83:626.

85. Dickerman SA, Rufler S: Mitral and tricuspid valve regurgitation in dilated cardiomyopathy. *Am J Cardiol* 1989;63:629.

86. Bayer R: Antibiotic prophylaxis and regurgitant murmurs. Letter. *Ann Intern Med* 1990;112:148.

87. Okell C, Eliot S: Bacteremia and oral sepsis with special references to the etiology of subacute endocarditis. *Lancet* 1935;2:869.

88. Elliott SE: Bacteremia following tonsillectomy. *Lancet* 1939;2:589.

89. Burman SO: Bronchoscopy and bacteremia. *J Thorac Cardiovasc Surg* 1960;40:635.

90. Pereira W, Kovnat DM, Kahn MA, et al: Fever and pneumonia after flexible fiberoptic bronchoscopy. *Am Rev Respir Dis* 1975;112:59.

91. Baltch AL, Buhac I, Agrawal A, et al: Bacteremia following endoscopy (Abstr). Presented at the 15th Interscience Conference on Antimicrobial Agents and Chemotherapy, September 1975, Washington, DC.

92. Dickman MD, Farrell R, Higgs, et al: Colonoscopy associated bacteremia. *Surg Gynecol Obstet* 1976;142:173.

93. LeFrock J, Ellis CA, Klainer AS, et al: Transient bacteremia associated with barium enema. *Arch Intern Med* 1975;135:835.

94. Marshall A: Bacteremia following retropubic prostatectomy. *Br J Urol* 1961;33:25.

95. Sullivan NM, Sutter VL, Mims MM, et al: Clinical aspects of bacteremia after manipulation of the genitourinary tract. *J Infect Dis* 1973;127:49.

96. McCormack WM, Rosner B, Lee YH, et al: Isolation of genital mycoplasmas from blood obtained shortly after vaginal delivery. *Lancet* 1975;1:596.

97. Peterson L, Peacock R: The incidence of bacteremia in pediatric patients following tooth extraction. *Circulation* 1976;53:676.

98. LeFroch J, Ellis C, Turchik J, et al: Transient bacteremia associated with percutaneous liver biopsy. *J Infect Dis* 1975;131(Suppl):104.

99. Sauerbruch T, Holl J, Ruckdeschel G: Bacteremia associated with endoscopic sclerotherapy of oesophageal varices. *Endoscopy* 1985;17:170.

100. Welsh JD, Griffiths WJ, McKee J: Bacteremia associated with esophageal dilatation. *J Clin Gastroenterol* 1983;5:109.

101. Ritvo R, Monroe P, Andriole VT: Transient bacteremia due to suction abortion: Implications for SBE prophylaxis. *Yale J Biol Med* 1977;50:471.

102. Denning K, Sedlmayr V, Seling B: Bacteremia with transesophageal echocardiography. Abstract 1882. *Circulation* 1989;80:473.

103. Karchmer A, Moellering R, Maki D, et al: Single antibiotic therapy for streptococcal endocarditis. *JAMA* 1978;241:1801.

104. Thompson R: Staphylococcal endocarditis. *Mayo Clin Proc* 1982;57:106.

105. Baltch A, Schaffer C, Hammer M: Bacteremia following dental cleaning in patients with and without penicillin prophylaxis. *Am Heart J* 1982;104:1135.
106. Goodman J, Kolhouse J, Koenig M: Recurrent endocarditis in an edentulous man. *South Med J* 1973;66:352.
107. American Society for Gastrointestinal Endoscopy: Infection control during gastrotinestinal endoscopy: Guidelines for clinical application. *Gastrointest Endosc* 1988;34:37S.
108. Endocarditis Working Party of the British Society for Antimicrobial Chemotherapy: Antibiotic prophylaxis of infective endocarditis. *Lancet* 1990;1:88.
109. Prevention of bacterial endocarditis. *Med Lett Drug Ther* 1989;31:112.
110. Garrod LP, Waterworth PM: The risks of dental extraction during penicillin treatment. *Br Heart J* 1962;24:39.
111. Geraci Je, Hermans PE, Washington JA II: *Eikenella corrodens* endocarditis: Report of a cure in two cases. *Mayo Clin Proc* 1974;49:950.
112. Parillo J, Borst G, Mazur M: Endocarditis due to resistant viridans streptococci during oral penicillin chemoprophylaxis. *N. Engl J Med* 1979;300:294.
113. Sprunt K: Role of antibiotic resistance in bacterial endocarditis, in Kaplan EL, Taranta AV (eds): *Infective Endocarditis.* AHA Monograph No. 52. Dallas, American Heart Association, 1977, p 17.
114. Bor DH, Himmelstein DU: Endocarditis prophylaxis for patients with mitral valve prolapse: A quantitative analysis. *Am J Med* 1984:76:711.
115. Goodman JS, Schaffner W, Collins HA: Infection after cardiovascular surgery: Clinical study including examination of antimicrobial prophylaxis. *N Engl J Med* 1968; 278:117.
116. Antunes M, Sanches M, Fernandes L: Antibiotic prophylaxis and prosthetic valve endocarditis. *J Heart Valve Dis* 1992;1:102.
117. Meier B, Luthy R, Siegenthaler W: Endokarditis-Prophylaxe mit Amoxycillin, Clindamycin oder Erythromucin. *Schweiz Med Wochenschr* 1984;114:1252.
118. Malinverni R, Overholser CD, Bille J, et al: Antibiotic prophylaxis of experimental endocarditis after dental extractions. *Circulation* 1988;182:7.
119. Caldwell RI, Hurwitz CA, Girod DA: Subacute bacterial endocarditis in children. *Am J Dis Child* 1971;122:312.
120. Kramer HH, Liersch R, Sievers G, et al: Pravention der bakteriellen Endokarditis in der Praxis. Ergebnisse einer Elternbefragung. *Monatsschr Kinderheilkd* 1982;13:504.
121. Sholler GF, Celermajer JM: Prophylaxis of bacterial endocarditis. *Med J Aust* 1984; 140:650.
122. Pitcher DW, Papouchado M, Channer KS, et al: Endocarditis prophylaxis: Do patients remember advice and know what to do? *Br Med J* 1986;293:1539.
123. Malinverni R, Bille J, Glauser MP: Single-dose rifampin prophylaxis for experimental endocaritis induced by high bacterial inocula of viridans streptococci. *J Infect Dis* 1987;156;151.
124. Malverni R, Francoli PB, Glauser MP: Comparison of single and multiple doses of prophylactic antibiotics in experimental streptococcal endocarditis. *Circulation* 1987;76(2): 376.

16

Experimental Models

Except for pigs and opposums, most animals do not develop infective endocarditis spontaneously.[1] Beginning in the 1880s various in vivo models of endocardial disease were developed. In one of these, the cardiac valves of dogs were traumatized surgically.[2–8] The need to understand the in vivo activity of antimicrobial agents within infected valves led to a search for an animal that was relatively cheap, readily available and easy to manipulate surgically. In 1970, Garrison and Freedman[9] developed a model of endocardial infection in rabbits in which the right side of the heart was traumatized by the insertion of a sterile catheter that was threaded through the femoral vein. A solution of *S. aureus* was then flushed over the damaged endothelium. This approach was modified to produce lesions in the left side of the heart by inserting a catheter into the right carotid artery[10] In an attempt to mimic the clinical situation in humans, Durack and Beeson[11] inserted the catheter through the right external jugular vein. A bolus of organisms was then injected into a vein in the ear. This procedure was thought to resemble closely the transient bacteremia of infective endocarditis.[12] Heralef et al:[13] and Santoro and Levison[13] adopted this approach to studies of rats. Overholser et al.[14] investigated the spontaneous bacteremia associated with poor dental hygiene by producing periodontal disease in rats. The first two molars were ligated with a silk string; then the animals were fed a diet containing a large quantity of sucrose. When a catheter was inserted into the carotid artery, 40% of the animals with periodontal disease developed infective endocarditis; only 7% of those that were not fed sucrose had valvular infection.

It is interesting to note that the valvular lesions described above closely resembled the early manifestations of infective endocarditis in humans.[15,16] Bacteria adhered to the fibrin-platelet thrombus covering the area of valvular trauma. As the infection progressed, the organisms were gradually covered by a layer of fibrin. The bacteria located superficially exhibited the highest level of metabolic activity; those that lay deeper in a vegetation were indolent.[17] As is the case in humans, persistent bacteremia developed as the valvular infection progressed.

Pathophysiology

Studies in rabbits have indicated that there are striking differences in the clinical course of infective endocarditis involving the right or left side of the heart. It has been noted that lesions in the right side heal spontaneously. This occurs more often when the intracardiac catheters are removed and the infection is caused by *S. aureus, Ps. aeruginosa,* or *S. viridans.*[18–20] Bayer and his colleagues[20] attributed this phenomenon to the high level of oxygen present in the left side of the heart which promoted the growth of the infecting bacteria within the vegetations. This difference in outcome appears to be especially marked in infections caused by *Ps. aeruginosa.* IVDA with infective endocarditis caused by this organism involving the right side of the heart are more responsive to treatment than are those with disease of the left side.[21]

The concentration of an antibiotic that is effective prophylactically in rabbits is usually too low to eliminate invading bacteria already established on the surface of a valve. This suggests that there are specific mechanisms preventing the development of infective endocarditis. Antibiotics administered prophylactically were found to prevent the attachment of an organism to a sterile vegetation. Probably more important is the ability of subbactericidal levels of an antibiotic to inhibit microbial growth and permit the defenses of the host to clear organisms that adhere to a fibrin thrombus.[22]

An understanding of the clinical importance of the factors involved in the adhesion of organisms has been derived from studies in animals (Table 16.1) Dextran has been noted to be effective.[23] Other bacteria utilize a number of substances that facilitate their attachment to valvular endothelium.[24,25]

Studies have been carried out to determine whether or not vaccines may be effective in preventing the development of infective endocarditis. The results of these studies in rabbits immunized with various organisms have been inconsistent[26–30] Type-specific immunization did not prevent the development of endocarditis caused by *Ps. aeruginosa* in rabbits. Van den Rijn[30] studied the protective activity of a whole-cell vaccine active against nutritionally variant streptococci. Although the results were positive, they did not appear to be related to the antibody but rather to other components of the immune system, most likely the complement cascade. It has been suggested that type-specific antibodies may interfere with the adhesion of organisms to a fibrin-platelet thrombus. This has been observed in animals vaccinated with *E. coli, S. epidermidis,* and *S. aureus.*[31–35]

The role of normal host defenses in protecting against infective endocarditis has been studied in animals treated with dexamethasone or nitrogen mustard.[34,35] These agents respectively, minimized the normal inflammatory response and led to the development of granulocytopenia. This interfered with spontaneous clearing of the infection of the right side of the heart even after the vascular catheter was removed.

In general, anticoagulation inhibits the development of a fibrin-platelet thrombus. Warfarin has been noted to interfere with the growth of vegeta-

Table 16.1. Microbial Adherence Factors Considered Important in the Pathogenesis of Experimental Endocarditis

Adherence Factor (references)	Infecting Organism	Evidence of Importance in Pathogenesis
Dextran (23)	Viridans streptococci	1. Dextran-positive strains were more virulent. 2. Dextran-positive strains were less virulent when grown without sucrose. 3. Dextranase pretreatment diminished virulence.
Slime (24)	S. epidermidis	The 50% infective dose was three times greater for the slime-negative variant strain (RP62A-NA) than for the slime-producing parent strain (RP62A).
Fibronectin (25)	S. aureus	The low-fibronectin-binding mutant strain was significantly less adherent to damaged heart valves than the parent strain, which bound fibronectin.

Source: Adapted from Baddour L, Christensen G, Lawrence J, et al: Pathogenesis of experimental endocarditis. *Rev Infect Dis* 1989;11:452.

tions.[36–38] Although this drug appears to improve the activity of antibiotics, the overall rate of survival was lower in animals treated with warfarin. This appears to be related to an increase in the incidence of embolization from the valvular vegetation. The behavior of streptokinase is similar to that of warfarin in rabbits.[39] Aspirin has no effect on the development of nonbacterial thrombotic endocarditis (NBTE).[40]

The importance of the integrity of the endothelium in the pathogenesis of endocarditis has been emphasized by Durack et al.[19] They noted that pressure produced by a vascular catheter on a valve leaflet for only 5 min set the stage for the development of infective endocarditis. Post-mortem study disclosed no evidence of NBTE. Ferguson et al.[41] confirmed these findings in the aorta of animals infected by staphylococci. Studies of valvular pathology after bacterial invasion of the bloodstream revealed small colonies of bacteria on the surface of the aorta. Although an inflammatory response was present, there was no deposition of platelets or fibrin. The results of these studies indicated that NBTE is the underlying factor in most patients with infective endocarditis. However, under certain conditions (e.g., insertion of a Swan-Ganz catheter), bacteria may directly infect an area of damaged endothelium.

Studies in rabbits have revealed that the negative relation between the susceptiblity of NBTE and the length of time a thrombus has been attached to a valve is significant.[42] The older the lesion, the less vulnerable it is to invasion by bacteria. Other studies[43] have indicated that the risk of infection decreases as endothelialization of the thrombus progresses. This begins as soon as the intravascular catheter is removed.

Therapy

Probably the most valuable data derived from studies in animals concern synergism in vivo, a concept presently poorly understood. Fantin and Carbon[8] defined synergism as "a bactericidal effect of the drug combination significantly more pronounced than the sum of the bactericidal effect of each agent alone in comparison with the effect in untreated animals." A classic example of this is the combination of a cell wall–active antibiotic (penicillin) and an aminoglycoside aimed at the enterococcus. The specific dose of each drug required to achieve this synergy in vivo is not clear. The level of penicillin in serum must be higher than the MIC of the antibiotic.[44] In vitro synergy has been demonstrated at both low or high doses of gentamicin.[45–47] A possible explanation for this discrepancy is the fact that the close-effect relationship of an aminoglycoside in vivo follows a sigmoidal curve. The same in vivo effect might be expressed by either the lowest or highest plateau of the sigmord-shaped dose response curve.[48] An increased interval between doses is associated with decreased activity of the antibiotic.[49] Penicillin facilitates the entry of an aminoglycoside into cells and leads to the death of enterococci. The interval between doses of this agent is not critical for the development of synergy for organisms killed by penicillin, such as *S. viridans* or *S. aureus*.[50]

Fantin and Carbon[8] have reported three methods for the production of synergy in animals: (1) the prevention of the development of bacterial resistance by treatment with a combination of antibiotics—for example, adding another antimicrobial agent to a quinolone[51]; (2) the use of two drugs to treat polymicrobial infections; and (c) pharmacokinetic synergism in vivo, which increases the killing of organisms by improving tissue penetration of one or more of the antibiotics administered.

Prophylaxis

Many antibiotics prevent the development of infective endocarditis caused by *S. viridans*, enterococci, and a number of other organisms in rabbits and rats.[52] A favorable outcome in animals does not predict success in humans. The in vivo models used to study synergism have been described in Chapter 5.

The following procedure has been carried out in animals to define the factors required to lessen or eliminate the risk of infection: A catheter is inserted into a peripheral vein and left in place for 1 day. Organisms are then injected 30 min after an antibiotic has been administered. The animal is then sacrificed. The level of protection is determined by histological study of the infected valve.[53] Early protocols suggested that 10^8 colony-forming units (cfu) should be administered intravenously. This concentration is 100 times larger than the minimal number of bacteria required to produce infection in 90% of rabbits (ID_{90}).[54,55] It was employed to ensure the development of infection in 100% of animals. Only cell wall-active antibiotics, such as penicillin and vancomycin, were noted to prevent the growth of *S. viridans*. Bacteriostatic agents did not inhibit the development of infective endocarditis.[56] A cell wall–active antibiotic plus an aminoglycoside was required for the successful prophylaxis of enterococcal endocarditis. This combination of drugs has been superior to penicillin or vancomycin in preventing valvular infection caused by nonenterococcal streptococci.[57] A single dose of a bactericidal agent failed to protect animals unless the drug had a prolonged half-life in serum. It appears that a high concentration of a drug for more than 12 hr is required to prevent infection of a cardiac valve by 10^8 cfu. This experience has led to the conclusion that effective prophylaxis rests on the complete elimination of organisms. The results of these studies were the basis for the recommendations for prophylaxis proposed by the AHA in 1977.[58]

When cfu are used, similar to human disease, 10^1 to 10^2, a single dose of a bacteriostatic or bactericidal drug prevents the development of infective endocarditis.[59–61] It is unlikely that interference with adherence of circulating organisms to a vegetation is the major target of antimicrobial prophylaxis.[62,63] The suppression of bacterial growth probably permits normal host defenses to remove the bacteria already attached to the vegetations.[64–67]

Certain features of animal models must be kept in mind when evaluating the data derived from such studies. Most important is information concerning the time when therapy is initiated in relation to the beginning of infection. The earlier this occurs, the more rapidly the valve is sterilized. The presence of a catheter decreases the possibilty of cure.[68] When it is in place for a prolonged period of time, a syndrome resembling infection of a prosthetic valve develops.[69–71]

There is considerable variation in the size and weight of vegetations. These features determine the ability of an antibiotic to prevent or eliminate endocardial infections.[72,73] The insertion of a catheter may perforate a valvular leaflet, alter the valvular hemodynamics, and increase the risk of the development of infective endocarditis.[74]

Concurrent infection of the endothelium of the carotid artery and cardiac valves has been documented.[75,76] The presence of a second valvular infection may decrease the effectiveness of treatment. It is not always clear whether or not the initial site of infection is a cardiac valve or the wall of an artery.

References

1. Sherwood B, Rowlands D, Vakilzadeh J: Experimental bacterial endocarditis in the opossum (*Didelphis virgnianna*). *Am J Pathol* 1971;69:513.
2. Murray B: The life and times of the enterococcus. *Clin Microb Rev* 1990;3:46.
3. Moellering R Jr, Wennersten C, Weinberg A: Studies on antibiotic synergism against enterococci. I. Bacteriologic studies. *J Lab Clin Med* 1971;77:821.
4. Moellering R Jr, Weinberg A: Studies on antibiotic synergism against enterococci. II.

Effect of various antibiotics on the uptake of ^{14}C-labelled streptomycin enterocci. *J Clin Invest* 1971;105:873.

5. Wynnokowitsch W: Beitrage zur Lehre von der Endokarditis. *Virchows Arch (Pathol Anat Physiol)* 1896;11:717.

6. Ribbert MWH: Beitrage zar Localization der infections krankheiten. *Dis Med Wochenschr* 1885;11:717.

7. Kinsella RA, Muether RO: Experimental streptococcal endocarditis. *Arch Intern Med* 1938;62:247

8. Fantin B, Carbon C: In-vivo antibiotic synergism: Contributions of animal models. *Antimicrob Agents Chemother* 1992;36:907.

9. Garrison PK, Freedman LR: Experimental endocarditis. I. Staphylococcal endocarditis in rabbits resulting from placement of a polyethylene catheter in the right side of the heart. *Yale J Biol Med* 1970;42:394.

10. Perlman BB, Freedman LR: Experimental endocarditis. II. Staphylococcal infection of the aortic valve following placement of a polyethylene catheter in the left side of the heart. *Yale J Biol Med* 1971;44:206.

11. Durack DT, Beeson PB: Experimental bacterial endocarditis. I. Colonization of a sterile vegetation. *Br J Exp Pathol* 1972;53:44.

12. Glauser MP, Franciolo P: Relevance of animal models to the prophylaxis of infective endocarditis. *J Antimicrob Chemother* 1987;20(Suppl A):87.

13. Haraief E, Glauser MP, Freedman LR: Vancomycin prophylaxis of streptococcal endocarditis in rats, in *Current Chemotherapy and Infectious Disease. Proceeding of the 11th ICC and the 19th Interscience Conference on Antimicrobial Agents and Chemotherapy.* Washington, DC, American Society of Microbiology, 1980, p 911.

14. Overholser CD, Moreillon P, Glauser MP: Experimental bacterial endocarditis after dental extractions in rats with periodontitis. *J Infect Dis* 1987;155:107.

15. McGowan D, Gillett R: Scanning electron microscopic observations on the initial lesions in experimental streptococcal endocarditis in the rabbit. *Br J Exp Pathol* 1980;61:164.

16. Ferguson P, McColm A, Ryan D: Experimental staphylococcal endocarditis and aortitis: Morphology of the initial colonization. *Virchow's Arch (A)* 1986;410:93.

17. Durack DT, Beeson PB: Experimental bacterial endocarditis. II. Survival of bacteria in endocardial vegetations. *Br J Exp Pathol* 1972;53:50.

18. Perlman BB, Freedman LR: Experimental endocarditis. III. Natural history of catheter induces staphylococcal endocarditis following catheter removal. *Yale J Biol Med* 1971;44:214.

19. Durack DT, Beeson PB, Petersdorf RG: Experimental bacterial endocarditis. III. Production and progress of the disease in rabbits. *Br J Exp Pathol* 1973;54:142.

20. Bayer AS, Norman D, Kim KS: Efficacy of amikacin and ceftazidime in experimental aortic valve endocarditis due to *Pseudomonas aeruginosa. Antimicrob Agents Chemother* 1985;28:781.

21. Chambers H, Korzeniowski O, Sande M, et al: *Staphylocoocus aureus* endocarditis: Clinical manifestations in addicts and non-addicts. *Medicine* 1983;62:170.

22. Francioli P, Moreillon P, Glauser MP: Comparison of single doses of amoxicillin-gentamicin for the prevention of endocarditis: Clinical manifestations in addicts and non-addicts. *Medicine* 1983;62:83.

23. Scheld WM, Valone JA, Sande MA: Bacterial adherence in the pathogenesis of endocarditis. Interaction of bacterial dextran, platelets and fibrin. *J Clin Invest* 1978;61:1394.

24. Christensen GD, Baddour LM, Simpson WA: Phenotypic variations of *Staphylococcus epidermidis* slime production in vitro and in vivo. *Infect Immun* 1987;55:2870.

25. Kuypers JM, Proctor RA: A low fibronectin (FN) binding mutant of Staphylococcus aureus (SA) shows reduced adherence to rat heart valves (Abstr.) *Program and Abstracts of the Twenty-seventh Interscience Conference on Antimicrobial Agents and Chemotherapy.* Washington, DC, American Society for Microbiology, 1987, p 185.

26. Durack DT, Gilliland BC, Petersdorf RG: Effect of immunization on susceptibility to experimental *Streptococcus mutans* and *Streptococcus sanguis* endocarditis. *Infect Immun* 1978;22:52.

27. Scheld WM, Thomas JH, Sande MA: Influence of preformed antibody on experimental *Streptococcus sanguis* endocarditis. *Infect Immun* 1979;25:781.

28. Alder SW II, Selinger DS, Reed WP: Effect of immunization on the genesis of pneumococcal endocarditis in rabbits. *Infect Immun* 1981;34:55.

29. Archer GL, Johnston JL: Effect of type-specific active immunization on the development and progression of experimental *Pseudomonas aeruginosa* endocarditis. *Infect Immun* 1979;24:167.

30. Van de Rijn I: Role of culture conditions and immunization in experimental nutritionally variant streptococcal endocarditis. *Infect Immun* 1985;50:641.

31. Thorig L, Thompson J, Van Furth R: Effects of immunization and anticoagulation on the development of experimental *Escherichia coli* endocarditis. *Infect Immun* 1980;28:325.

32. Thorig L, Thompson J, Van Furth R: Effect of immunization on the induction and course of experimental *Streptococcus sanguis* and *Staphylococcus epidermidis* endocarditis. *Infection* 1980;8:267.

33. Greenberg DP, Ward JI, Bayer AS: Influence of *Staphylococcus aureus* antibody on experimental endocarditis in rabbits. *Infect Immun* 1987;55:3030.

34. Franciolo PB, Freedman LR: Streptococcal infection of endocardial and other intravascular vegetations in rabbits: Natural history and effect of dexamethasone. *Infect Immun* 1979;24:483.

35. Yersin BR, Glauser MP, Freedman LR: Effect of nitrogen mustard on natural history of right-sided streptococcal endocarditis in rabbits: Role for cellular host defenses. *Infect Immun* 1982;35:320.

36. Hook EW III, Sande MA: Role of vegetation in experimental *Streptococcus viridans* endocarditis. *Infect Immun* 1974;10:1433.

37. Thompson J, Eulderink F, Lemkes H, et al: Effect of warfarin on the induction and course of experimental endocarditis. *Infect Immun* 1976;14:1284.

38. Thorig L, Thompson J, Eulderick F: Effect of warfarin on the induction and course of experimental *Staphylococcus epidermidis* endocarditis. *Infect Immun* 1977;17:504.

39. Johnson CE, Dewar HA, Aherne WA: Fibrinolytic therapy in subacute bacterial endocarditis: An experimental study. *Cardiovasc Res* 1980;14:482.

40. Dewar HA, Jones MR, Barnes WSF, et al: Fibrinolytic therapy in bacterial endocarditis; experimental studies in dogs. *Eur Heart J* 1986;7:520.

41. Ferguson D, McColm A, Savage T: Amorphologic study of experimental rabbit staphylococcal endocarditis and aortitis: Formation and effect of infected and uninfected vegetations on the aorta. *Br J Exp Pathol* 1986;67:667.

42. Freedman LR, Valone J: Experimental endocarditis. *J Prog Cardiovasc Dis* 1979;22:169.

43. Pujadad-Capmany R, Permanyer-Miralds G, Foz-Sala M, et al: Reduction of the susceptibility to infective endocarditis with time in animals with endocavitary catheters. *Br J Exp Pathol* 1984;65:683.

44. Vogelman B, Gudmundson S, Turnidge J, et al: In vivo postantibiotic effect in a thigh infection in neutropenic mice. *J Infect Dis* 1988;157:287.

45. Matsumoto JY, Wilson WR, Wright AJ, et al: Synergy of penicillin and decreasing concentrations of aminoglycoside against enterococci from patients with infective endocarditis. *Antimicrob Agents Chemother* 1980;18:944.

46. Henry NK, Wilson WR, Geraci JE: Treatment of streptomycin-susceptible enterococcal experimental endocarditis with combinations of penicillin and low-or-high dose streptomycin. *Antimicrob Agents Chemother* 1986;30:725.

47. Wright AJ, Wilson WR, Matsumoto JY, et al: Influence of gentamicin dose size on the efficacy of combinations of gentamicin and penicillin in experimental streptomycin-resistant enterococcal endocarditis. *Antimicrob Agents Chemother* 1982;22:972.

48. Carrizosa J, Levison M: Minimal concentration of aminoglycoside that can synergize with penicillin in enterococcal endocarditis. *Antimicrob Agents Chemother* 1981;20:405.

49. Fantin B, Carbon C: Importance of the aminoglycoside dosing regimen in the penicillin–netilmicin combination for treatment of *Enterococcus faecalis*–induced experimental endocarditis. *Antimicrob Agents Chemother* 1990;34:2387.

50. Thauvin C, Lemeland J, Humbert G, Fillastre J: Efficacy of Pefloxacin-fosfomycin in experimental Endocarditis caused by methicillin-resistant *Staphylococcus aureus*. *Antimicrob Agents Chemother* 1988;32:919.

51. Michea-Hamzehpour M, Pechere JC, Marchou B, et al: Combination therapy: A way to limit emergence of resistance? *Am J Med* 1986;80(Suppl 6B):138.

52. Glauser MP, Francioli P: Relevance of animal models to the prophylaxis of infective endocarditis. *J Antimicrob Chemother* 1987;20(Suppl A):87.

53. Durack DT, Petersdorf RG: Chemotherapy of experimental streptococcal endocarditis. I. Comparison of commonly recommended prophylactic regimens. *J Clin Invest* 1973; 52:592.

54. Pelletier Ll, Durack DT, Petersdorf RG: Chemotherapy of experimental streptococcal endocarditis. IV. Further observations on prophylaxis. *J Clin Invest* 1975;56:319.

55. James J, Macfarlane T, McGowan D, Mackenzie D: Failure of Post-bacteremia delayed antibiotic proplylaxis of expermental rabbit endorcarditis. *J Antimicrob Chemother* 1987;20:883.

56. Southwick FS, Durack DT: Chemotherapy of experimental streptococcal endocarditis. III. Failure of a bacteriostatic agent (tetracycline) in prophylaxis. *J Clin Pathol* 1975; 27:261.

57. Durack DT, Starkebaum MK, Petersdorf RC: Chemotherapy of experimental streptococcal endocarditis. VI. Prevention of enterococcal endocarditis. *J Lab Clin Med* 1977; 90:171.

58. Durack DT: Experience with prevention of experimental endocarditis. *Am Heart Assoc Monogr* 1977;52:28.

59. Malinverni R, Overholser C, Bille J: Antibiotic prophylaxis of experimental endocarditis after dental extractions. *Circulation* 1988;77:183.

60. Fluckiger U, Francioli P, Blaser J, et al: Role of amoxicillin serum levels for sucessful prophylaxis of experimental endocarditis due to tolerant streptococci *J Inf Dis* 1994;169:1397.

61. Everett ED, Hirschman JV: Transient bacteremia and endocarditis prophylaxis. A review. *Medicine (Baltimore)* 19077;56:61.

62. Moreillon P, Francioli P, Overholser D, et al: Mechanisms of successful amoxicillin prophylaxis of experimental endocarditis due to *Streptococcus intermedius*. *J Infect Dis* 1986;154:801.

63. Berney P, Glauser MP, Francioli P: Successful prevention of experimental streptococcal endocarditis with single dose amoxicillin administrated after bacterial challenge (Post-phylaxie) (Abstr.). In *Program and Abstracts of the Twenty-sixth Interscience Conference on Antimicrobial Agents and Chemotherapy, New Orleans,* 1986, p 279.

64. Horne D, Tomasz A: Hypersusceptibility of penicillin-treated group B streptococci to bacterial activity of human polymorphonuclear leukocytes. *Antimicrob Agents Chemother* 1981;19:745.

65. Meddens MJ, Thompson J, Eulderink F, et al: Role of granulocytes in experimental *Streptococcus sanguis* endocarditis. *Infect Immun* 1982;36:325.

66. Meddens MJ, Thompson J, Leigh PC, et al: Role of granulocytes in the induction of an experimental endocarditis with a dextran-producing *Streptococcus sanguis* and its dextran-negative mutant. *Br J Exp Pathol* 1984;65:257.

67. Moreillon P, Francioli P, Overholser D, et al: Mechanism of successful amoxicillin prophylaxis of experimental endocarditis due to *Streptococcus intermedius*. *JIO* 1986;154: 801.

68. Carrizosa J, Kaye D: Antibiotic synergism in enterococcal endocarditis. *J Lab Clin Med* 1976;88:132.

69. Carrizosa J, Kaye D: Antibiotic concentrations in serum, serum bactericidal activity, and results of therapy of streptococcal endocarditis in rabbits. *Antimicrob Agents Chemother* 1977:124:79.

70. Pelletier LL, Petersdorf RG: Chemotherapy of experimental streptococcal endocarditis. V. Effect of duration of infection and retained intracardiac catheter on response to treatment. *J Lab Clin Med* 1976;87:692.

71. Malinverni R: Past and present recommendations for prophylaxis of bacterial endocarditis. Their acceptance and failure. In Horstkotte D, Bodnar E, (eds): *Infective Endocarditis*. London, ICR Publishers, 1991, p 291.

72. Ferguson DJP, McColm AA, Ryan DM, et al: A morphological study of experimental staphylococcal endocarditis and aortitis. I: Formation and effect of infected and uninfected vegetations on the aorta. *Br J Exp Pathol* 1986;67:667.

73. Friedrichs W, Horstkotte D, Pippert H: Prevention of experimental endocarditis in the rat model: Influence of methodical factors on results in infective endocarditis. in Horstkotte D, Bodnar E, (eds): *Infective Endocarditis*. London, ICR Publishers, 1991, p 277.

74. Gersony WM, Hayes CJ: Bacterial endocarditis in patients with pulmonary stenosis, aortic stenosis, or ventricular septal defect. *Circulation* 1977;56(Suppl 1):84.

75. Ferguson DJP, McColm AA, Ryan DM, et al: A morphological study of experimental staphylococcal endocarditis and aortitis. II. Interrelationship of bacteria, vegetation and cardiovasculature in established infections. *Br J Exp Pathol* 1986;67:679.

76. Santoro J, Levison ME: Rat model of experimental endocarditis. *Infect Immun* 1978;19:915.

Index